Trauma
Resuscitation
The team approach

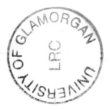

First published 1993 by
THE MACMILLAN PRESS LTD
Houndmills, Basingstoke, Hampshire RG21 2XS
and London
Companies and representatives
throughout the world

ISBN 0–333–54538–9

A catalogue record for this book is available
from the British Library

Printed in China

17/7/96

1114427°

Trauma Resuscitation

The team approach

Edited by
Peter A. Driscoll
Carl L. Gwinnutt
Cindy LeDuc Jimmerson
Olive Goodall

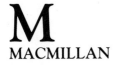

MACMILLAN

Contents

Editors

Peter A. Driscoll BSc FRCS
ATLS Instructor; Senior Lecturer in Emergency Medicine.
University Department of Emergency Medicine, Hope Hospital, Manchester, UK.

Carl L. Gwinnutt MB BS FRCA
ATLS Instructor; Consultant Anaesthetist.
Hope Hospital, Manchester, UK.

Cindy LeDuc Jimmerson RN CEN
Trauma System Design Consultant.
Oregon, USA.

Olive Goodall RGN
Clinical Nurse Manager in Emergency Medicine.
University Department of Emergency Medicine, Hope Hospital, Manchester, UK.

Contributors

Simon Brook BA RGN
ATNC Instructor; Charge Nurse in A/E Medicine.
St. Mary's Hospital, London, UK.

Alison Brown RGN
Senior Sister in Trauma Care.
The Trauma Unit, Johannesburg General Hospital, Johannesburg, Republic of South Africa.

Terry Brown DA FRCS
Registrar in Emergency Medicine.
University Department of Emergency Medicine, Hope Hospital, Manchester, UK.

Mark Doyle FRCS
Consultant in Emergency Medicine.
Department of Accident and Emergency Medicine, Ardkeen Hospital, Waterford, Ireland.

Gill Ellison RGN
Bereavement Counsellor; Sister in Emergency Medicine.
University Department of Emergency Medicine, Hope Hospital, Manchester, UK.

Abigail Hamilton RGN
ATNC Instructor; Staff Nurse in Intensive Care.
Southampton General Hospital, Southampton, UK.

Robert Harvey FRCS
ATLS Instructor; Senior Registrar in Orthopaedic Surgery.
Hope Hospital, Manchester, UK.

Tim Hodgetts MRCP DipIMC RCSEd RAMC
BASICS Instructor; Senior Registrar in Emergency Medicine.
Royal Army Medical College, London, UK.

David Hodgkinson BMedSc MRCP FRCS
Lecturer in Emergency Medicine.
University Department of Emergency Medicine, Hope Hospital.
Manchester, UK.

Bridgett Landon MB ChB
Anatomy Demonstrator.
Department of Anatomy,
St. Bartholomew's Hospital, London, UK.

Gabby Lomas RGN
TNCC Instructor; Sister in Emergency Medicine.
University Department of Emergency Medicine, Hope Hospital,
Manchester, UK.

Joahre Niener MB ChB
Medical Officer.
Maun Hospital, Botswana.

Kevin Mackway-Jones MA MRCP FRCS
ATLS Instructor; Senior Registrar in Emergency Nursing.
Withington Hospital, Manchester, UK.

Corrine Siddall RGN
Sister in Emergency Medicine.
University Department of Emergency Medicine, Hope Hospital,
Manchester, UK.

Joanne Walker RGN
Sister in Emergency Medicine.
University Department of Emergency Medicine, Hope Hospital,
Manchester, UK.

Steven Walker RGN
Staff Nurse in Emergency Medicine.
University Department of Emergency Medicine, Hope Hospital,
Manchester, UK.

Marilyn Woodford
Co-ordinator of the Major Trauma Outcome Study (UK).
North West Injury Research Centre, Hope Hospital, Manchester, UK.

Boxes

Figures

Tables

Journals

Title	Abbreviation
Acta Neurochirurgica Supplement	Acta Neurochir. Supp.
American College of Emergency Physicians	ACEP
American College of Surgeons' Bulletin	Am. Coll. Surgeons Bull.
American Journal of Diseases of Children	Am. J. Dis. Child
American Journal of Surgery	Am. J. Surg.
Anaesthesia	–
Anaesthesic Society Journal	Anaesth. Soc. J.
Anaesthesiology	–
Annals of Emergency Medicine	Ann. Emerg. Med.
Annals of Neurology	Ann. Neurol.
Annals of the Royal College of Surgeons (England)	Ann. R. Coll. Surg.
Annals of Surgery	Ann. Surg.
34th Annual Proceedings of the Association for the Advancement of Automotive Medicine	34th Ann. Proc. AAAM
Archives of Emergency Medicine	Arch. Emerg. Med.
Archives of Surgery	Arch. Surg.
British Journal of Hospital Medicine	Br. J. Hosp. Med.
British Journal of Intensive Care	Br. J. Int. Care
British Journal of Medicine	Br. Med. J.
British Journal of Surgery	Br. J. Surg.
Canadian Anaesthesiology Society Journal	Can. Anaesth. Soc. J.
Canadian Journal of Anaesthesiology	Can. J. Anaesth.
Canadian Journal of Surgery	Can. J. Surg.
Canadian Medical Association Journal	Can. Med. Assoc. J.

Title	Abbreviation
Chest	–
Circulatory Shock	*Cir. Shock*
Clinical Anaesthesiology	*Clin. Anaesthesiol.*
Clinical Intensive Care	*Clin. Int. Care*
Clinical Orthopaedics and Related Research	*Clin. Ortho. Rel. Res.*
Clinics in Medicine	*Clin. Med.*
Clinics in Plastic Surgery	*Clin. Plast. Surg.*
Critical Care Clinics	*Crit. Care Clinics*
Critical Care Medicine	*Cr. Care Med.*
Critical Care Nursing	*Crit. Care Nurs.*
Emergency	–
Emergency Medical Clinics of North America	*Em. Med. Clinics N. Am.*
Emergency Medical Reports	*Em. Med. Repts*
Emergency Medical Services	*Emerg. Med. Serv.*
Emergency Medicine	*Em. Medicine*
Health Trends	–
Heart Lung	–
Hospital Update	–
Infectious Disease Clinics of North America	*Infect. Dis. Clin. N. Am.*
Injury	–
Intensive Care	*Int. Care*
Intensive Therapy	*Int. Ther.*
Intensive Therapy and Clinical Monitoring	*Int. Ther. Clin. Mon.*
Journal of the American College of Emergency Physicians	*JACEP*
Journal of the American Medical Association	*JAMA*
Journal of Burn Care and Rehabilitation	*J. Burn Care Rehabil.*
Journal of Emergency Nursing	*J. Emerg. Nursing*
Journal of Environmental Injuries	*J. Environ. Inj.*
Journal of Hospital Infection	*J. Hosp. Infec.*
Journal of Neurosurgery	*J. Neurosurg.*
Journal of the Royal College of Surgeons (Edinburgh)	*J. R. Coll. Surg. Edinb.*
Journal of Trauma	*J. Trauma*
Lancet	–
Military Medicine	*Mil. Medicine*
Morbidity and Mortality Weekly Report	*MMWR*
New England Journal of Medicine	*N. Eng. J. Med.*
The Nursing Clinics of North America	*Nurs. Clin. N. Am.*

Title	Abbreviation
New York State Journal of Medicine	*NY State J. Med.*
Nursing	–
Nursing Research	–
Nursing Standard	–
Nursing Times	–
Paediatrics	–
Paraplegia	–
Patient Care	–
Perspectives in Shock Research	*Perspec. Shock Res.*
Pharmacology and Therapeutics	*Pharmac. Ther.*
Quarterly Journal of Experimental Physiology	*Q. J. Exp. Physiol.*
Radiology	–
Seminars in Orthopaedics	*Seminars in Ortho.*
Southern Medical Journal	*S. Med. J.*
The Surgical Clinics of North America	*Surg. Clin. N. Am.*
Topics in Emergency Medicine	*Top. Emerg. Med.*
Trauma Nursing	–
Trauma Quarterly	–

Foreword

In 1988 the Royal College of Surgeons of England published its report on the Management of Patients with Major Injuries. The report contained data from a survey of 1 000 trauma deaths and concluded that at least one in five patients, presenting to hospitals in the United Kingdom alive, subsequently died unnecessarily. These avoidable deaths were due to medical mismanagement at every level and throughout the specialties. The report confirmed suspicions held by many in the front line of trauma management, and served as a catalyst for a variety of initiatives designed to reduce this appalling toll, often of the youngest and most productive members of our society. Amongst other suggestions the Royal College of Surgeons of England proposed an improvement in medical and paramedical education.

The Advanced Trauma Life Support Course (ATLS) for doctors was introduced late in 1988, followed by the Advanced Trauma Nursing Course (ATNC). More recently the Pre Hospital Trauma Life Support (PHTLS) programme was initiated for paramedics. These educational packages have truly changed behaviour in ambulances and resuscitation rooms nationally and have resulted in better early care.

As well as these educational initiatives, a pilot Trauma Centre has been established in Stoke and nationwide Accident and Emergency Consultants have established Trauma Teams to initiate rapid assessment and resuscitation of trauma victims.

There has not, as yet, however, been a comprehensive text providing all the information necessary to mount an optimum management response to a patient with major injuries. This excellent text will admirably fill this gap.

This volume is the result of the commitment of a group of nurses and doctors who strongly believe that the early care of the multiply injured should, and can, be improved. The authors are well-known to those working with trauma during the 'Golden Hour'. They have been key individuals in raising the profile of the trauma patient and advocating speedy and efficient patient management by optimal team organisation and training. The value of the book is enhanced by the multi-disciplinary nature of the contributors.

It will be obvious from reading the text that not only is the advice on patient management sensible and practical but it has been carefully put together by those directly involved in patient care. The environment in which critically injured patients are initially managed is, without doubt, demanding and highly stressful. For doctors and nurses in this situation the combination of the need for urgent action, together with concern about their own performance within a highly charged situation, can easily lead to chaos. This potential for chaos can only be reduced by pre-planning, together with theoretical and practical preparedness.

This book, edited by four trauma care workers, provides sound information for all team members and will, therefore, take its place in the front line as a factor in the reduction of death and disability from this modern epidemic – trauma.

L. Hadfield
London

D. V. Skinner
Oxford

Preface

The evolution of trauma care in developed countries around the world has created new and exciting roles for all the personnel involved in the resuscitation and recovery of critically injured patients. The stress on strict, separate roles for the nurse, the doctor, the paramedics and the ancillary staff is now being replaced by a greater emphasis on the 'team approach'. This acknowledges the interactive nature of the procedures undertaken by the trauma team and the need for close co-operation at all stages of the resuscitation. It is an approach at its most successful when based on a formally organized team structure which incorporates the concept of task allocation. This enables procedures to be undertaken simultaneously, thereby reducing resuscitation times. In addition, it puts *each* member of the trauma team in the position of being responsible for evaluating the patient and the situation, anticipating the next most appropriate action even as one is being performed, and communicating with each member of the team to provide the best care.

This book has been created with this new vision of the multi-member trauma team in mind. The objective of the authors is to present a comprehensive view of trauma management and its sequelae that relates to both nurses and doctors involved with trauma resuscitation. The general approach to the clinical management of the patient is similar to that espoused by the Advanced Trauma Nursing Course (ATNC) and the Trauma Nursing Core Course (TNCC), both of which have been adopted as a standard of training by the Royal College of Nursing. It also follows the principles of the American College of Surgeons' Advanced Trauma Life Support Course (ATLS), now adopted by the Royal Colleges of Surgeons in the UK.

In addressing both nurses and doctors, the book emphasizes the importance of all personnel involved having a good understanding of the pathophysiological changes underlying a trauma resuscitation. This enables greater co-operation between personnel and facilitates the anticipation of the patient's needs. Consideration is therefore given to the relevant mechanisms of injury, the physiological response to injury, and a practical system of identifying and addressing life-threatening conditions. Trauma care is reviewed in a systematic way, body system by body system. In addition, in the chapters concerned with areas where injury is commonly life-threatening, particular attention is paid to the applied anatomy and physiology of the normal system. Following this, the pathophysiological changes due to trauma and the clinical management of these patients is reviewed. For further information, the interested reader is referred to the section at the end of each chapter: this lists both nursing and medical literature which can be used to follow up on particular aspects of trauma care.

No attempt has been made to highlight either the nurses' or doctors' allocated tasks since the aim of the book is to emphasize the need for an *integrated team* approach. At certain points in the text, however, the nurse's role has been stressed, and technical procedures that in the UK would be mainly undertaken by doctors have been highlighted for easy reference. The extent to which nurses and doctors carry out particular tasks will depend on training and local policy. With limitations in medical personnel – as seen in developing countries, for example – the trauma nurse could be expected to take over more of the doctor's role. In *every* situation, though, the philosophy of the trauma team should be understood by *all* members, so that consistent good care can be achieved.

The authors recognize that trauma care is delivered in a growing variety of settings. It is our desire to equip all personnel, no matter what the environment in which they practise, with information that can assist them in developing the appropriate decision-making skills required in managing the injured patient. We are confident that *Trauma Resuscitation: the team approach* will help nurses and doctors reach their potential as members of the trauma team; and, by doing so, improve each patient's chances of returning to a full and active life.

Peter Driscoll
Carl Gwinnutt
Cindy LeDuc Jimmerson
Olive Goodall

April 1993

A note about gender

For the sake of clarity, throughout this book the trauma victims and doctors are always assumed to be male and the trauma nurses to be female. In reality, of course, each can be of either sex.

Acknowledgements

All the authors would like to thank the following experts who have taken the time and trouble to read and correct particular sections of this book:

Chapter 10

Professor J. Ryan
Professor of Military Surgery.
RAMC, London, UK.

Chapter 15

Dr I. W. McAndrew
Medical Officer.
*British Nuclear Fuels Ltd,
Sellafield, UK.*

Mr S. Morris
Senior Nursing Officer.
*British Nuclear Fuels Ltd,
Sellafield, UK.*

Photography

Dept. Medical Illustration.
Hope Hospital, Manchester, UK.

Figures

The authors gratefully acknowledge the permission granted by those listed for the reproduction of the following figures: American College of Surgeons, 12.4; British Medical Journal, 8.4, 11.2; Butterworth Heinemann, 6.1; Butterworths, 8.5, 8.6; Churchill Livingstone, 8.1, 8.3b; D. Fawcett, 10.1; R. Harvey, 9.3, 9.8; Oxford University Press, 2.1, 3.1, 3.4, 5.1, 5.3; Parthenon Publishing, 1.1, 2.9, 2.10, 2.13, 3.12, 3.13, 4.6, 4.7, 9.1; S. Royal, 9.7; J. Ryan, 5.4, 10.2, 10.3; Smith & Nephew, 12.2; J. Waterlow, 1.9; Williams & Wilkins, 3.6.

Special thanks to Dr C. Wells, Staff Nurse S. Rose and District Resuscitation Training Officer D. Wallis, who suffered above and beyond the bounds of friendship to proofread the whole manuscript.

In 1988–89 the Smith & Nephew Foundation awarded Fellowships to Peter Driscoll, Simon Brook and Abigail Hamilton to study trauma care in Europe, North America and South Africa. This book is but a small repayment to the Foundation's generosity.

Abbreviations

a	arterial
A	alveolar
ABG	arterial blood gases
ACCOLC	access overload control
ADH	antidiuretic hormone
A/E	accident and emergency department
AIDS	acquired immune-deficiency syndrome
AIO	Ambulance Incident Officer
AIS	Abbreviated Injury Scale
AP	antero-posterior view
ARDS	adult respiratory distress syndrome
ATLS	Advanced Trauma Life Support Course
ATNC	Advanced Trauma Nursing Course
BASICS	The British Association for Immediate Care
BLS	basic life support
BP	blood pressure
bt	beat
CaO_2	content of oxygen in arterial blood
CI	cardiac index; confidence interval
CNS	central nervous system
CO	carbon monoxide; cardiac output
CO_2	carbon dioxide
COHb	carboxyhaemoglobin
CPP	cerebral perfusion pressure
CSF	cerebrospinal fluid
CT	computerized tomography
CvO_2	content of oxygen in venous blood
CVP	central venous pressure

DAI	diffuse axonal injury
DO_2	oxygen delivery
DPG	diphosphoglycerate
DPL	diagnostic peritoneal lavage
DTPA	diethylenetriaminepentaacetic acid
ECG	electrocardiograph
ECV	emergency control vehicle
ECM	external cardiac massage
EDH	extradural haematoma
EDP	end diastolic pressure
EDTA	ethylenediaminetetraacetic acid
ENT	ear, nose and throat
ET	endotracheal
GCS	Glasgow Coma Scale
GMC	General Medical Council
Hb	haemoglobin
Hct	haematocrit
HIV	human immunodeficiency virus
HPPF	human plasma protein fraction
IC	intercostal
ICH	intracerebral haematoma
ICP	intracranial pressure
IDH	intradural haematoma
ISS	Injury Severity Score
ITU	intensive care unit
IV	intravenous
IVC	inferior vena cava
JVP	jugular venous pressure
KE	kinetic energy
LA	local anaesthetic
LSP	life-saving procedures
LVEDP	left ventricular end diastolic pressure
MAP	mean arterial pressure
MIO	Medical Incident Officer
mmHg	millimetres of mercury
MMT	mobile medical team
MOF	multiple organ failure
MTOS	Major Trauma Outcome Study
NAIR	National Arrangements for Incidents Involving Radiation
NG	nasogastric

NIO	Nursing Incident Officer
NIPB	non-invasive blood-pressure monitor
OER	oxygen extraction ratio
P	partial pressure
PA	posterior-anterior view
PAC	pulmonary artery catheter
$PaCO_2$	partial pressure of arterial carbon dioxide
PaO_2	partial pressure of arterial oxygen
PASG	pneumatic anti-shock garment
PHTLS	Pre Hospital Trauma Life Support
PM	post-mortem
POWP	pulmonary artery occlusion (wedge) pressure
PR	rectal examination
Ps	probability of survival
PVC	polyvinyl chloride
PvO_2	partial pressure of oxygen in venous blood
Q	volume of blood
RHA	Regional Health Authority
RTS	Revised Trauma Score
SaO_2	oxygen saturation of arterial blood
SAH	subarachnoid haemorrhage
SDH	subdural haematoma
SvO_2	mixed venous oxyhaemoglobin saturation
SVR	systemic vascular resistance
TBSA	total body surface area
TNCC	Trauma Nursing Core Course
TRISS	Trauma Score and ISS
UKCC	United Kingdom Central Council for Nursing, Midwifery and Health Visiting
v	venous
V	volume of gas
VO_2	oxygen consumption
WHO	World Health Organization

Introduction

Peter Driscoll

■ The size and extent of the problem

The 'developed' world is at war. In the UK alone, the annual number of deaths from trauma is 14 500–18 000; in the USA the figure is approximately ten times greater. A third of the victims are killed on the road, and just under a third in incidents at home. As in all wars, it is the youth of the country which takes the heaviest losses. Trauma remains the most common cause of death in industrialized nations, in people under 35.

In the USA there are 70 million non-fatal injuries per annum. These patients go on to occupy 12 per cent of all hospital beds in that country. In the UK annually, 60 000 are admitted to hospital following road traffic accidents, and 26 000 from industrial incidents. Overall, casualties from this 'trauma war' occupy more hospital beds, and cause the loss of more working days, than cancer and cardiac patients combined. For the British taxpayer, the cost of this slaughter is high – £2.22 billion per annum, that is around 1 per cent of the gross national product (WHO estimation). In the USA, the figure is put at $75–100 billion – approximately equal to one and a half times the total military expenditure on the Gulf war. The final cost is even higher because there is also a loss of national talent and tax revenue, in addition to the emotional and material consequences suffered by each family affected. The cumulative effect of trauma patients who survive, but in a crippled state, adds to this financial nightmare.

□ National ignorance

In the UK the medical and nursing professions appear to accept a broad standard of 'appropriate care' for trauma patients. This is not based on any serious debate or research, contrary to the situation relating to other

1

diseases. It required a Royal College investigation on eleven health districts to find out that one-third of the trauma deaths that occurred after arrival in hospital were preventable. These deaths resulted from missed diagnosis, hypoxia, continuing haemorrhage and lack of timely surgery.

■ The trimodal distribution of death following trauma

The first peak in mortality occurs at, or shortly after, the time of injury. These patients die of major neurological or vascular injury and most cannot be resuscitated with present-day technology. However, 40 per cent of the deaths in this group could be avoided by various prevention programmes.

The second peak occurs several hours after the injury. These patients commonly die from airway, breathing or circulatory problems. The majority of these cases are potentially treatable. This period is known as the 'golden hour' to emphasize that this is the time following injury when re-suscitation and stabilization are critical.

The final peak occurs days or weeks after the injury. These victims die from multiple organ failure (MOF), acute respiratory disease syndrome (ARDS) or overwhelming infection. It is now known that inadequate resus-citation in the immediate or early post-injury period leads to an increased mortality rate during this phase.

■ Injury patterns

In the developed world trauma is usually caused by a blunt mechanism. This leads to multiple injuries, with usually one system severely affected and one or two others areas damaged to a lesser degree. Overall, the incidence of life-threatening injuries to different systems is as follows: head, 30–70 per cent; chest, 20–35 per cent; abdomen, 10–35 per cent; and spine, 5 per cent. In excess of 40 per cent of the trauma victims also have orthopaedic injuries but these are not usually life-threatening.

■ Problems with current management of trauma victims

☐ Prevention

There are few cases which are true 'accidents' – 'events without apparent cause'. For example, the man who crashes his car after drinking alcohol has *not* had an accident. All traumatic events are an interaction between the host, the agent, the social culture and the legal system. The Transport and

Road Research Laboratory (UK) estimated that 65 per cent of road traffic 'accidents' were due to human error. About 80 per cent of the pedestrians injured were themselves at fault, with children and the elderly being the worst offenders.

The link between alcohol abuse and many types of injury has been well documented. In the UK it is a factor in at least 28 per cent of all fatal car crashes, and in the USA 40–50 per cent of the people dying following trauma have a blood-alcohol level greater than 100 mg%. Alcohol can also affect the clinical course of the patient by affecting the diagnostic signs and physiological and immunological response to trauma.

Prevention by legislation has been used effectively in various countries over the past years, with laws on smoke alarms, flame-resistant clothing, drink/driving, seatbelts, child car seats, car design and motorcycle helmets being introduced. Education has also been used to some effect. Unfortunately trauma, like all diseases, is more common among the socially deprived, and would be improved by material changes in the social conditions.

☐ Pre-hospital care

The standard of care in the pre-hospital phase varies significantly between countries as well as between districts inside the same country. In the UK there is a definite need for improvement because the ambulance personnel are trained to be competent at following protocols. This applies equally to the current UK paramedic training. Unlike the North American system, once 'extended trained' they receive little audit and feedback on their management of the patients, so there is no accumulation of knowledge and experience. This situation is perpetuated by there being little medical input into the service and by the very limited communications between the hospital and the on-site team. The result is a profession which is not utilizing its post-training learning experiences.

☐ On admission

In Britain, trauma victims frequently arrive late at night when the A/E departments are staffed by inexperienced junior doctors. This can lead to delays in getting senior help once the clinician realizes there is a problem. There are also difficulties in priortizing patients' injuries. A laparotomy or inserting a pelvic external fixer may form part of the initial resuscitation if the patient is haemodynamically unstable. Delays in carrying out the life-saving procedures (LSP) have to be prevented as such delays have a strong (negative) correlation with physiological changes in the patient in the resuscitation room. The time for the LSP also affects the overall survival of the trauma patient.

Trauma teams are not exclusive to Trauma Centres. Indeed many District General Hospitals (and their equivalents in Europe and the USA) have such teams. This has the theoretical advantage of bringing together a group of people with the appropriate expertise to manage the multiply injured patient. In the UK, however, the teams usually comprise junior doctors with limited experience in handling the complex problem of trauma management. The organization of the team is informal, with members arriving at different times and carrying out procedures in an *ad hoc* manner. There is no overall coordination and no allocation of duties to the team members. There is also no national guidance on the organization of the ideal trauma team, its structure and who should be in charge.

Once resuscitation starts the next problem encountered is the poor knowledge base for the management of the pathophysiological changes after trauma. It has been found that shocked patients have an increased chance of survival if certain therapeutic goals in the cardiac index, oxygen delivery and oxygen consumption are reached. This requires aggressive oxygen and fluid resuscitation with early recourse to surgery if the haemorrhage cannot be controlled. The expensive and invasive monitoring systems required to do this safely are rarely used in resuscitation rooms. Instead, reliance is put on clinical skills and inadequate monitoring devices recording variables such as blood pressure and heart rate. This leads to lesser degrees of hypoxia and hypovolaemia not being recognized, resulting in too little oxygen and fluid being given, and too late. It is therefore not surprising that hypoxia and hypovolaemia are the chief causes of preventable death in the middle and final mortality peaks in industrialized nations.

☐ Definitive care

In the Royal College of Surgeons (England) report, 170 of 514 hospital deaths were considered preventable. Of the 170 patients, 105 required an operation but 83 (79 per cent) had either no operation or an inadequate one. In 113 of the preventable cases, the patients died from injuries other than to the head, with the majority being under the province of the general surgeon.

The general lack of trauma expertise in Britain is further demonstrated in the poor management of those patients requiring inter-hospital transfer.

☐ Rehabilitation

For every trauma death resulting from a road traffic accident there are two or three people who are permanently injured. It follows that there is a pressing need for all types of rehabilitation care.

☐ Quality assurance

In the 1970s the United States government funded the Major Trauma Outcome Study (MTOS) to evaluate major trauma care in the USA. This has since ended, but a similar system has been set up in Manchester to evaluate UK trauma care. The essential data upon which MTOS is based are the Injury Severity Score (ISS), the Revised Trauma Score (RTS), and the patient's age. The ISS is an anatomical description of the injury; the RTS is a physiological assessment of the patient on arrival at the hospital.

MTOS allows assessment of three aspects of care. Firstly, it identifies unexpected deaths and survivors in the hospital. In so doing it highlights specific areas for clinical and administrative review. Secondly, by creating a national database, it allows centres to compare their results. This allows the weaknesses and strengths of trauma care in this country to be identified. Finally, it allows international comparisons.

■ The role of the team in trauma care

It can be seen from the previous discussion that there is considerable scope for improvement in all aspects of trauma care. A fully integrated team of trained nurses and doctors needs to be present to deal with the trauma victim when he arrives at the hospital. An efficient, organized resuscitation needs to be commenced which leads to initial stabilization, diagnosis and definitive management.

It has been shown that the most efficient team organization is achieved by having each team member carrying out individual tasks simultaneously. This process is known as 'horizontal organization'. (The *least* efficient technique, in which each task is carried out sequentially, is known as 'vertical organization'.) If tasks are to be performed simultaneously, precise allocation of tasks to team members is essential, or there is chaos. Each procedure is divided into manageable units and allocated to individual team members by a designated nursing and medical team leader. These tasks must be divided evenly among the team to prevent overloading of any particular member.

When these organizational changes are introduced, significant reductions in resuscitation times can be achieved (Figure I.1). In particular, the time to carry out the life-saving procedures is shortened; this is known to correlate with the short- and long-term survival of the patient.

The initial management of the trauma victim can be a difficult and stressful time which can easily become overwhelming without prior planning. The allocation of staff to specific roles within the team relieves the stress and ensures that the department functions safely, whilst the injured patient receives immediate assessment and life-saving intervention.

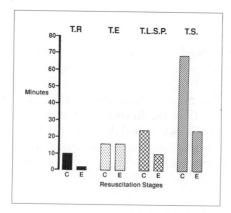

Figure I.1 Changes in resuscitation times following organizational alteration of the trauma team: TR = time taken to record the vital signs; TLSP = time taken to complete the life-saving procedures (i.e. primary survey); TE = time taken to examine the patient fully (i.e. secondary survey); TS = time taken to complete the whole resuscitation

To enable these organizational changes to be introduced, the team members have to have the skills to carry out the particular tasks. This can be facilitated by having all the nursing staff dealing with trauma victims complete an Advanced Trauma Nursing Course (ATNC) or a Trauma Nursing Core Course (TNCC). Similarly, each team doctor should have successfully completed an Advanced Trauma Life Support Course (ATLS).

This certainly should be the aim for the future. Until this is achieved, however, the necessary organizational changes required for the team approach can still be made with appropriate departmental training. The following chapters provide information on which these changes can be based. For those who have already completed the above courses, the following chapters will reinforce the knowledge and skills acquired; we hope that it will also spur others to undertake similar training.

■ References and further reading

American College of Surgeons Committee on Trauma 1993. *Advanced Trauma Life Support Course for Physicians: course manual.* Chicago: American College of Surgeons.

Anderson I D, Woodford M, de Dombal F T, *et al.* 1988. Retrospective study of 1000 deaths from injury in England and Wales. *Br. Med. J.* **296**: 1305.

Anderson I D, Woodford M & Irving M H 1989. Preventability of death from penetrating injury in England and Wales. *Injury* **20**(2): 69.

Association of Chief Ambulance Officers 1990. *Proposals for the Future of the Ambulance Service.*

Baker C, Oppenheimer L, Stephens B, *et al*. 1980. Epidemiology of trauma deaths. *Am. J. Surg.* **140**(1): 144.

Boyd C, Tolson M A & Copes W S 1987. Evaluating trauma care: the TRISS method. Trauma Score and Injury Severity Score. *J. Trauma* **27**(4): 370.

Cales R & Trunkey D D 1985. Preventable trauma deaths. A review of trauma care systems development. *JAMA* **254**(8): 1059.

Castille K 1991. Trauma training for nurses. *Nursing* 4: 22.

Committee on Trauma 1986. Hospital and prehospital resources for optimal care of the injured patient. *Am. Coll. Surgeons Bull.* 71.

Dearden C & Rutherford W 1985. The resuscitation of the severely injured in the accident and emergency department – a medical audit. *Injury* **16**(4): 249.

Driscoll P 1992. Trauma: today's problems, tomorrow's answers. *Injury* **23**(3): 151.

Driscoll P & Vincent C 1992a. Organizing an efficient trauma team. *Injury* **23**(2): 107.

Driscoll P & Vincent C 1992b. Variation in trauma resuscitation and its effects on patient outcome. *Injury* **23**(2): 111.

Driscoll P & Wells C 1991. Trauma care since 1988. *Health Trends* **22**: 118.

Emergency Nurses Association 1988. *TNCC Course Manual*, 2nd edn. Chicago: Award Printing Corporation.

Fisher R & Dearden C 1990. Improving the care of patients with major trauma in the accident and emergency department. *Br. Med. J.* **300**: 1560.

Gentleman D & Jennett B 1981. Hazards of inter-hospital transfer in comatosed head-injured patients. *Lancet* **2**: 853.

Irving M 1989. The evolution of trauma care in the United Kingdom. (Gissane memorial lecture 1989.) *Injury* **20**(6): 317.

McCoy G, Johnstone R, Nelson I, *et al*. 1989. A review of fatal road accidents in Oxfordshire over a 2-year period. *Injury* **20**(2): 65.

Roy P 1987. The value of trauma centres: a methodologic review. *Can. J. Surg.* **30**(1): 17.

Royal College of Surgeons of England 1988. *The Management of Patients with Major Injuries: report of a working party*. London: Royal College of Surgeons of England.

Sharples P, Storey A, Aynsley-Green A, *et al*. 1990. Causes of fatal childhood accidents involving head injury in northern region, 1979–86. *Br. Med. J.* **301**: 1193.

Sheehy S, Marvin J & Jimmerson C 1989. *Manual of Clinical Trauma Care: the first hour*. St. Louis: C V Mosby.

Shoemaker W, Kram H 1988. Crystalloid and colloid therapy in resuscitation and subsequent ICU management. *Clin. Anaesthesiol.* **2**: 509.

Spencer J D 1985. Why do our hospitals not make more use of the concept of a trauma team? *Br. Med. J.* **290**: 136.

Trunkey D D 1984. Trauma care systems. *Em. Med. Clinics N. Am.* **2**(4): 913.

West J, Trunkey D & Lim R 1979. Systems of trauma care. A study of two countries. *Arch. Surg.* **114**(4): 455.

Westerby S 1989. Trauma: the problem and some solutions. In Westerby S (ed.): *Trauma: pathogenesis and treatment*. London: Heinemann Medical Books.

Yates D 1989. Injury scoring system. *Int. Ther. Clin. Mon.* **10**: 38.
Yates D, Woodford M & Hollis S 1992. Preliminary analysis of the care of injured patients in 33 British hospitals: first report of the United Kingdom major trauma outcome study. *Br. Med. J.* **305**: 737.

Chapter 1

Resuscitation and stabilization of the severely injured patient

Peter Driscoll and Simon Brook

Objectives

The objectives of this chapter are to help members of a trauma team:

- to understand the structure and function of a trauma team;
- to gain an overview of the whole of the management of the patient in the resuscitation room.

Many of the points mentioned will be reinforced and described in greater detail in the ensuing chapters. The reader may find it useful, therefore, to concentrate initially on the team's structure and function. After studying Chapters 2, 3 and 4, this chapter should then be reread so that the clinical issues described can be considered.

■ Introduction

The efficient management of the severely injured patient is dependent on a team approach and on a predetermined system to guide the personnel through the initial assessment and life-saving procedures. These two essential elements will enable each member to carry out their allotted tasks simultaneously. In so doing, the time to resuscitate the patient is reduced, and his chances of surviving increased. (See the Introduction for details.)

It is important, therefore, that each member of the team is familiar both with their own roles and with those of their colleagues. Accordingly, a comprehensive view of the medical and nursing management of the trauma patient is given here so that the trauma nurse can:

- see where her role fits into the overall organization;
- appreciate the importance of her role;

- anticipate what may be required as the resuscitation progresses;
- extend her role in an emergency.

■ Pre-hospital information and communication

Direct communication between the ambulance crew and hospital remains rare in the United Kingdom, but most Accident & Emergency (A/E) departments do have a dedicated telephone link to ambulance control. The ambulance personnel can therefore give a few details to the control centre, which are then relayed to the hospital by land-line. Thus the A/E department usually receives some prior warning that a severely injured patient in about to arrive. This time is best spent marshalling, briefing and preparing the trauma team.

In the United States and other advanced industrialized nations, communication systems are in place which enable those attending the patient to talk directly with the trauma team. The paramedical staff can therefore receive advice while the hospital staff obtain essential information (Box 1.1). Without such a system, the team has to wait until the paramedics arrive at the department with the patient. The ideal set-up would be to have a communications system which would also permit the transmission of monitored data.

BOX 1.1   Essential pre-hospital information

The incident:
- The nature of the incident
- The number, age and sex of the casualties

For each patient:
- The patient's complaints, priorities and injuries
- The airway, ventilatory and circulatory status
- The conscious level
- The management plan and its effect
- The estimated time of arrival

It is crucial to determine the *mechanism* of the injury. This gives invaluable information about the forces the patient was subjected to and the direction of impact. Further help comes from a description of the damage to the car, for example, or of the weapon used (see Chapter 10).

Patterns of injuries occur following certain accidents. For example, a frontal impact (Figure 1.1) can result in damage to the head, face, airway, neck, heart, lungs, thoracic aorta, main bronchi, liver, spleen, knee, shaft of

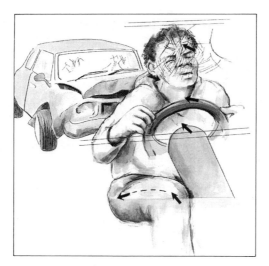

Figure 1.1 A frontal road traffic accident
Source: © Landon B, Driscoll P & Goodall J 1993. *The Atlas of Trauma Management*.
Carnforth, Lancashire: Parthenon. Reproduced by kind permission.

femur and hips! Another serious situation is one where an occupant of a car
is ejected following a collision: this victim has a 300 per cent greater chance
of a sustaining a serious injury than those who remained in the car.

In the cases of road traffic accidents, it is important also to note whether
any persons were dead at the scene. If so, this would imply that considerable
forces where generated and that any survivors also could potentially have
serious injuries.

Should the patient arrive without prior warning, it is the nurse's responsibility to assess the patient, including the mechanism of injury, and to alert
other members of the trauma team if she considers it appropriate.

■ The trauma team

The group of nurses and doctors who make up the trauma team need to be
summoned once it has been decided that the patient requires resuscitation-
rom facilities. As any time delay can be so important, these people must be
immediately available and pre-organized to ensure that the right person gets
to the right place at the right time.

The objectives of the team are shown in Box 1.2.

BOX 1.2   Objectives of the trauma team

The team has five objectives:
- to resuscitate and stabilize the patient
- to determine the nature and extent of the injuries
- to categorize the injuries in order of priority
- to prepare and transport the patient to a place of definitive care (e.g. theatre or another hospital)
- to treat the patient holistically and humanistically, being conscious of the crisis being faced by the patient and his relatives

---

☐ Team members

The trauma team should comprise the following nursing, medical and radiological staff:

Nursing staff

- A nursing team leader.
- An 'airway nurse'.
- Two 'circulation nurses'*.
- A 'relatives' nurse'.

Medical staff

- A medical team leader.
- An 'airway doctor'.
- Two 'circulation' doctors*.

In view of the potential airway problems which may present, it is preferable that the airway doctor is a skilled anaesthetist or intensive-care clinician.

In all cases, the nursing and medical personnel chosen for the respective roles must be appropriately trained. Seniority *per se* is no guarantee of competence!

Radiographer

At least one radiographer must be a member of the trauma team.

On first sight it appears that a lot of personnel will be taken away from the department for a long time. However, the aim is to achieve an efficient and rapid correction of all the immediately life-threatening conditions. Once this has been completed, only the core personnel need to remain, and those marked with an asterisk (*) can return to their normal duties.

☐ Team members' roles

Each member has to be thoroughly familiar with her or his respective duties so that tasks can be performed simultaneously for the maximum benefit of the patient in the shortest possible time. It is also essential that problems are anticipated rather than reacted to once they have already developed.

When nurse and doctors pair up to tackle the various tasks, the efficiency of the team improves. Therefore examples of paired roles and tasks are listed below. However, assignments may vary between units, depending on the resources available.

Team leaders

Nursing team leader

- Co-ordinates the nursing team.
- Prepares sterile packs for procedures.
- Assists the circulation nurses and brings extra equipment as necessary.
- Records clinical findings, laboratory results, IV and drug infusion, and the vital signs as called out by the circulation nurse. (In several units this particular duty is delegated to a junior nurse, thereby freeing the nursing team leader for her other responsibilities.)

Medical team leader

- Coordinates the specific tasks of the individual team members.
- Checks breathing and assimilates the clinical findings.
- Lists the investigations in order of priority.
- Liaises with specialists who have been called.
- Questions the ambulance personnel to ascertain the mechanism of injury, the pre-hospital findings, and the treatment given so far.
- Depending on the skill of the rest of the team members, carries out particular procedures, such as pericardiocentesis and thoracotomy.

Airway personnel

Airway nurse

- Assists in securing the airway and stabilizing the cervical spine.
- Establishes a rapport with the patient, giving psychological support throughout his ordeal in the resuscitation room. Ideally, all information to the patient should be fed through her.

Airway doctor

- Clears and secures the airway whilst taking appropriate cervical spine precautions.
- Inserts central and arterial lines if required.

Circulation personnel

Circulation nurses

- Assist with the removal of the patient's clothing.
- Assist with starting IV infusions, chest drain insertion and catheterization.
- Assist in special procedures such as thoracotomies.
- Measure the vital signs and connect the patient to the monitors.
- Monitor the fluid balance.

Circulation doctors

- Assist in the removal of the patient's clothes.
- Establish peripheral IV infusions and take blood for investigations.
- Carry out certain procedures such as urinary catheterization and chest drain insertion.
- Carry out other procedures, depending on their skill level.

Relatives' personnel

Relatives' nurse

- Cares for the patient's relatives when they arrive.
- Liaises with the trauma team to provide the relatives with appropriate information and support.

Radiological personnel

Radiographer

- Takes three standard x-rays for each patient subjected to blunt trauma: chest, pelvis and lateral cervical spine. A more selective approach is used with victims of penetrating trauma.

To avoid chaos and disorganization, there should be no more than six people physically touching the patient. The other team members must keep well back.

■ Preparation

It is the nurse's responsibility at the beginning of every shift to ensure that the resuscitation room is fully stocked and the equipment in working order and ready for use. When the room is actually needed, only minimum preparation is then necessary.

Prior to the patient's arrival, the trauma team should assemble in the resuscitation room and put on protective clothing. Ideally universal precautions should be taken by each member (see Chapter 19 for details). However, if these are not available, rubber gloves, plastic aprons and glasses must be worn. **All blood and body fluids should be assumed to carry HIV and hepatitis viruses.**

Trauma victims often have sharp objects such as glass and other debris in their clothing, in their hair and on their skin. Ordinary surgical gloves give no protection against this, so the personnel undressing the patient must initially wear more robust gloves.

Whilst protective clothing is being put on, the team leaders should brief the personnel, ensuring that each member knows the task for which he or she is responsible. A final check of the equipment can then be made by the appropriate team members (see Chapter 20 for further details).

■ Reception and transfer

If there is a long distance between the ambulance bay and the resuscitation room, the airway personnel should assess the patient in the back of the ambulance. Provided that there is no urgent airway problem which requires immediate intervention, the patient can be moved.

Once the trauma victim arrives in the resuscitation room the nursing team leader should start the stop-clock so that accurate times can be taken.

In the UK the patient will usually be on a scoop stretcher, with or without some form of short spinal board. In North America the trauma victim invariably arrives on a long backboard. This device facilitates the transfer of the patient from the stretcher to the trolley. Such a procedure must be coordinated so that there is no rotation of the spinal column or exacerbation of pre-existing injuries. Team members should also check that lines and leads are free so that they do not become disconnected or snagged.

Five people are required for transfer if the victim is not on any lifting device. The team must be well drilled in this technique and coordinated by a team leader experienced in the safe transfer of patients with possible spinal trauma. One of the airway personnel should stabilize the head and neck, as three people lift from the side and the fifth removes the ambulance trolley (Figure 1.2).

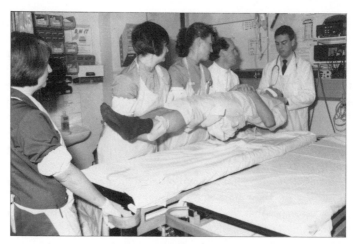

Figure 1.2 A patient being lifted onto a trolley

■ Primary survey and resuscitation

The objective of this phase in the resuscitation is to hunt out and treat any immediately life-threatening condition.

Although each patient is nursed as an individual, the team must follow a strict routine in order to perform efficiently. Though the following tasks are described sequentially, they should be carried out simultaneously. Whilst the medical team leader is gaining information from the ambulance personnel (see later), the activities listed in Box 1.3 are being performed.

BOX 1.3   The primary survey and resuscitation phase

Checks made by the trauma team:
- *A* – Airway and cervical spine control
- *B* – Breathing
- *C* – Circulation
- *D* – Dysfunction of the CNS
- *E* – Exposure

☐ **(A) Airway and cervical spine control**

If the patient is a victim of blunt trauma or if the mechanism of injury indicates that this region may have been damaged (see Chapter 8) the airway personnel must initially assume the presence of a cervical spinal instability. Consequently, none of the activities described to clear and secure the airway must involve movement of the neck.

The airway nurse must manually immobilize the cervical spine at the same time as the airway doctor talks to the patient. Talking not only establishes supportive contact, but can also be used to assess the airway. If the patient replies with a normal voice, giving a logical answer, then the airway can be assumed to be patent and the brain adequately perfused.

Airway

An impaired or absent reply indicates that the airway could be obstructed, most commonly by the tongue. This must be pulled forward in such a way that the cervical spine is not moved – that is, using either the chin lift or the jaw thrust technique (see Chapter 2).

If this does not improve the situation the airway must be checked for obstruction. The mouth should be opened and vomitus or other liquid debris removed with a rigid sucker. Pliable suckers are contraindicated since they are more likely to obstruct. If they are passed nasally (see Chapter 2), they can also pass into the cranial vault, through a fractured cribriform plate.

The complications of alcohol ingestion and possible injuries of the chest and abdomen increase the chance of the patient vomiting. Since it is impractical to nurse the trauma victim on his side, constant supervision in the supine position is required. If vomiting starts, no attempt should be made to turn the patient's head to one side unless a cervical spine injury has been ruled out radiologically and clinically. However, if a spinal (back) board is in place, the whole patient can be turned (Figure 1.3). In the absence of this piece of equipment, the trolley should be tipped head-down by 20° and the vomit sucked away as it appears in the mouth.

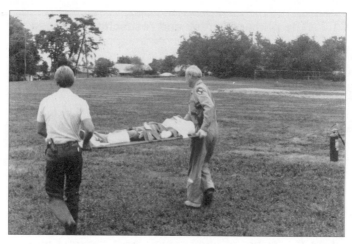

Figure 1.3 A patient on a backboard

If the patient has a pharyngeal (gag) reflex, he is capable of maintaining his own airway. Consequently, no attempt must be made to insert a Guedel airway as this can precipitate vomiting, cervical movement, and a rise in intracranial pressure. A nasopharyngeal airway is recommended in these situations because it is less likely to stimulate a gag reflex.

Trauma victims rarely have empty stomachs, and so have a significant chance of vomiting following gastric distension with air. This can follow even a good mask ventilation technique using a non-rebreathing circuit. Therefore, in the absence of a gag reflex, the patient needs early endotracheal intubation to maximize ventilation and to prevent bronchopulmonary aspiration (see Chapter 2 for details). A nasogastric tube should also be inserted to limit distension of the stomach.

Once the airway has been cleared and secured, the patient is given a high flow (12–15 l/min) of 100% oxygen.

Cervical spine

Once the airway has been secured, the neck is inspected quickly for:

- Swellings and wounds, which can indicate that there are local injury, damaged blood vessels or interstitial emphysema from a pneumothorax.
- Tracheal deviation, indicating a tension pneumothorax (see below).
- Distended neck veins, which indicate that there is a rise in the central venous pressure. This can result from a tension pneumothorax, cardiac tamponade or damage to the great vessels (see Chapter 3).

To enable the airway nurse now to safely release the patient's head and neck, the cervical spine needs to be secured using either a semi-rigid collar, sandbags and tape (Figure 1.4), or a commercially available spine support (Figure 1.5). The only exception to this rule is the restless patient who will not keep still. In this case, the cervical spine can be damaged by immobilizing the head and neck whilst allowing the rest of the patient's body to keep moving. A suboptimal level of immobilization is therefore accepted, comprising a semi-rigid collar on its own.

Motorcycle helmets should be removed only by two skilled operators. One needs to expand the helmet laterally as it is taken off the head, whilst the other immobilizes the neck from below. The cervical spine is then secured in the manner described previously.

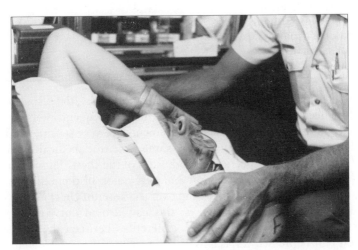

Figure 1.4   Neck stabilization with a semi-rigid collar, sandbags and tape

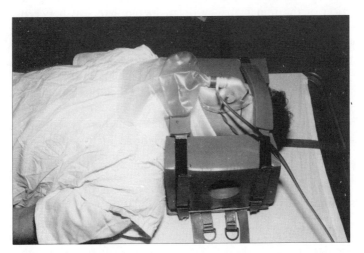

Figure 1.5   Neck stabilization with a commercial apparatus

☐ **(B) Breathing**

There are six immediately life-threatening thoracic conditions which must be searched for, and treated, during the primary survey and resuscitation phase (Box 1.4).

BOX 1.4   Immediately life-threatening thoracic conditions

- Airway obstruction
- Tension pneumothorax
- Cardiac tamponade
- Open chest wound
- Massive haemothorax
- Flail chest

To determine whether any of these conditions exist, the respiratory rate and effort need to be monitored and recorded at frequent intervals by one of the circulation nurses – these measurements are very sensitive indicators of underlying lung pathology. At the same time, the medical team leader should make a visual inspection of both sides of the chest. This examination should be followed by auscultation and percussion of the axillae to assess ventilation of the periphery. Listening over the anterior chest mainly detects air movement in the large airways: this can drown out sounds of pulmonary ventilation. In consequence, differences between the two sides of the chest can be missed, especially if the patient is being artificially ventilated.

If there is no air entry to either side then there is either a complete obstruction of the upper airway or an incomplete seal between face and mask. The maintenance of an effective seal is by no means simple, so the airway personnel need to be skilled in the use of a bag and facemask if the patient requires ventilation but is not intubated. Ideally a two-person technique should be used, with one holding the mask on and pulling the patient's chin forward with both hands, whilst the other person squeezes the bag.

There is usually a local thoracic problem if there is a difference in air entry and percussion note between the right and left sides of the patient's chest. Examples of this are a pneumo- or haemothorax.

If a pneumothorax is suspected, it is vital to determine whether it is under tension because a build-up in pressure in the pleural cavity can rapidly embarrass the heart, lungs and circulation with fatal consequences (see Chapter 3). If the findings support this diagnosis, a 16 g cannula connected to a syringe is inserted into the second intercostal space in the midclavicular line. The aim is to release the positive pressure in the chest. If there is sudden release of air, the diagnosis is confirmed and a chest drain can be inserted on that side. Alternatively, if there is no rapid decompression of the pleural cavity, then an urgent chest x-ray must be taken before a chest drain is placed.

A haemothorax is defined as being massive if it is over 1.5 litres in volume or collects at greater than 200 ml per hour for four hours. Initial treatment consists of a chest drain, however there is usually enough time to confirm the clinical suspicion with a chest x-ray before this procedure is carried out.

The heart is potentially involved with any penetrating injury which enters the area indicated in Figure 3.12 (page 84). This can lead to a pericardial tamponade due to the blood collecting in the pericardial sac. If it is suspected, the medical team leader and one of the circulation nurses should aspirate the blood using the subxiphoid percutaneous approach (see Chapter 3).

Open chest wounds need to be covered with an occlusive dressing, taped on three sides, and a chest drain inserted to prevent the development of a tension pneumothorax.

The immediate treatment of a flail segment of chest wall is dependent on the underlying pulmonary contusion. If there is a low arterial concentration of oxygen, or if he is becoming exhausted, then the patient will require intubation and positive pressure ventilation (see Chapter 3).

☐ (C) Circulation

Any overt bleeding must be controlled by direct pressure using appropriate sizes of absorbent sterile dressings. Tourniquets are only used when the affected limb is deemed unsalvageable.

One of the circulation nurses should measure the blood pressure and note the rate, volume and regularity of the pulse. An automatic blood-pressure recorder and ECG monitor should also be connected to the patient at this time, along with a pulse oximeter.

At the same time, the medical team leader should determine whether the patient demonstrates any clinical evidence of shock – that is, inadequate oxygen delivery to vital organs (see Chapter 4). This requires the assessment of skin colour, clamminess, capillary refill time, heart rate, blood pressure, pulse pressure and conscious level.

Simultaneously, two wide-bore (14–16 g) peripheral lines must be inserted, preferably in the antecubital fossa. If peripheral vasoconstriction makes this impossible, another means of venous access is required. This can be either by a venous cutdown, or by the insertion of a short wide-bore central line (see Chapter 4). Traditionally the medial basilic and distal long saphenous veins are chosen for venous cutdowns. This procedure is recommended because cannulation of a central vein can produce significant injury if it is carried out by unskilled hands.

Once the first cannula is in-position, 10 ml of blood is drawn for group, typing or full cross-matching. A further 10 ml is taken for a full blood count and analysis of the urea and electrolytes. However, the cannula should not be jeopardized if it is difficult to aspirate blood. Instead, it should simply be connected to the blood administration set and the infusion started. The required blood sample can then be taken from the femoral vein or artery. An arterial sample also needs to be obtained for blood gas and pH analysis. This can wait, however, until the end of the primary survey.

In the UK colloids are usually given as the initial intravenous fluid, in preference to Ringer's lactate (see Chapter 4). A litre must be given rapidly in the hypovolaemic patient and the patient's signs monitored. If he is still haemodynamically unstable, a further litre is given as typed or universal donor blood is prepared.

In North America and parts of Africa, Ringer's lactate is usually the initial intravenous fluid. If this is used, two litres must be given and the response monitored. This can be repeated, but again blood should be administered early if the patient remains haemodynamically unstable.

To reduce the incidence of hypothermia, all fluids must be warmed before use.

☐ (D) Dysfunction of the CNS

A rapid and gross assessment of the conscious level is made by asking the patient to put his tongue out, to wiggle his toes, and to squeeze the clinician's fingers. It should be noted whether the trauma victim carries out these activities spontaneously, following verbal command, to pain, or not at all. This is known as the AVPU system (Box 1.5). Pupil size and reactivity must also be assessed. These tests will need to be augmented with a more detailed examination during the secondary survey.

BOX 1.5   Assessing conscious level: the AVPU system

A – **A**lert
V – responding only to **V**erbal stimulus
P – responding only to **P**ain
U – **U**nresponsive to any stimulus

☐ (E) Exposure

While the patient's dignity must be respected, it is essential that all clothing is removed so that the entire skin surface can be examined. In the nontrauma patient it is often easier to slide clothing off by sitting the patient forward and manoeuvring the limbs. The presence of injuries and the possibility of spinal instability prohibits this in trauma patients. Consequently, with this type of patient garments must be cut along seams using large bandage scissors which facilitate their removal with minimal patient movement. If the patient is conscious an explanation can be given and permission sought.

It is important to note that the rapid removal of tight clothing can precipitate sudden hypotension due to the loss of the tamponade effect in the hypovolaemic patient. These garments should only be removed at the team leaders' discretion and when two, large-bore peripheral intravenous lines are running.

Exposed trauma patients can lose body heat rapidly no matter what the season is. This leads to a fall in the core temperature, particularly if the patient has a spinal injury. Studies have also shown that resuscitative measures are impaired, and the prognosis reduced, if hypothermia is allowed to develop (see Chapter 13). The resuscitation room should therefore be kept warm and the patient covered with blankets between examinations.

The well-practised trauma team should complete the objectives of the primary survey and resuscitation phase within seven minutes (Box 1.6). Prearrangement with the laboratory for rapid processing and reporting will facilitate the team leaders' evaluation of the patient's state.

BOX 1.6 Objectives of the primary survey and resuscitation phase

- Assessment and stabilization of the airway
- Stabilization of the cervical spine
- Assessment and correction of any ventilatory problems
- Assessment of the patient's haemodynamic state
- Control of any overt haemorrhage
- Insertion of two large-bore peripheral infusions
- Blood samples taken and sent to the laboratory
- Assessment of the patient's conscious level
- Establishment of supportive contact
- Removal of the patient's clothes
- Covering of the patient with warm blankets
- Initial vital signs recorded and monitors connected
- Insertion of a gastric tube, if appropriate

The vital signs should be recorded every five minutes so that the patient's progress or deterioration can be determined. An important question to ask is, 'Is the patient getting better or worse?' This helps to determine whether the team needs to move rapidly to definitive care. For example, the patient should be taken directly to theatre to gain control of a source of bleeding if there is no response to aggressive intravenous resuscitation.

Only when all the ventilatory and hypovolaemic problems have been corrected can the team continue the more detailed secondary survey.

As the primary survey and resuscitation phase is under way, the relatives' nurse should greet any of the patient's friends or relatives who arrive. She can then take them to a private room which has all necessary facilities and stay there, so that she will be able to provide support and information (see Chapter 16). Periodically, therefore, she will have to go to the resuscitation room to receive an update from the nursing team leader as well as to give information to both team leaders about the relatives.

Once the primary survey has been completed, the leaders can release the non-essential members of the team so that they can return to their normal activities in the department.

■ Secondary survey

The objectives of this phase are:

- to examine the patient from head to toe to determine the full extent of his injuries;
- to take a complete medical history;
- to assimilate all clinical, laboratory and radiological information;
- to formulate a management plan for the patient.

It is important to note that should the patient deteriorate at any stage, the team leader must abandon the secondary survey and reassess the trauma victim's airway, breathing and circulatory state in the manner described in the primary survey.

As with the primary survey, a well-coordinated team effort is required in which each member has a specific task. Procedures by individual team members are followed according to a precise protocol and again tasks are performed simultaneously rather than sequentially.

The detailed assessment of the patient is usually carried out by the medical team leader who calls out his findings which are recorded by the nursing team leader. The common error of being distracted before the whole body has been inspected must be avoided as potentially serious injuries could be missed, especially in the unconscious patient.

During the secondary survey the airway nurse must maintain verbal contact with the patient. At the same time, one of the circulation nurses

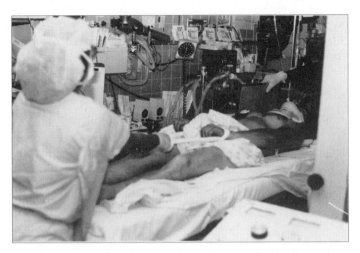

Figure 1.6 Pulling the arms down for a cervical radiograph

must continue to measure the vital signs regularly and also take responsibility for monitoring the intravenous fluids.

All blunt-trauma patients require cervical spine, chest and pelvic radiographs in the resuscitation room. Unless the chest x-ray has already been taken during the primary survey, the first to be taken should be of the lateral cervical spine. This can be taken immediately after the secondary survey, or during it, if the team members are protected. This x-ray is used to exclude 85 per cent of the cervical abnormalities, but to do so it needs to show all seven cervical vertebrae as well as the C7-T1 junction. To facilitate this, one of the team members should pull the patient's arm towards the feet as the radiograph is taken, whilst another member of the team maintains inline stabilization (Figure 1.6). A 'swimmer's view' can be used if this fails to give an adequate view.

At the end of the secondary survey further cervical radiographs will need to be taken to help exclude a skeletal abnormality. This process is described in detail in Chapter 8.

☐ Examination

The scalp

This must be examined for lacerations, swellings or depressions. Its entire surface must be inspected, but the occiput will have to wait until the patient is turned or the cervical spine 'cleared' both clinically and radiologically. Visual inspection may discover fractures in the base of the lacerations. However, wounds should not be blindly probed as further damage to underlying structures can result. If there is major bleeding from the scalp, digital pressure or a self-retaining retractor should be used. It is important to remember that in small children scalp lacerations can bleed sufficiently to cause hypovolaemia, so haemostasis is crucial in these cases.

Neurological state

The medical team leader can now carry out a 'mini-neurological' examination of the patient. This comprises an assessment of the conscious level (using the Glasgow Coma Scale), the pupillary response, and the presence of any lateralizing signs (see Chapter 6). One of the circulation nurses should then continue to monitor these parameters. If there is any deterioration, hypoxia or hypovolaemia must be ruled out before an intracranial injury is considered.

Base of skull

Fractures to this structure will produce signs along a diagonal line demonstrated in Figure 1.7. Bruising can develop over the mastoid process (Battle's sign) but this usually takes 12–36 hours to appear; it is therefore of limited use in the resuscitation room. A cerebrospinal fluid (CSF) leak may be missed as the CSF is invariably mixed with blood. Fortunately its presence in this bloody discharge can be detected by noting the delay in clotting of the blood and by the double-ring pattern that results when it is dropped onto an absorbent sheet. In this situation nothing, including an auroscope, should be inserted into the external auditory canal, because of the risk of introducing infection and hence causing meningitis. As there is a small chance of a nasogastric tube passing into the cranium through a base-of-skull fracture, these tubes should be passed orally when this type of injury is suspected.

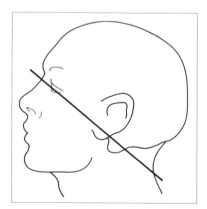

Figure 1.7 Diagonal line demonstrating the level of the base of the skull

Eyes

Inspection of the eyes should be carried out before significant orbital swelling makes examination too difficult. The assessor must look for haemorrhages, both inside and outside the globe; for foreign bodies under the lids (including contact lenses); and for the presence of penetrating injuries. If the patient is conscious, the visual acuity can be tested by having him read a name badge or fluid label. If he is unconscious, the pupillary response and corneal reflexes are tested.

The face

This should be palpated symmetrically for deformities and tenderness. The assessor must also check for lost teeth and stability of the maxilla by pulling the latter forward to see whether the middle third of the face is stable (see Chapter 7). Middle-third fractures can be associated with an airway obstruction in conjunction with a base-of-skull fracture. However, only those injuries coexisting with an airway obstruction need to be treated immediately.

Mandibular fractures can also cause airway obstruction, because of the loss of stability of the tongue.

The neck

This must always be carefully examined if a cervical injury is suspected. Once the airway nurse has restored manual inline stabilization, the team leader can remove the sandbags, tape and semi-rigid collar so that the neck can be assessed. It should be inspected for any deformity (rare), bruising and lacerations. Each of the cervical spinous processes can then be palpated for tenderness or a 'step off' deformity. The posterior cervical muscles should also be palpated for tenderness or spasm. The conscious patient can assist by indicating if there is pain or tenderness in the neck and locating the site.

Lacerations should be inspected only: they should *never* be probed with metal instruments or fingers. If laceration penetrates platysma, definitive radiological or surgical management will be needed. The choice depends on the clinical state of the patient (see Chapter 3).

The thorax

The priority at this stage is to identify those thoracic conditions which are potentially life-threatening, along with any remaining chest injuries (see Chapter 3).

The chest wall must be reinspected for bruising, signs of obstruction, asymmetry of movement, and wounds. Acceleration and deceleration forces can produce extensive thoracic injuries. However, these invariably leave marks on the chest wall which should lead the team to consider particular types of injury. For example, the diagonal seatbelt bruise may overlap a fractured clavicle, a thoracic aortic tear, pulmonary contusion or pancreatic laceration. Good pre-hospital information is vital to determine the mechanism of injury.

The assessor should next palpate the sternum and then each rib, starting in the axillae and proceeding caudally and anteriorly. The presence of any crepitus, tenderness or subcutaneous emphysema must be noted. Auscultation and percussion of the whole chest can then be carried out to determine whether there is any asymmetry between the right and left sides of the chest.

Pulmonary and cardiac contusions are potentially life-threatening and should be considered when the chest wall has received a significant direct blow. An example of this is the collision between a driver's thorax and a steering wheel following a road traffic accident. The intensive management these patients' requirements is discussed in detail in Chapter 3.

The thoracic aorta can be torn when the patient has been subjected to a rapid deceleration force, as for example in a road traffic accident or a fall from a height. A high index of suspicion, along with a thorough examination and an erect chest x-ray, are essential in these cases (see Chapter 3).

A ruptured diaphragm and a perforated oesophagus can follow both blunt and penetrating trauma. However, diagnosis is made usually on the appearance of the chest radiograph. Their management is described in Chapter 3. The management of a pneumothorax or haemothorax has been discussed previously.

The abdomen

The objective of this part of the secondary survey is simply to determine whether the patient requires a laparotomy. A precise diagnosis of which particular viscus has been injured is time-consuming and of little relevance at this stage.

A thorough examination of the whole abdomen is required, therefore the pelvis and perineum must be assessed. All bruising, abnormal movement and wounds must be noted and any exposed bowel covered with warm saline-soaked swabs. Lacerations should be inspected but not probed blindly as further damage can result. It is not possible to determine the actual depth of the wound if underlying muscle is penetrated; such cases will require further investigations (see Chapter 5).

The abdomen needs to be palpated in a systematic manner so that areas of tenderness can be detected. The gross stability of the pelvis should then be assessed and a rectal examination carried out. The latter provides five pieces of information:

- Sphincter tone – this can be lost after spinal injuries.
- Direct rectal trauma.
- Pelvic fractures.

- Prostatic position – this can be disrupted after posterior urethral injury.
- Blood in the lower alimentary canal.

The rate of urine output is an important indicator in assessing the shocked patient (see Chapter 4). It should therefore be measured in all trauma patients, and in most cases this will require catheterization. If there is no evidence of urethral injury, the catheter is passed transurethrally in the normal way. However, if urethral trauma is suspected (Box 1.7), and the patient is unable to urinate, a suprapubic catheter may be necessary. The urine that is voided initially should be tested for blood and saved for microscopy and subsequent possible drug analysis.

BOX 1.7   Signs of urethral injury in a male patient

- Bruising around the scrotum
- Blood at the end of the urethral meatus
- High-riding prostate

Marked gastric distension is frequently found in crying children, adults with head or abdominal injuries, and patients who have been ventilated with a bag-and-mask technique. The insertion of a gastric tube facilitates the abdominal examination of these patients and reduces the risks of aspiration.

An intra-abdominal bleed should be suspected if the ribs overlying the liver and spleen are fractured (5–11), if the patient is haemodynamically unstable, or if there are seatbelt marks, tyre marks or bruises over the abdominal surface. However, the detection of abdominal tenderness is unreliable if there is a sensory defect due to neurological damage or drugs, or if there are fractures of the lower ribs or pelvis. In these cases, a diagnostic peritoneal lavage should be carried out to help rule out an intraperitoneal injury (see Chapter 5). Ideally this should be performed by the general surgeon who would be responsible for any subsequent laparotomy.

Extremities

The limbs are examined by inspection, palpation and then movement. All the long bones must also be rotated and, if the patient is conscious, he should be asked actively to move each limb.

Upon completion of the examination, the presence of any bruising, wounds and deformities must be noted, along with any crepitus, instability, neurovascular abnormalities or soft-tissue damage (see Chapter 9).

As time delays can result in tissue loss, gross limb deformities need to be corrected and the pulses and sensation rechecked before any radiographs are taken.

Any wounds associated with compound fractures must be swabbed and covered with a non-adherent dressing. As different surgeons will need to examine the limb, a Polaroid™ photograph of the wound before it is covered will reduce the number of times the dressings have to be removed.

All limb fractures need splintage to reduce fracture movement and hence pain, bleeding, the formation of fat emboli, and secondary soft-tissue swelling and damage. In the case of shaft-of-femur fractures, a traction splint should be used (see Chapter 9).

The spinal column

A detailed neurological examination needs to be carried out at this stage to determine whether there are any abnormalities in the peripheral nervous system. Motor and sensory defects, and in male patients the presence of priapism, can help indicate the level and extent of the spinal injury.

If the cord has been transected above the spinal origin of the sympathetic nervous system, hypotension results due to peripheral vasodilatation. The degree of vasodilatation depends on how little sympathetic tone remains. A cervical transection of the cord removes all vasoconstrictor tone and so leads to profound hypotension. However, this neurogenic shock is not associated with a tachycardia because the sympathetic innervation of the heart has been lost (see Chapter 4).

A detailed description of the diagnosis, treatment and nursing care of this type of condition is described in Chapter 8.

Soft-tissue injuries

A detailed inspection of the whole of the patient's skin is needed to determine the number and extent of the soft-tissue injuries. Each breach in the skin needs to be inspected to determine its site, depth and the presence of any underlying structural damage that will require surgical repair during the definitive care phase. However, once the clinical state of the patient stabilizes, superficial wounds can be cleaned, irrigated and dressed. A detailed description of the management of soft-tissue injuries is given in Chapter 10.

The back

If a spinal injury is suspected, the patient should be moved only by a well-coordinated log-rolling technique (Figure 1.8) or a vertical lift. Usually the former is used, and the patient is turned away from the examiner, who takes this opportunity to clear away all the debris from under the patient. He or she should then assess the whole of the back, from occiput to heels, looking for bruising and open wounds. The back of the chest must be auscultated; the area between the buttocks inspected; and the vertebral column palpated for boggy swellings, malalignment and deformities in contour. The exami-

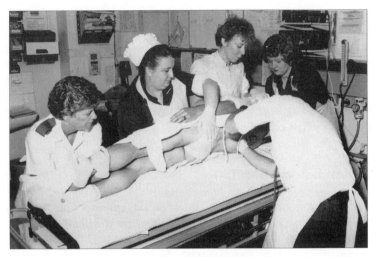

Figure 1.8 A patient being 'log-rolled'

WATERLOW PRESSURE SORE PREVENTION/TREATMENT POLICY
RING SCORES IN TABLE, ADD TOTAL. SEVERAL SCORES PER CATEGORY CAN BE USED

BUILD/WEIGHT FOR HEIGHT	★	SKIN TYPE VISUAL RISK AREAS	★	SEX AGE	★	SPECIAL RISKS	★
AVERAGE	0	HEALTHY	0	MALE	1	TISSUE MALNUTRITION	★
ABOVE AVERAGE	1	TISSUE PAPER	1	FEMALE	2		
OBESE	2	DRY	1	14 - 49	1	e.g.: TERMINAL CACHEXIA	8
BELOW AVERAGE	3	OEDEMATOUS	1	50 - 64	2	CARDIAC FAILURE	5
		CLAMMY (TEMP↑)	1	65 - 74	3	PERIPHERAL VASCULAR	
CONTINENCE	★	DISCOLOURED,	2	75 - 80	4	DISEASE	5
		BROKEN/SPOT	3	81+	5	ANAEMIA	2
COMPLETE/						SMOKING	1
CATHETERISED	0						
OCCASION INCONT	1	MOBILITY	★	APPETITE	★	NEUROLOGICAL DEFICIT	★
CATH/INCONTINENT							
OF FAECES	2	FULLY	0	AVERAGE	0	eg: DIABETES, M.S, CVA,	
DOUBLY INCONT	3	RESTLESS/FIDGETY	1	POOR	1	MOTOR/SENSORY	
		APATHETIC	2	N.G. TUBE/		PARAPLEGIA	4 - 6
		RESTRICTED	3	FLUIDS ONLY	2		
		INERT/TRACTION	4	NBM/ANOREXIC	3	MAJOR SURGERY/TRAUMA	★
		CHAIRBOUND	5				
						ORTHOPAEDIC -	
						BELOW WAIST,SPINAL	5
SCORE 10+ AT RISK 15+ HIGH RISK 20+ VERY HIGH RISK						ON TABLE > 2 HOURS	5
						MEDICATION	★
© J Waterlow 1991 Revised March 1992						CYTOTOXICS,	4
						HIGH DOSE STEROIDS	
OBTAINABLE FROM: NEWTONS, CURLAND, TAUNTON, TA3 5SG						ANTI-INFLAMMATORY	

Figure 1.9 The Waterlow scoring system
Source: © Waterlow J 1992. Reproduced by kind permission.

nation finishes with palpation of the longitudinal spinal muscles for spasm and tenderness. The patient is then log-rolled back into the supine position.

The nursing team leader will need to make an initial assessment of the skin using a pressure-sore scoring system, such as the Waterlow system

(Figure 1.9). In the elderly, and other high-risk patients, there must be meticulous attention from the outset to prevent pressure sores. The patient may have spent a considerable time in one position before being rescued, and if he requires surgery he may have to remain in the same position for several more hours. It is therefore important to note how long the trauma victim remains in one position and to move whatever can be moved every thirty minutes, using hip lifts for example. This factor needs to be taken into consideration when compiling the nursing plans.

☐ Medical history (AMPLE)

At the end of the secondary survey, the medical team leader must fully assess the patient's medical history. Part of this information will already have been acquired from the ambulance personnel by the medical team leader.

The team needs to be familiar with the mechanism of the injury and to take account of the pre-morbid state of the patient. A witness's history of the event (usually collected by the ambulance personnel), and the past medical history from the family and friends, can also be important in planning the care of the individual.

The important elements of the medical history can be remembered by the mnemonic *AMPLE* (Box 1.8):

BOX 1.8   Important elements of the medical history (AMPLE)

A – Allergies
M – Medicines
P – Past medical history
L – Last meal
E – Events leading to the incident

■ Assimilation of information

As the condition of the patient can change quickly, repeated examinations and constant monitoring of the vital signs are essential. The circulation nurse, responsible for recording the latter at 15-minute intervals, must be vigilant and must bring any deterioration in the respiratory rate, pulse, blood pressure, conscious level or urine output to the immediate attention of the team leaders.

By the end of the secondary survey, the answers to the following questions must be known:

☐ **Is the patient's respiratory function satisfactory?**

If it is not adequate, then the cause must be sought and corrected as a priority.

☐ **Is the patient's circulatory status satisfactory?**

It is essential that the trauma team recognizes shock early in its progress and intervenes aggressively. It is equally important to evaluate the patient's response to the resuscitative measures (see Chapter 4).

If less than 20 per cent of the blood volume has been lost, the vital signs usually return to normal after less than two litres of colloid. If they then remain stable this implies that the patient is not actively bleeding. However, care and constant supervision are needed in these cases because these trauma victims may deteriorate later.

Transient responders are patients who are actively bleeding or recommence bleeding during the resuscitation. Their vital signs improve initially but then decline. Usually they have lost over 30 per cent of their blood volume and require an infusion with typed blood. Control of the bleeding source invariably requires an operation.

In a shocked patient, the total lack of response to a colloid infusion suggests either that the condition is not due to hypovolaemia, or that the patient has lost over 40 per cent of his blood volume and continues to bleed faster than the rate of the fluid infusion. The history, the mechanism of injury and the physical findings will help to determine which is the most likely (see Chapter 3). The former needs invasive techniques to monitor the pulmonary and central venous pressures. In the case of major haemorrhage, an operation and a blood transfusion are urgently required. The source of the bleeding is usually in the chest, abdomen or pelvis.

☐ **Are any further radiological investigations required?**

This depends on the condition of the patient. If he is hypoxic or haemodynamically unstable then these problems must be addressed first. Once his condition stabilizes, radiographs of particular sites of injury can be performed along with other, specialized investigations. It is an important part of the team leaders' responsibilities to determine the priorities of these investigations.

☐ **What are the extent and priorities of the injuries?**

The team leaders must categorize all the injuries so that the most dangerous is treated first.

☐ **Have any injuries been overlooked?**

The mechanism of injury and the injury pattern must be considered to avoid overlooking sites of damage. It is important to remember that trauma rarely 'skips' areas. For example, if injuries have been found in the thorax and the femur, but not in the abdomen, then probably injury there has been missed. The patient must be re-examined.

☐ **Are tetanus toxoid, human antitetanus immunoglobulin (Humotet™) or antibiotics required?**

This will depend on both local and national policies, which should be known by the team leaders.

☐ **Is analgesia required?**

Severely injured patients need analgesia. Contraindications (i.e. pneumothorax and head and abdominal injuries) apart, Entonox can be given until the baseline observations are recorded. Intravenous morphine can then be titrated against the patient's pain level. Narcotics are contraindicated in head-injured patients and those with abdominal trauma until the respective surgeons have examined the patient.

■ Definitive care

Once the patient has been adequately assessed and resuscitated, definitive care can start. In many cases this will require either one or more operations, or intensive care management, or both. It is therefore very important that the transition from the resuscitation room to these areas is made as smoothly as possible.

The medical notes must be written up at the end of the resuscitation by the medical team leader; whilst the charts, vital signs, fluid input and output information, drug administration and preliminary nursing care documentation are all collated by the nursing team leader. A purpose-designed single trauma sheet can facilitate this process (Figure 1.10 – see pages 36–7).

The relatives' nurse can then brief the team leaders about the condition of any relatives or friends who are in the department on the patient's behalf. The medical team leader should accompany her back to the relatives' room, to talk to them. If this doctor has instead had to go urgently with the patient, another clinician, fully conversant with the situation, should be sent in his place.

If the patient is unconscious, his clothing and belongings may provide essential information. Usually the rescue personnel will have sought the trauma victim's identity before arrival at hospital. However, whether the patient's name is known or not, some system of identification is required, not least so that drugs and blood can be administered safely. This becomes more important when there are several patients in the resuscitation room. If identity bracelets are impractical, then indelible markers can be used to write a number on the patient's skin.

The patient must not leave the department without identification.

Any possessions brought in with the patient must be handed over to the nursing staff by the rescue personnel. These must be kept safely, along with the patient's clothing and property. At the end of the secondary survey, or during it if there are hands to spare, all these articles must be searched. A check is needed for any medical alert card or disc, any suicide note, and any medicine bottles or tablets.

Jewellery, and if relevant dentures, need to be removed from the patient and stored in a labelled valuables bag or envelope. This should be with his permission if he is conscious. Rings and other constrictive jewellery must also be removed as the fingers may swell. If this is not possible, they should be cut off. At an appropriate moment, and preferably by nurses outside the trauma team, the property is collected, checked, recorded, signed for and locked away. Whatever the outcome of the resuscitation, relatives take a dim view of items of property being misplaced. Nurses are legally responsible for this property and protracted problems can result if the patient's seemingly unimportant effects are disregarded in the heat of the moment.

If a criminal case is suspected, all clothing and possessions, and any loose debris, bullets or shrapnel, are required for forensic examination. These too must be collected, labelled, placed in waxed bags and signed for prior to releasing them to the appropriate authorities according to established procedures (see Chapter 17).

If a delay in transfer is anticipated, the patient can be given a gentle, preliminary wash to remove any blood, mud or other contaminating material.

☐ Preparation for transfer of the patient

Communication

To facilitate a smooth transfer, it is important to ensure that the receiving facility and personnel have been contacted directly by the medical team leader. If an inter-hospital transfer is envisaged, the clinicians must also

Name — — — — — — Age/D.O.B.— — — —
Address — — — — — — — — — — — — — —
— — — — — — — — — — — — — —
— — — — — — — — A/E No:— — — —

Date— — — — Time of arrival — — — —
Drugs— — — — Allergies — — — — —
PMH — — — — — — — — — — — —
— — — — — — Last ate — — — — —

BLOODS	RESULTS	BLOODS	RESULTS
☐ Hb		☐ WCC	
☐ Hct		☐ PLTS	
☐ Na		☐ BS	
☐ K		☐ Urea	
☐ BM			

	Time	% O₂			
☐ ABG	pO²				
	pCO²				
	pH				
	BE				
☐ Other					

PRIMARY SURVEY

ASSESSMENT

☐ **AIRWAY**
- ☐ Normal   Gag Y/N
- ☐ Unconscious
- ☐ Facial fractures

CERVICAL SPINE
- ☐ Normal ☐ Suspect injury ☐ Firm collar ☐ In line traction

☐ **BREATHING**
- *RR ON ARRIVAL................../min*
- ☐ Trauma   (blunt/penetrating)
- ☐ Pneumothorax (open / closed / tension)
- ☐ Haemothorax
- ☐ Flail segment

☐ **CIRCULATION**
- *SYSTOLIC BP ON ARRIVAL ....mmHg*
- ☐ Haemorrhage
  - ☐ External
  - ☐ Internal   ☐ Chest
    - ☐ Abdomen
    - ☐ Pelvis

☐ **DYSFUNCTION**
- *GCS ON ARRIVAL...................*
- ☐ Alert
- ☐ Responds to verbal commands
- ☐ Responds to pain
- ☐ Unresponsive
  - Pupils equal : Y / N

RESUSCITATION

- ☐ Spontaneous
- ☐ Mask/mask + airway   — — — %O²
- ☐ Ventilated   ☐ ETT - size — — —
- ☐ N-G tube

- ☐ Chest drain
  - Left   Right
  - Size — — — Size — — — —

- IV (1)-site — — — — Size — — — — —
- IV (2)-site — — — — Size — — — — —
- **Blood ordered**   ☐ 0 Neg
  - Time — — hrs   ☐ Grouped
    - ☐ X-match
    - ☐ G + S
- ☐ Pressure dressings
- ☐ Arterial blood gases
- ☐ ECG monitor

- ☐ In line stabilisation of
  - whole spine

X-RAYS	Findings
☐ C-spine	
☐ CXR	
☐ Pelvis	
☐ SXR	
☐ Long bones	
☐ Spine	
☐ C.T. scan	

DRUGS	Dr. sig.	Sig. given
☐ Tet. tox.		
0.5 ml		
☐ Humo. Tet.		
250 units		
☐ Analgesics		
☐ Antibiotic		
☐ Anaesthetic drugs		

SECONDARY SURVEY   Tick pulses present
Summary of Injuries

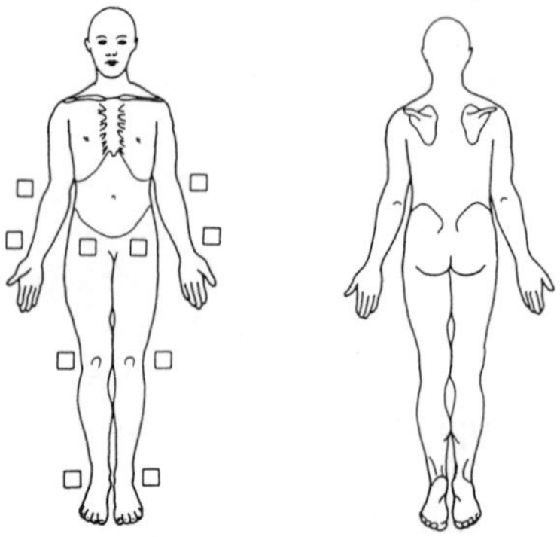

PERITONEAL LAVAGE			
RBC — — — — /mm³	WBC — — — /mm³		
Bacteria — — — Y/N	Food — — — Y/N		
Performed by — — — —	Time — — — —		

USS abdo — — — — — — — — — — —

URINE   (Cath / MSU / Other)
Blood — — — — — Ketones — — — —
Sugar — — — — — Protein — — — —

REFERRALS

	Grade	Time Called	Time Arrived
☐ Anaesthetist			
☐ Gen.surgeons			
☐ Orthopaedic			
☐ Neurosurg.			
☐ Thoracic			
☐ Plastic			
☐ Max. fac.			
☐ Other			

DISPOSAL TIME
Ward — — — — — — — — hrs
ITU — — — — — — — — hrs
Theatre — — — — — — hrs
CT scan — — — — — — hrs
Died — — — — — — — hrs
Transfer — — — — — — hrs

Resuscitation led by :
Initially : — — — — — — — — — —
Finally : — — — — — — — — — —

Chart compiled by :
Name — — — — — Signature — — — —

Figure 1.10 A trauma sheet

INCIDENT DETAILS : Time
- Mechanism

- Pre-hospital care

Vital signs at scene :
BP [ ] Pulse [ ] RR [ ] GCS [ ]

NURSING DETAILS
Relatives   Name _ _ _ _ _ _ _ _ _ _ Phone no. _ _ _ _
Address _ _ _ _ _ _ _ _ _ _ _ _ _ _ _ _
_ _ _ _ _ _ _ _ _ _ _ _ _ _ _ _ Contacted Y/N
Other details

VITAL SIGNS

Blood pressure

Pulse ●

| Hour |
| Minute |
| 180 |
| 160 |
| 140 |
| 120 |
| 100 |
| 80 |
| 60 |
| 40 |
| 20 |
| 0 |
| Respiratory rate |
| Temperature °C |
| Arterial oxygen saturation (%) |

James Driscoll McCabe 1991

Pupil scale (mm)
- •1
- ●2
- ●3
- ●4
- ●5
- ●6
- ●7
- ●8

ACTIONS / EVENTS

| Hour |
| Minute |

PUPILS
+ Reacts
- No reaction
C Closed by swelling

R   Size
    Reaction
L   Size
    Reaction

G.C.S.

VERBAL	Orientated	5
	Confused	4
	Inappropriate words	3
	Incomprehensible sounds	2
	None	1
MOTOR	Obeys commands	6
	Localises pain	5
	Flexion to pain	4
	Decorticate movement	3
	Extension to pain	2
	None	1
EYE	Spontaneous	4
	To speech	3
	To pain	2
	None	1

G.C.S. Total Score

HAEMACCEL

I.V. Site 1				I.V. Site 2			
Time	Fluid	Vol.	Given	Time	Fluid	Vol.	Given

Total input IV site 1= [ ] ml   Total input IV site 2 = [ ] ml
TOTAL IV INPUT = [ ] ml

URINE OUTPUT		OTHER LOSSES	
Catheter / voided		Specify : _ _ _ _ _ _ _	
Time	Vol.	Time	Vol.

TOTAL URINE OUTPUT	TOTAL OTHER LOSSES
= [ ] ml	= [ ] ml

Department of Medical Illustration, S.H.A. H91071270

decide on the most suitable method of transportation and how the patient should be prepared for the journey. For example, it is difficult to subdue patients in the confined space of an aircraft: if air transport is required and the patient is confused or aggressive, the use of restraints (physical or pharmacological) should therefore be considered prior to leaving.

Assessment

All aspects of the primary survey must be reassessed before the patient leaves, and appropriate adjustments made. For example, the patient who tolerates an oropharyngeal airway should be intubated and ventilated so that the airway can be protected and hypoxia and hypercarbia prevented. All cannulae, catheters, tubes and drains must be secured.

Monitoring

If a parameter needs to be monitored *before* transfer, it also needs to be monitored *during* transfer.

Carl Gwinnutt 1992

Monitoring during the transfer period must be continued to ensure that ventilation and tissue perfusion are adequate. Therefore a fully-charged ECG monitor, an automatic BP recorder and a pulse oximeter are essential.

Equipment and drugs

The trolley carrying the patient during intra-hospital transfer must also transport the suction system, the oxygen supply, the ventilator, the portable BP monitor and the defibrillator-monitor. Airway adjuncts, needles and drugs are usually carried separately by one of the medical team.

The same principles apply for inter-hospital transfers, however it is important to remember that portable ventilators use their gas supply as their power source: an adequate amount of oxygen must therefore be taken (see Chapter 22).

Transfer personnel

During transit, the patient needs to be accompanied by appropriately trained staff who can monitor the patient and intervene with any ventilatory or perfusion problems. If he is intubated, the most suitable personnel are the airway nurse and doctor.

Records

All the medical and nursing notes, radiographs, blood tests, identifying labels and, if necessary, consent forms must be taken with the patient.

Relatives and friends

The nurse dealing with these people must inform them about the transfer. When the trauma victim is to be moved to another hospital, this nurse should also help the friends and relatives in their own transportation arrangements.

Final check

Before moving off, the team must ensure that the patient is appropriately covered and, for intra-hospital transfers, that the lift, if needed, has been reserved.

Upon arrival

The transfer team must hand over to the doctor and nurse who will be in charge of the patient's definitive care. In this way important events during transfer as well as a summary of the initial resuscitation can be given to the personnel directly responsible for the patient. All documentation can be handed over at this stage and the transfer equipment retrieved.

☐ Preparation of the resuscitation room

As the transfer is under way, the remaining staff can begin preparing the area for the arrival of the next trauma victim. Throughout the resuscitation the team should have kept the area as tidy and organized as possible, with sharps, open packs and instruments being disposed of as they are used. This is essential for both safety and efficiency. Wet, greasy floors need to be wiped or covered immediately after spillage to avoid accidents to staff.

Once the patient has been transferred and the resuscitation area restocked, checked and made ready, the team can get together for a preliminary or definitive debriefing session.

■ Summary

To enable the patient to receive the most efficient resuscitation, a group of nurses and doctors must be ready to meet him when he arrives at the A/E department. These people must be coordinated by nursing and medical team leaders so that they are all aware of the tasks they have to perform, and so that these are carried out simultaneously.

The first priority is to detect and treat all the immediately life-threatening conditions. Following this, a detailed head-to-toe assessment can be completed. The team leaders can then list the patient's injuries and their priorities for both further investigations and definitive treatment.

■ References and further reading

American College of Surgeons Committee on Trauma 1993. *Advanced Trauma Life Support for Physicians*. Chicago: American College of Surgeons.

Beaver B M 1990. Care of the multiple trauma victim. The first hour. *Nurs. Clin. N. Am.* **25**(1): 11.

Braverman A 1990. Eliciting assessment data from the patient who is difficult to interview. *Nurs. Clin. N. Am.* **25**: 743.

Committee on Trauma of the American College of Surgeons 1986. Hospital and pre-hospital resources for optimal care of the injured patient. *Am. Coll. Surgeons Bull.* **71**: 4.

Cowley R 1976. The resuscitation and stabilisation of major multiple trauma patients in a trauma centre environment. *Clin. Med.* **83**: 14.

Driscoll P & Vincent C 1992a. Organizing an efficient trauma team. *Injury* **23**(2): 107

Driscoll P & Vincent C 1992b. Variation in trauma resuscitation and its effects on patient outcome. *Injury* **23**(2): 111.

Dunham C & Cowley R 1986. *Shock Trauma – critical care handbook*. Royal Tunbridge Wells: Aspen.

Holbrook J 1990. Honing physical diagnostic skills. *Patient Care* **24**: 123.

Huggins B 1990. Trauma physiology. *Nurs. Clin. N. Am.* **25**(1): 1.

Jeffries N & Bristow A 1991. Long-distance inter-hospital transfers. *Br. J. Int. Care.* Nov.: 197.

Kinney B 1989: Assessment: the key to qualify patient care. *Emerg. Med. Serv.* **18**: 30.

Lazear S 1992. Aeromedical transport. In Sheehy S, Marvin J & Jimmerson C (eds): *Emergency Nursing, Principles and Practice*, 3rd Edn. St. Louis: C V Mosby.

Myers C, Brown A, Dunjey S, *et al.* 1993. Trauma teams: order from chaos. *Em. Medicine* **5**: 28.

Rice M & Abel C 1992. Triage. In Sheehy S, Marvin J & Jimmerson C (eds): *Emergency Nursing, Principles and Practice*, 3rd Edn. St. Louis: C V Mosby.

Ridley S, Wright I & Rogers P 1990. Secondary transport of critically ill patients. *Hospital Update* **16**: 289.

Salvatores S 1992. Interfacility transport. In Sheehy S, Marvin J & Jimmerson C (eds): *Emergency Nursing, Principles and Practice*, 3rd Edn. St. Louis: C V Mosby.

Shatney C H 1988. Initial resuscitation and assessment of patients with multisystem blunt trauma. *S. Med. J.* 81(4): 501.

Sheehy S 1992. Multiple trauma. In Sheehy S, Marvin J & Jimmerson C (eds): *Emergency Nursing, Principles and Practice*, 3rd Edn. St. Louis: C V Mosby.

Simoneau J 1992. Physical assessment. In Sheehy S, Marvin J & Jimmerson C (eds): *Emergency Nursing, Principles and Practice*, 3rd Edn. St. Louis: C V Mosby.

Weight J 1986. The initial management of the trauma patient. *Crit. Care Clinics* 2: 705.

Chapter 2

Management of the airway with cervical spine control

Carl Gwinnutt, Peter Driscoll and Olive Goodall

Objectives

The objectives of this chapter are to teach the personnel allocated to manage the trauma patient's airway:

- how to assess and secure the airway;

- basic airway management;

- the use of simple airway adjuncts;

- artificial ventilation;

- advanced airway management;

- the use of drugs to aid intubation;

- the use of surgical airways in the resuscitation room.

■ Introduction

Airway control is an essential prerequisite for successful resuscitation of the trauma patient. It is therefore the first feature of the patient that is assessed and secured. It needs to be remembered that the cervical spine may be at risk during these activities if they are not performed in a controlled way. This chapter will describe how the airway can be assessed, cleared and secured without jeopardizing an unstable cervical spine.

■ Applied anatomy

Figure 2.1 demonstrates the important structures and surface landmarks of the upper airway.

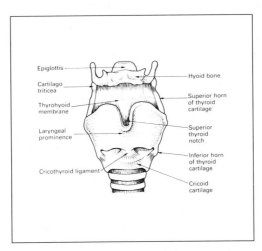

Figure 2.1a   Anterior view of the upper airway
Source: © Romanes G J (ed.) 1969. *Cunningham's Manual of Practical Anatomy*, Vol. 2, 13th edn. Oxford: Oxford University Press. By permission of Oxford University Press.

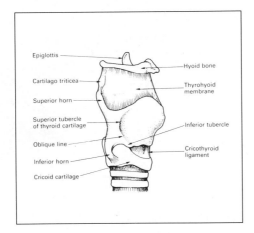

Figure 2.1b   Lateral view of the upper airway
Source: © Romanes G J (ed.) 1969. *Cunningham's Manual of Practical Anatomy*, Vol. 2, 13th edn. Oxford: Oxford University Press. By permission of Oxford University Press.

■ Standby preparation

All equipment must be checked regularly (see Box 2.6 and Figure 2.6). The team leader must allocate the responsibility of the airway and cervical spine to the most appropriate doctor and nurse. They should then complete a final check of equipment whilst awaiting the arrival of the patient.

■ Transfer of the patient to the resuscitation room

As soon as the ambulance arrives the trauma victim's airway should be assessed, cleared and secured before he is moved to the resuscitation room. Simultaneously the neck should be secured: if not already stabilized with a rigid cervical collar, sandbags and tape, the nurse should secure it with her hands and forearms (Figure 2.2).

A minimum of five people will be required to transfer the patient unless he is already on a spinal board or scoop stretcher (see Chapter 8). The doctor and nurse responsible for the airway must ensure that there is no uncontrolled movement of the spine and that any artificial airway, previously inserted, is not displaced.

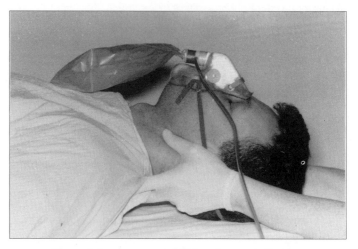

Figure 2.2   A nurse stabilizing the cervical spine

■ Assessing and securing the airway

The quickest way of evaluating the airway is to ask the patient 'Are you all right?' If he replies in a lucid manner then the airway personnel will know:

1 that the airway is clear;

2 that the patient has a reasonable vital capacity breath;

3 that cerebral perfusion is sufficient to maintain consciousness.

An impaired response may be due to acute severe airway obstruction (Box 2.1). There may be noisy breathing (stridor), a rapid respiratory rate (tachypnoea), and agitation due to cerebral hypoxia, or any combination of these. There may be associated use of the accessory muscles (e.g. sterno-mastoids and scalenes) and indrawing of the intercostal, supraclavicular and suprasternal spaces. If the situation persists, carbon dioxide will accumulate in the blood (hypercapnia) and this may cause the patient's conscious level to deteriorate.

BOX 2.1   Problems with the airway

Sign	Common cause in trauma victims
Stridor	Obstructed airway
Tachypnoea	Obstructed airway
	Intrathoracic pathology
	Hypovolaemia
Poor ventilation	Obstructed airway
	Severe cerebral hypoxia

If there is no attempt at a reply, the patient is usually unconscious (Box 2.2).

BOX 2.2   Causes of an altered conscious level

T – Trauma to the brain	*A* – Alcohol
I – Insulin/diabetes	*E* – Epilepsy
P – Poisons	*I* – Infection
P – Psychiatric	*O* – Opiates
S – Shock	*U* – Urea/metabolic

These causes can be remembered by the mnemonic *Tipps on the vowels.*

Profound hypoxia from any cause can reduce the conscious level.

The airway personnel must assess the adequacy of the patient's airway if they suspect that he is unconscious. This is carried out using the 'look, listen and feel' method:

- *Look* – to see whether the chest is rising and falling.
- *Listen* – close to the patient's mouth for breathing or gurgling sounds.
- *Feel* – with the side of one's face for expired air.

If the patient is not breathing, then this may be because the airway is obstructed.

☐ **Alleviating airway obstruction**

The tongue is the most common cause of airway obstruction. As a patient's conscious level deteriorates, a loss in submandibular muscle tone allows the tongue to slide back and occlude the oropharynx. At the same time the epiglottis may obstruct the larynx. Other causes are unstable maxillary or mandibular fractures, haemorrhage in the mouth obstructing the oropharynx, and direct obstruction of the larynx.

In most cases an airway can be provided by pulling the tongue forward. This is most commonly achieved using the chin lift or jaw thrust technique. In the case of facial injuries, providing other injuries permit, gravity can also be employed by placing the patient semi-prone. It is important that the effectiveness of these manoeuvres is assessed using the 'look, listen and feel' method.

Chin lift

The index and middle fingers pull the mandible forward, as the thumb assists and pushes down the lower lip and jaw (Figure 2.3).

Jaw thrust

The fingers of both hands are placed behind the angles of the jaw, with the thumbs placed over the malar prominences. Downward pressure is exerted on the thumbs as the fingers lift the mandible forward (Figure 2.4).

In all unconscious patients, and particularly those in whom these manoeuvres fail to provide an airway, the mouth should then be opened and inspected for foreign bodies, vomit and teeth. Solid, loose debris is best removed manually with a pair of Magill's forceps. The angulation of this instrument allows objects to be removed without occluding the view of the airway. Good illumination and care are also necessary to ensure that the posterior wall of the pharynx is not damaged. Liquid debris should be removed with a rigid sucker (Yankauer type).

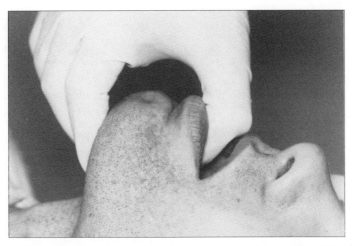

Figure 2.3   The chin lift: the index and middle fingers pull the mandible forward as the thumb assists and pushes the lower lip and jaw downwards

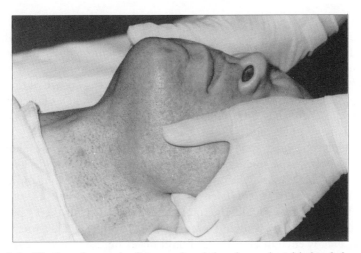

Figure 2.4   The jaw thrust: the fingers of each hand are placed behind the angles of the jaw, with the thumbs placed over the malar prominences; downward pressure is exerted on the thumbs as the fingers push the mandible forward

Simple airway devices

The doctor or nurse must ascertain whether the pharyngeal reflex ('gag') is present. If the protective reflexes are adequate, then pulling the tongue forward may be all that is required to clear the airway.

If these reflexes are absent or depressed then an oropharyngeal (Guedel) airway should be inserted. This will help keep the airway patent by prevent-

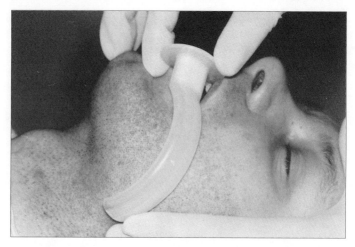

Figure 2.5 Determining the appropriate size of Guedel airway

ing the tongue from falling back into the pharynx. Although the different-sized airways are numbered (2–4, for small to large adults respectively), these numbers do not need to be remembered as an approximate guide is given by the distance from the angle of the jaw to the corner of the mouth (Figure 2.5). The airway should be inserted 'upside down', as far back as the hard palate, then rotated through 180° and fully inserted until the flange lies in front of the upper and lower incisors.

If a pharyngeal reflex is present in an adult, then a nasopharyngeal airway may be better tolerated. The size of this airway relates to its internal diameter in millimetres, with recommended sizes being 7 mm for an adult male and 6 mm for an adult female. Once lubricated, the tube is inserted through the nostril – usually the right, unless obviously blocked – parallel to the hard palate, using a slight rotatory action, until it reaches the pharynx. **If resistance is encountered force should *never* be used, as this can precipitate haemorrhage.** Instead, the other nostril is tried. Once in place, the tube is secured by inserting a safety pin through the expanded end to prevent the tube being inhaled. **This device should never be used if a basal skull fracture is suspected.**

The patency of the airway is then reassessed by repeating the 'look, listen and feel' method. Clear breath sounds on auscultation of the chest indicate that the chosen airway is appropriate and in the correct place, and that no complications have occurred (Box 2.3). If until now the cervical spine has been immobilized manually, the assisting nurse can now stabilize the neck with a rigid collar, two sandbags and tape, or with a commercially available apparatus (see Figures 1.4 and 1.5).

BOX 2.3   Complications from airway insertion

- Trauma to all structures encountered
- Partial or complete airway obstruction
- Laryngeal spasm because the device is too long
- Vomiting because the patient has a gag reflex
- Gastric dilatation and hypoventilation because air is directed into the oesophagus

---

BOX 2.4   Actions required to assess and secure the airway

- Cervical spine stabilization and 'Are you all right?'
- Look, listen and feel
- Chin lift or jaw thrust
- Look, listen and feel
- Clear the mouth
- Oral or nasal airway
- Look, listen and feel

■ Breathing

In all trauma patients, the aim should be to achieve an inspired oxygen concentration of 100%.

□ Spontaneous ventilation

A close-fitting mask should be placed over the patient's nose and mouth and connected to oxygen at a flow rate of 15 l/min. This is necessary to compensate for leaks around the mask and to minimize the rebreathing of exhaled air, both of which will reduce the concentration of oxygen the patient receives; the latter may also raise the carbon dioxide levels and jeopardize patients with a head injury (see Chapter 6). Whenever possible, a reservoir bag should also be used as this will raise the inspired oxygen concentration to around 85% (Figure 2.2).

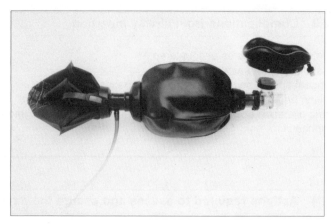

Figure 2.6   A self-inflating bag, a one-way valve, a mask, a reservoir bag, and an oxygen source

☐ Artificial ventilation

If the patient is not breathing (apnoeic) or has inadequate ventilation, a bag-valve-facemask apparatus should be used to provide artificial ventilation (Figure 2.6). A one-way valve prevents expired gas from entering the self-inflating bag. An oxygen supply of 15 l/min should be connected appropriately and this will increase the inspired oxygen concentration to approximately 50%. Whenever possible a reservoir bag should also be attached. This ensures that the bag refills with a greater proportion of oxygen than room air. With a tight-fitting mask this method allows the delivery of virtually 100% oxygen.

The mask is applied to the trauma victim's face with the thumb and index finger, whilst the three other fingers are carrying out a jaw thrust manoeuvre (Figure 2.7). The commonest problem with this procedure is inadequate ventilation due to a leak between the patient's face and the mask. It is well recognized that a two-person technique, with one person holding the mask on the face with both hands, and the other squeezing the bag with both hands, is more efficient than a single-person technique. If the situation and space allow, the doctor and nurse should use the two-person technique. Whichever technique is used, the bag should be squeezed at 12–15 breaths/minute and the chest auscultated bilaterally to ensure ventilation.

☐ Cricoid pressure

This procedure is usually reserved for use during intubation. However, it

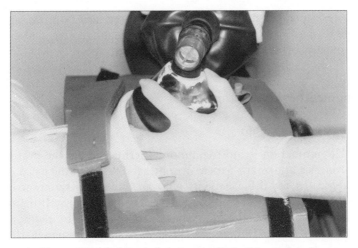

Figure 2.7 A facemask being applied with one hand

can minimize gastric distension during ventilation with a facemask and thereby reduce the chance of aspiration (see page 62).

■ Advanced airway control

In certain situations it may be inappropriate or prove impossible to maintain a patent airway by basic airway techniques (Box 2.5). In these situations an advanced technique – either tracheal intubation or a surgical airway – should be used. The preferred method of airway control is tracheal intubation, using either the nasal or oral route, depending upon the circumstances and experience of the airway personnel. Once completed, tracheal intubation provides several advantages: it facilitates ventilation and allows a high concentration of oxygen to be delivered; the airway is isolated and the risk of aspiration of gastric contents reduced; the airway can be suctioned to remove secretions or inhaled debris; and the tracheal route can be used for the administration of certain drugs.

BOX 2.5   Reasons for advanced airway techniques

■ Unconscious with loss of protective reflexes
■ Poor airway with basic techniques (e.g. severe facial trauma)
■ Specific need for ventilation (e.g. head injury)
■ Compromise of normal respiratory mechanism (e.g. chest injury)
■ Anticipation of airway obstruction (e.g. inhalational injury)

It must be remembered that before the advanced airway procedure, and if possible during it, the patient should continue to receive a high flow of 100% oxygen by the basic techniques described above.

☐ Endotracheal intubation

Oral or nasal intubation?

In the UK intubation is most commonly performed via the oral route. In North America and South Africa, in contrast, the use of the nasal route has been advocated for those patients who are breathing spontaneously and where there exists the possibility of a cervical spine injury. If the patient is apnoeic or a cervical spine injury has been ruled out by the appropriate specialist, then orotracheal intubation is warranted. Ultimately, the skill of the airway doctor or nurse and the urgency of the situation will need to be considered.

Endotracheal intubation: procedure

Before starting, the airway doctor and nurse must ensure that they have everything they require (Figure 2.8 and Box 2.6), that the equipment is functioning, and that it is laid out appropriately. This applies particularly to

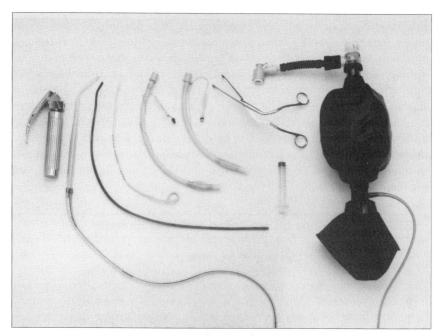

Figure 2.8 Equipment required for endotracheal intubation

laryngoscopes and suction. The assisting nurse will have to maintain inline cervical spine stabilization throughout this procedure if there is suspicion of a cervical injury. (Remember that a normal lateral cervical x-ray does not by itself totally rule out a cervical spine injury.)

BOX 2.6   Equipment required for endotracheal intubation

- Endotracheal tube:
  - Male: 8–9 mm internal diameter, length 23 cm
  - Female: 7–8 mm internal diameter, length 21 cm
  - Check cuff has no leak
  - Check proximal end has a standard 15 mm connector
- Functional laryngoscope
- 10 ml syringe
- Magill forceps
- Water-soluble lubricant
- Functional Yankauer sucker
- Bag-valve apparatus with oxygen and reservoir bag
- Catheter mount
- Gum elastic bougie
- Stylet
- Bandage for securing the tube

Whenever possible, intubation should be preceded by a period of pre-oxygenation with cricoid pressure (see also rapid sequence induction, page 61). The optimal position for intubation is with the patient's neck flexed and the head extended at the atlanto-occipital joint (often likened to 'sniffing the morning air'). Unfortunately, this is rarely achievable in the trauma patient due to the presence of a rigid collar protecting the cervical spine.

The laryngoscope is always held in the *left* hand, and the mouth opened using the index finger and thumb of the right hand in a scissor action. The blade of the laryngoscope is inserted along the right side of the tongue, displacing it to the left, until the tip fits into the gap between the base of the tongue and the epiglottis (vallecula; Figure 2.9). Force is then applied in the direction in which the handle is pointing (Figure 2.9), thereby lifting the tongue and epiglottis to expose the larynx. There should be *no* wrist movement: instead, all the force comes from the upper arm. If the wrist is allowed to move, the widest, most proximal part of the laryngoscope blade can lever on the patient's upper teeth and damage them.

Frequently only the lower part of the cords or arytenoids are seen, because the inline cervical spine stabilization prevents extension of the head. Nonetheless it is possible, with experience, to intubate the trachea using a gum elastic bougie as an introducer. With this suboptimal view of the cords, the bougie is inserted at laryngoscopy with its tip pointing anteriorly so that

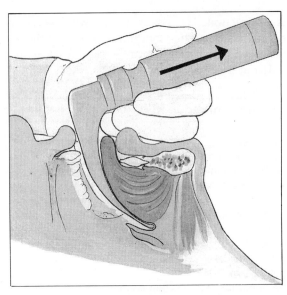

Figure 2.9 Intubation: profile of the face with the laryngoscope inserted
Source: © Landon B, Driscoll P & Goodall J 1993. *The Atlas of Trauma Management*.
Carnforth, Lancashire: Parthenon. Reproduced by kind permission.

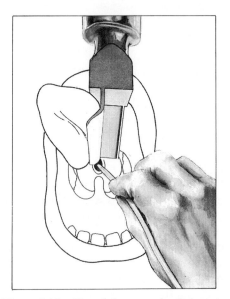

Figure 2.10 Use of the gum elastic bougie
Source: © Landon B, Driscoll P & Goodall J 1993. *The Atlas of Trauma Management*.
Carnforth, Lancashire: Parthenon. Reproduced by kind permission.

it passes behind the epiglottis into the larynx (Figure 2.10). The person carrying out the intubation should not take his or her eyes off the target area until the bougie is safely inserted – a momentary lapse could result in the bougie being placed in the oesophagus. The appropriate endotracheal tube is then slid over the bougie, into the larynx, and the bougie withdrawn.

Once in place, the cuff should be inflated and the endotracheal tube connected to the bag-valve circuit (Figure 2.8). The tube position is checked by looking for symmetrical movement of the chest wall, and listening over both axillae and stomach when the bag is squeezed. The best method of confirming correct positioning of the tube is to measure the carbon dioxide concentration in expired gas. Oesophageal intubation should be suspected if the end tidal carbon dioxide is less than 0.1%. Less sensitive indicators are 'burping' sounds, diminished air entry over the lung fields, gastric noise, or absence of chest expansion on squeezing the bag.

Wherever an incorrect tube placement is suspected, the rule is 'if in doubt, take it out'. The cuff is deflated and the tube withdrawn completely. The patient should be oxygenated using a bag-valve-mask device before reattempting intubation. It is essential not to persist in the attempt at intubation without intermittently oxygenating the patient. A tip is to take a deep breath when picking up the laryngoscope: once *you* feel the need to breathe again, so will the patient.

If the tube has been inserted too far into the trachea, it will pass into a main bronchus (usually the right). This will produce poor ventilation of the opposite side, and hence decreased chest movement and reduced breath sounds over the axilla. The cuff should be deflated and the tube withdrawn 1–2 cm. Following reinflation of the cuff the position can be rechecked. It is important that this situation is not confused with a developing pneumothorax, when unilateral breath sounds are heard (see Chapter 3). Only when the tube is in the correct place and secured should cricoid pressure be released and only on the instruction of the person carrying out the intubation.

If the patient arrives with an endotracheal tube in place, its position, adequacy and need should be assessed in the manner described above. On no account should it be assumed that intubation has been carried out correctly or that the tube is still in the trachea.

If a prolonged period of intubation is expected then a tube with a high-volume, low-pressure cuff should be used in order to reduce damage to the tracheal muscosa. However, the absence of this specific type of tracheal tube should not delay intubation if required urgently.

Complications

Endotracheal intubation does have well-recognized complications (Box 2.7). The airway personnel must be aware of these. Proper training and preparation can minimize their occurrence.

BOX 2.7   Complications following endotracheal intubation

- *Trauma* – lips, teeth, tongue, jaw, pharynx, larynx, cervical spine
- *Vomiting* – degree of unconsciousness misjudged
- *Hypoxia* – prolonged attempt; intubation of the right main bronchus or oesophagus; failed intubation

---

On occasion it may prove impossible to intubate the patient, for example if there is pharyngeal oedema or trauma deranging the anatomy. Having failed to maintain an adequate airway using more basic techniques, then the creation of a surgical airway should be considered (see page 63).

Breathing

Once the patient has been successfully intubated, he should be ventilated with 100% oxygen. Initially the bag-valve system can be used, with the reservoir attached and connected to a flow of oxygen of 15 l/min. The patient should be ventilated at a rate of 12–15 breaths/minute. If a mechanical ventilator is available, a tidal volume of 10 ml/kg at a rate of 12 breaths/minute can be used.

A chest x-ray and arterial blood-gas tensions (ABG) should be measured as soon as possible following intubation. The former allows identification of chest injuries and demonstrates the position of the tracheal tube. The ABG is used to check the adequacy of the ventilation. A large-bore gastric tube should be also be inserted to deflate and empty the stomach. A nasal approach for this tube is contraindicated if a base-of-skull fracture is suspected.

If the airway is soiled by blood or vomit, tracheo-bronchial suction can be carried out using a flexible tube passed down the endotracheal tube. This should be less than half the diameter of the tracheal tube and the procedure preceded by pre-oxygenating the patient.

Using a sterile technique, the catheter is threaded down the endotracheal tube. Once in place, suction is commenced in an intermittent fashion as the tube is withdrawn with a rotatory motion. The patient should not be deprived of oxygen for longer than 15 seconds and on no account must the suction be connected directly to the tracheal tube. Once the suction catheter has been removed, the patient must be ventilated for at least 1 minute before the procedure is repeated.

The most serious complication following suction is hypoxia from a decrease in lung volume, particularly if suction is prolonged. Dysrhythmias, sympathetic stimulation, vagal stimulation, mucosal damage and rises in intracranial pressure are all well-recognized problems. Consequently, the patient's ECG needs to be monitored throughout this procedure and a pulse oximeter used if available.

☐ Drugs used to facilitate intubation

In certain situations the patient will need to be rendered unconscious and paralysed prior to intubation. This is achieved by the administration of an intravenous anaesthetic agent, followed by a muscle relaxant. **The use of these agents must be restricted to those with anaesthetic training, because of the potential problems associated with their use.**

The decision to use these drugs will depend upon several factors:

- the presence of airway obstruction;
- any predicted difficulties with intubation;
- the presence of specific injuries.

A specific group of patients for whom drugs are widely used prior to intubation is the head-injured. Intravenous anaesthetic agents can be used to modify the rise in intracranial pressure (ICP) that accompanies intubation as a result of an increase in cerebral blood flow (see Chapter 6).

In those patients requiring intubation where there is no evidence of airway obstruction and no reason to expect difficulty with intubation, then it is appropriate to administer an intravenous anaesthetic agent followed by a muscle relaxant, to provide optimal conditions for intubation. The technique used is a 'rapid sequence induction' in an attempt to maximize oxygenation and minimize the risk of aspiration (see below).

When considering the use of drugs, however, it is imperative to identify any patient in whom the airway is compromised and ventilation impaired (e.g. because of several facial trauma and laryngeal oedema), or where any difficulty with intubation is predicted (e.g. because of a short neck, or an immobilized cervical spine). In these circumstances, the use of drugs to anaesthetize and paralyse the patient is *not* recommended. This is because after their administration, the patient would become apnoeic and totally dependent on the airway nurse or doctor to secure the airway and maintain ventilation. If either of these proved difficult or impossible, the patient would become hypoxic, thereby forcing the airway doctor to create a surgical airway under poor and hurried conditions, and unnecessarily. Under these circumstances, there are two alternatives, but both require the skill of an experienced anaesthetist.

Firstly, anaesthesia can be induced by an inhalational agent (e.g. halothane in oxygen), using the patient's own respiratory efforts. The inspired concentration of anaesthetic is gradually increased until the patient is rendered unconscious and the pharyngeal reflexes are suppressed. Direct laryngoscopy can then be performed to assess the lower airway and the ease of intubation. If the larynx can be seen, then either a tracheal tube can be passed (which may provoke coughing) or a muscle relaxant can be administered, knowing that intubation will be possible.

The alternative technique is to use fibre-optic bronchoscopy with topical anaesthesia only. The lower airway can be examined and, in experi-

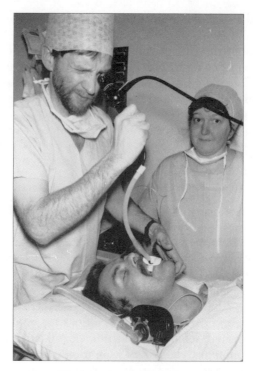

Figure 2.11   Fibre-optic bronchoscopy with intubation

enced hands, intubation performed using the bronchoscope as a guide over which the tube is passed into the larynx (Figure 2.11). This technique can be used in awake patients provided that they are co-operative.

Whichever technique is used, difficulty in performing intubation should be expected and the airway doctor should be prepared to create a surgical airway. Ideally an experienced clinician should be standing by with the necessary equipment to undertake a surgical cricothyroidotomy.

Pharmacology

The patient's vital signs must be continuously monitored whenever the following drugs are used.

Induction agents

The drugs used to induce loss of consciousness in patients are generally short-acting anaesthetic agents. They are occasionally referred to as hypnotics, although they do not induce true sleep. Strictly speaking, only a muscle relaxant is needed to facilitate intubation. However, relaxants are always preceded by an anaesthetic agent, as paralysis alone would be extremely unpleasant and associated with potentially harmful reflexes, such as hypertension, tachycardia, or increase in intracranial pressure (ICP).

Most intravenous anaesthetic agents affect the cardiovascular system, causing hypotension by either, depressing myocardial contractility, causing vasodilatation or both. These actions would obviously be detrimental to trauma patients, particularly those who are hypovolaemic, where the response would be exaggerated. The exception to this rule is ketamine, which may actually *stimulate* the cardiovascular system. Unfortunately, it also increases cerebral blood flow, which may endanger patients with head injuries.

Etomidate is the induction agent of choice in trauma patients as it is associated with a greater degree of cardiovascular stability compared to other agents. This leads to maintenance of vital organ perfusion with less hypotension. The cerebral blood flow is also reduced as a result of a decreased oxygen demand by the brain, thereby helping to control ICP, particularly if raised. The risk of allergic reaction is low. The disadvantages are that etomidate causes pain on injection, hiccups and involuntary muscle movement in some patients.

Following the IV administration of 0.2–0.3 mg/kg, consciousness will be lost within 30–45 seconds for a duration of 6–10 minutes. Etomidate is compatible with the other drugs mentioned and comes in ampoules of 10 ml (2 mg/ml), ready for use. This eliminates the risk of dilutional errors.

Midazolam is a short-acting benzodiazepine which can be given intravenously to induce and maintain anaesthesia. The time to loss of consciousness is longer than with etomidate, but this is partly due to the fact that there is considerable variation in the dose required and therefore it has to be titrated against the patient's response.

The normal dose is 0.15–0.2 mg/kg, although this may be dramatically reduced in the critically ill and elderly. Repeat doses of 2–4 mg can be given to maintain anaesthesia during ventilation.

Muscle relaxants

These drugs are administered to facilitate laryngoscopy and to abolish laryngeal reflexes, allowing intubation. This would not otherwise be possible without deeply anaesthetizing the patient, which would cause severe cardiovascular depression. It must be remembered that once these drugs have been given the patient will become apnoeic and at risk of regurgitation and aspiration of gastric contents. Therefore their administration commits the airway doctor and nurse to carrying out intubation.

Muscle relaxants are divided into two groups, depolarizing and non-depolarizing, according to their pharmacological action.

Depolarizing relaxants

Suxamethonium is known as a depolarizing agent because it attaches to the same receptors as acetylcholine and causes depolarization of the muscle membrane. This produces a transient, generalized fasciculation (twitching) prior to full relaxation. Its action is normally short-lived because it is broken down by naturally produced pseudocholinesterase.

The advantage of suxamethonium is that it produces complete relaxation within 30–45 seconds following intravenous injection. It is given as a bolus of 1.5 mg/kg and has a duration of action 3–5 minutes. It comes in 2 ml ampoules containing 50 mg/ml.

Unfortunately there are a number of problems associated with its use:

1   Repeated boluses of suxamethonium can lead to vagal stimulation and bradycardia. Therefore atropine should be readily available, and always administered prior to a second dose.

2   Suxamethonium may cause hyperkalaemia after major crush injuries, burns more than 24 hours old, massive denervation injury, and in certain cases of pre-existing neuromuscular disorders.

3   Suxamethonium may provoke an acute rise in intra-ocular pressure, which in penetrating eye injuries can cause vitreous humour to be expelled.

4   Suxamethonium may result in prolonged apnoea (3–24 hours) in patients who do not have pseudocholinesterase (1 in 2800 of the population).

5   There is a risk of suxamethonium triggering malignant hyperpyrexia, a rare disorder of muscle metabolism.

6   Suxamethonium needs to be stored at 4 °C (i.e. in a fridge), as it breaks down at room temperature.

Despite all these problems, suxamethonium remains the relaxant of choice in an emergency situation because of its rapid onset of action.

Non-depolarizing relaxants

Although there are a number of drugs in the non-depolarizing category, it is the authors' preference to use atracurium.

Atracurium competes with acetylcholine for the same receptors on the muscle surface, but it does not depolarize the membrane. Consequently, no fasciculations are seen following injection.

Full relaxation occurs more slowly than with suxamethonium, intubation being possible around 120 seconds after administration of 0.6 mg/kg; with smaller doses the time is progressively longer. Duration of action is also dose-dependent, 0.6 mg/kg lasting about 30–40 minutes. Repeated doses of 0.1–0.2 mg/kg can be given to maintain relaxation and facilitate controlled ventilation. There is no effect on the cardiovascular system at these doses and atracurium can be used safely in all patients. It comes in 2.5 ml and 5 ml ampoules containing 10 mg/ml, and it should be stored in the fridge as it undergoes very slow spontaneous degradation at room temperature. Its main use in trauma patients should be for the maintenance of relaxation following intubation with suxamethonium, or for use in those situations where suxamethonium is contraindicated.

☐ Rapid sequence induction

An important potential complication of emergency anaesthesia is vomiting or regurgitation of the gastric contents, followed by aspiration pneumonitis. Normally the patient's own reflexes protect the airway, but once these have been removed by the administration of anaesthetic and muscle-relaxant drugs, the patient is at risk. As all trauma patients should be assumed to have a full stomach, steps must be taken to minimize the chances of this potentially fatal complication.

Preparation

Whenever possible, a nasogastric tube (or orogastric, if there is a fractured base of skull) should be passed and aspirated to remove any liquid stomach contents prior to intubation. This manoeuvre does not guarantee an empty stomach, however.

Before starting, it is important to check the availability and function of all the equipment and monitors (Box 2.8). All drugs should be drawn up into labelled syringes. Suction is vital and should be switched on and positioned at the side of the patient's head.

The patient should be on a tipping trolley, have adequate intravenous access, and be attached to an ECG monitor, an automated blood-pressure monitor (such as a Dinamap™) and a pulse oximeter, with baseline recordings taken.

The patient is then oxygenated for 2 minutes by administering high-flow oxygen. At the same time, if he is conscious, a warning is given that he will become dizzy and sleepy following the injection of the induction agent.

The appropriate dose of etomidate is then injected into a fast-running intravenous infusion, followed by the correct dose of suxamethonium. As the patient loses consciousness (which can be assessed by the loss of the eyelash reflex), cricoid pressure is applied (see below). After a period of 30–45 seconds, the patient will be maximally relaxed, a point indicated by cessation of fasciculations, and intubation can be performed in the manner previously described.

Once the tube is in the trachea, the cuff is inflated, the lungs are ventilated manually using a bag-valve attached to the endotracheal tube,

---

BOX 2.8   Checks before pharmacologically paralysing the patient

---

- Equipment:
  - As for endotracheal intubation
  - Bag-valve-facemask system and reservoir bag
  - Oxygen delivery apparatus
  - Ventilator
- Monitors:
  - BP, ECG, pulse oximeter
  - End tidal CO_2
- Drugs:
  - Suxamethonium and atropine
  - Atracurium
  - Midazolam
  - Etomidate
- Patient:
  - Airway in place
  - Oxygenated
  - Vital signs being monitored
  - IV access in place

---

and air entry is assessed in both axillae. If everything is satisfactory, cricoid pressure can now be released. Ultimately the patient can be connected to a mechanical ventilator, as previously described. If by chance everything fails, use expired-air ventilation and blow down the endotracheal tube!

Long-term unconsciousness and ventilation can be achieved, when required, with the appropriate doses of midazolam and atracurium. The patient must be continuously monitored, with particular emphasis being placed on skin colour, chest movement, blood pressure, heart rate, temperature, cardiac rhythm and ventilation.

☐ Cricoid pressure

The airway nurse should stand facing the patient's head. The tips of the thumb and index finger should be placed on the cricoid ring. This structure must be identified beforehand if the nurse is uncertain. Direct pressure in the midline is applied as the patient loses consciousness. This occludes the oesophagus by squeezing it between the cricoid ring and the 6th cervical vertebra, and thereby prevents regurgitation and passage of air into the stomach. Cricoid pressure is still effective even if a naso- or orogastric tube is in place.

This technique is not without its own complications. If incorrectly applied, the trachea can be deviated, making intubation more difficult. It should also be discontinued if the patient begins actively to vomit, otherwise the oesophagus is at risk of rupturing. In this situation the patient must be quickly tipped head-down, the airway cleared of vomit, the pressure released, and cervical spine stabilization maintained. If enough personnel are present, the patient can be turned in a controlled way onto his side.

Occasionally, premature cessation of the pharmacological paralysis is required in the resuscitation room. However, this should only be carried out by trained staff because reversal of the neuromuscular blocking agent by the intravenous administration of neostigmine can lead to complications.

☐ Surgical airway

In certain cases it may be impossible to intubate a patient. This may result from complete obstruction of the airway due to oedema (e.g. inhalation burns) and trauma (e.g. laryngeal damage). In these situations a surgical airway is required.

As with the endotracheal procedure, it is important that all the equipment is checked and in place before this procedure is commenced. In addition, a high flow of oxygen to the upper airway should be maintained throughout the surgical procedure: it is unlikely there is complete obstruction.

A complex situation arises when the patient is conscious but has an obstructed airway. He will tend to move around in a desperate desire to breathe. In cases where there is facial trauma the patient may wish to sit forward to stop the blood running down his throat and to allow his unstable face to fall forward and so partially clear his airway. On no account should these patients be restrained, sedated or paralysed without an experienced anaesthetist being present and the trauma team being ready to create a surgical airway. The reason for this precaution is that once the patient's respiratory drive has been removed an airway has to be provided immediately. This may be impossible to achieve in the case of severe airway obstruction. In this situation the airway must be cleared and secured as best as possible, and a high flow rate of oxygen provided, whilst a surgical airway is created.

Needle cricothyroidotomy

This is the surgical airway of choice for patients under 12 years old and as a stopgap before surgical cricothyroidotomy in patients who are older. The restriction on the younger trauma victim is because of the undeveloped airway. The cricoid ring is the only complete ring and so is structurally very important in the child. In view of the risk of damaging the ring during a surgical cricothyroidotomy, the needle method is recommended.

Needle cricothyroidotomy: procedure

A 5 ml syringe is required, attached to a 12 g or 14 g cannula. A length of oxygen tubing, with either a 'Y' connector fitted or a side hole cut in it, is also needed.

The trachea and larynx of the patient with an obstructed airway are usually moving vertically upwards and downwards because of the respiratory effort. Following skin preparation, the operator should hold the thyroid cartilage in one hand and insert the cannula through the cricothyroid membrane in a caudal direction (Figure 2.12), whilst aspirating on the syringe. A free flow of air into the syringe indicates that the cannula is in the trachea. It is then advanced a few more millimetres before threading the cannula down the needle into the trachea. Once in place the cannula is connected to the oxygen tubing, which is delivering this gas at 15 l/min. A ratio of 1 second inspiration to 4 seconds to allow expiration should be maintained. Most of the expired air goes out through the upper airway and not through the cannula, which has a high resistance. This is why this procedure is contraindicated if there is a complete airway obstruction. Due to the inefficiency of the system carbon dioxide accumulates, so the procedure should not be continued for longer than 45 minutes. By this point a definitive surgical airway should have been created.

Complications following this procedure include air entrapment and pneumothorax due to the high airway pressure required during ventilation. This is most marked during spontaneous ventilation that requires a large respiratory effort. In these cases, sedation and muscle paralysis is therefore recommended. Needle insertion can produce haemorrhage or oesophageal damage if the needle is positioned incorrectly. The cannula is relatively small and thin and so kinks easily and does not allow the suctioning of

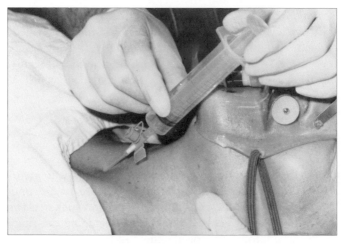

Figure 2.12 Needle cricothyroidotomy

secretions. Each of these features can lead to obstruction. Finally, subcutaneous and mediastinal emphysema can develop.

Surgical cricothyroidotomy

As with all procedures, check the equipment and connections before commencing. As a tracheostomy tube is passed through the cricothyroid membrane a tube of smaller diameter is used than would be used for a standard tracheostomy. An adult male would require a 5–6 mm size and an adult female a 4–5 mm size.

This procedure is contraindicated if there is trauma to the larynx or if there is an expanding haematoma within the operating field, as a torrential haemorrhage may result from the surgical incision. A tracheostomy is the technique of choice in the case of laryngeal trauma.

Surgical cricothyroidotomy: procedure

Following skin preparation and local infiltration with 1% lignocaine (with adrenaline 1:100 000 to minimize cutaneous bleeding), the thyroid cartilage is held as described previously. The operator makes a longitudinal incision down to the cricothyroid membrane (Figure 2.13). A finger is then inserted into the wound to reassess the membrane's position. This structure is then incised transversely and a channel created either with the scalpel handle held vertically or with a self-retaining retractor. The assisting nurse will need to maintain this channel in a moving larynx at this stage. The tracheostomy

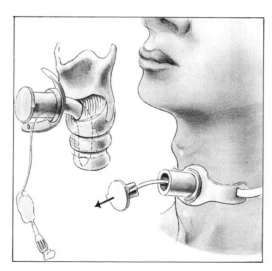

Figure 2.13 Surgical cricothyroidotomy
Source: © Landon B, Driscoll P & Goodall J 1993. *The Atlas of Trauma Management.*
Carnforth, Lancashire: Parthenon. Reproduced by kind permission.

tube is then inserted, making sure it is going into the lumen of the trachea and not just running down its anterior aspect.

Once in place, the central trocar of the tube is removed and the tube connected to a bag-valve or ventilatory circuit. The cuff can then be inflated and the air entry to each side of the chest checked. The tube should then be tied in, and the trachea sucked out.

A chest x-ray and an arterial blood gas sample should be taken as soon as possible after the surgical airway has been inserted. Care must also be taken to reassess the airway and breathing whenever the patient is moved or if there is a deterioration in his clinical state.

■ Summary

As the establishment of a patient airway is so fundamental to the management of the trauma patient, and the procedures potentially so varied, it is vital that only an experienced nurse is given the responsibility of managing the airway.

The patient's airway must be cleared and secured, and the cervical spine stabilized, as soon as possible. Initially basic techniques are used, with more advanced procedures being carried out only if basic techniques prove to be inadequate.

■ References and further reading

American College of Surgeons Committee on Trauma 1993. *Advanced Trauma Life Support Course for Physicians.* Chicago: American College of Surgeons.

Atkinson R, Rushman G & Lee J 1987. *A Synopsis of Anaesthesia.* Bristol: John Wright.

Benumof J L 1991. Management of the difficult adult airway. *Anaesthesiology* 75: 1087.

Crosby E 1992. Tracheal intubation in the cervical spine-injured patient. *Can. J. Anaesth.* 39: 105.

Dallen L, Wine R & Benumof J 1991. Spontaneous ventilation via transtracheal large-bore intravenous catheters is possible. *Anesthesiology* 75: 531.

Watson D 1991. Management of the upper airway. In Skinner D, Driscoll P & Earlam R (eds): *ABC of Major Trauma.* London: BMJ Publications.

Wood P & Lawler P 1992. Managing the airway in cervical spine injury: a review of the advanced trauma life support protocol. *Anaesthesia* 47: 792.

Chapter 3

Thoracic trauma

Peter Driscoll, Carl Gwinnutt and Olive Goodall

Objectives

The objectives of this chapter are to teach members of the trauma team:

- relevant anatomy of the chest wall and thoracic contents;

- basic physiology of ventilation, diffusion and perfusion;

- recognition and primary treatment of six immediately life-threatening thoracic conditions;

- recognition and primary treatment of six potentially life-threatening thoracic conditions;

- recognition and primary treatment of neck wounds;

- principles of definitive thoracic trauma care.

■ Introduction

Injuries to the thorax are responsible for 25 per cent of all trauma deaths, usually as a result of acute tissue hypoxia or hypovolaemia. Around 85 per cent of cases can be treated without the need for a thoracic surgeon. It is therefore extremely important that the trauma team develops the expertise to recognize and manage thoracic injuries as well as being aware of those problems that require expert help.

■ Applied anatomy

Figure 3.1 demonstrates several anatomical features which are clinically important.

Chest wall

The lungs and chest wall are each lined by a fibrous layer called the pleura. Normally there is only a *potential* cavity between these linings, but it expands when air (*pneumothorax*) or blood (*haemothorax*) is introduced.

The pleural cavity and the apex of the lung project above the clavicle. Consequently a pneumothorax or lung injury can occur following penetrating injuries to the lower neck.

The chest wall and the lungs are elastic structures which are pulling in opposite directions. The chest wall is trying to open out whereas the lungs are trying to collapse. The interface between these two opposing forces results in a vacuum (negative pressure) in most of the intrapleural space. Therefore, if there is a breach either in the lungs or in the chest wall, then air is sucked into this vacuum.

During inspiration the diaphragm descends and the intercostal muscles contract causing the ribs to move upwards and outwards. This increases the intrathoracic volume, which decreases the pressure inside the airways. Air is therefore drawn into the lungs.

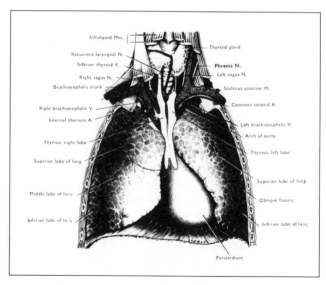

Figure 3.1 The chest wall with the thoracic contents and diaphragm
Source: © Romanes G J (ed.) 1969. *Cunningham's Manual of Practical Anatomy*, Vol. 2, 13th edn. Oxford: Oxford University Press. By permission of Oxford University Press.

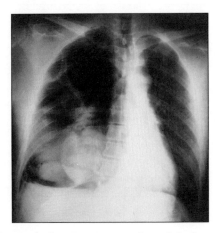

Figure 3.2 Radiograph showing compression of the heart due to a tension pneumothorax

Following trauma a 'one-way valve' may develop on the lung surface. During inspiration air leaks through the 'valve' into the pleural cavity, but fails to escape during expiration as the valve closes. With subsequent respiratory cycles, the volume and pressure of air in the pleural cavity increases, resulting in the collapse of the ipsilateral lung, causing profound hypoxia. Furthermore, the mediastinum is displaced towards the opposite hemithorax, impeding venous return and diminishing cardiac output. This condition is known as a *tension pneumothorax* (Figure 3.2), and if not rapidly relieved, it is fatal.

When a rib is fractured in two places, the middle section can move independently from the relatively fixed end-pieces. Consequently, due to the negative intrapleural pressure, this section will be drawn in during inspiration and pushed out during expiration. This is known as *paradoxical movement*. A *flail chest* results when two or more ribs are fractured in two or more places (Figure 3.3). It also applies to the situation in which the clavicle and first rib are similarly affected. In the early stages, however, the spasm of the chest wall musculature will splint these fractures, and so eliminate paradoxical movement. This spasm leads to an increased energy expenditure for breathing. Over time the muscles become fatigued and abnormal movement becomes apparent.

This can be a life-threatening condition, particularly if there is an underlying pulmonary contusion (see later), which adds to the hypoxia already produced as a result of the impaired ventilation. This is demonstrated in the mortality rates for these two conditions:

- Mortality for pulmonary contusion is 16 per cent.
- Mortality for a flail chest is 16 per cent.
- Mortality for both is 42 per cent.

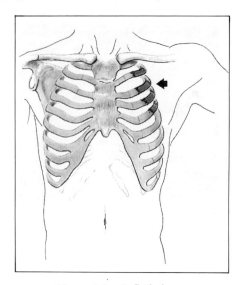

Figure 3.3   A flail chest
Source: © Landon B, Driscoll P & Goodall J 1993. *The Atlas of Trauma Management.*
Carnforth, Lancashire: Parthenon. Reproduced by kind permission.

The lower six ribs overlie the abdominal cavity when the diaphragm is elevated during expiration. Therefore a penetrating wound in this area may enter the peritoneal cavity as well as causing pulmonary injury. Furthermore, a fracture of these ribs can be associated with injury to the underlying liver and spleen. It follows that these 'mid-section' injuries should be considered indicators of both abdominal and chest damage.

☐   **Mediastinum**

The trachea, the oesophagus and the major blood vessels lie in close proximity to one another in the neck. In the chest they are contained, along with the heart, within the mediastinum (Figure 3.4). The surface landmarks of the mediastinum are medial to the nipple line anteriorly, or medial to the medial edges of the scapulae posteriorly. Consequently, penetrating injuries in this area may damage one or more of these structures.

The distal part of the arch of the aorta is anchored just inferior to the left subclavian artery. Following rapid deceleration in patients who have fallen from a great height, or who have crashed a car at high speed, the unanchored section of the aortic arch moves freely with the forward momentum. The result is a tearing of the inner two layers of the descending aorta just distal to the left subclavian artery. Blood escapes, but is contained by the outer (adventitial) layer of the aorta in 10 per cent of cases. This is known as a *dissecting thoracic aortic aneurysm*. If this outer layer is also

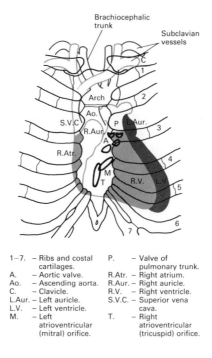

Figure 3.4 The surface anatomy landmarks of the mediastinum
Source: © Romanes G J (ed.) 1969. *Cunningham's Manual of Practical Anatomy*, Vol. 2,
13th edn. Oxford: Oxford University Press. By permission of Oxford University Press.

breached in the injury then the patient rapidly exsanguinates and does not
reach hospital alive (90 per cent of cases).

☐ Heart

The right border is formed by a line joining the 3rd to the 6th costal
cartilage, 1 cm from the right of the sternum (Figure 3.4). Inferiorly, the
border extends from the right 6th costal cartilage to the apex beat. Finally,
the left border is formed by a line joining the apex beat to the left 2nd costal
cartilage, 2.5 cm lateral to the sternum.

The heart is covered with a tough, inelastic fibrous sac called the
pericardium. In the healthy state, even a small collection of blood within the
pericardium could create enough pressure to act as a constricting jacket on
the heart. This compromises ventricular filling and hence cardiac output
(see Chapter 4). This condition is known as a *pericardial tamponade*, and
usually follows penetrating trauma of the heart.

■ Respiratory pathophysiology

This section will concentrate on normal and abnormal pulmonary function. An explanation of partial pressures of gases, the symbols used and the normal arterial blood gas (ABG) values is given in Appendix 3.1 (page 99).

The main functions of the lungs are oxygen uptake and carbon dioxide elimination. To do this air has to get to the alveoli (*ventilation*, V), blood has to reach the pulmonary capillaries (*perfusion*, Q), and oxygen and carbon dioxide have to cross the gas–blood interface (*diffusion*). Finally the balance between ventilation and perfusion (the V/Q ratio) has to be correct. Impairment of any of these processes can lead to *hypoxaemia* (a low level of oxygen in the blood) and *hypercapnia* (a high level of carbon dioxide in the blood).

☐ Ventilation

The various normal ventilatory volumes and rates are described in Figures 3.5 and 3.6.

Tidal volume is the amount of air taken into the chest with each breath. It is normally equal to 7–8 ml/kg (500 ml in a 70 kg patient). The *minute volume* is the volume of air inspired each minute: it can be calculated by multiplying the tidal volume by the respiratory rate. This gives a value normally around 7.5 l/min for a 70 kg patient at rest (500 ml × 15).

Only 70 per cent (350 ml) of each tidal volume reaches a point distal to the terminal bronchi where gas exchange occurs. The remaining 150 ml fill the airways proximal to this point and are therefore not involved in gas

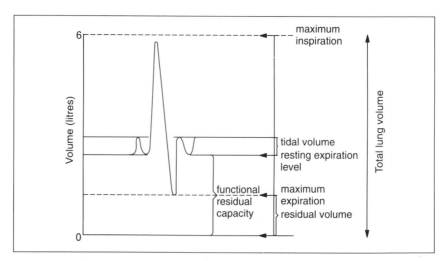

Figure 3.5 Normal ventilatory volumes as measured by spirometry

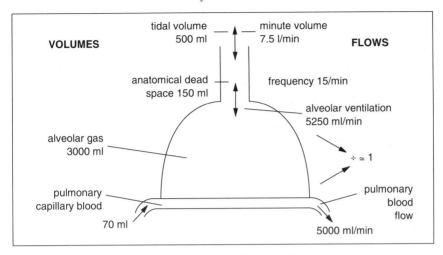

Figure 3.6 Normal volumes and flows
Source: © West J 1990. *Respiratory Physiology – the essentials*, 4th edn. Baltimore:
Williams & Wilkins. Reproduced by kind permission.

transfer. This volume is known as the *anatomical dead space*. Failure of gas transfer also occurs in areas of the lung which are ventilated but not perfused with blood. When these areas are added to the anatomical dead space, a volume known as the *physiological dead space* is produced. In healthy individuals the physiological and anatomical dead spaces are approximately the same, as ventilation and perfusion are well matched.

The amount of air remaining in the lungs at the end of normal expiration is termed the *functional residual capacity*. It is normally 2.5–3.0 litres. As 350 ml of each tidal volume is available for gas transfer, only 12–16 per cent of the functional residual capacity is replaced with fresh alveolar air at each breath. This leads to a slow replacement of gas and prevents sudden changes in the amount of the various gases dissolved in the blood.

☐ **Pulmonary perfusion**

The cardiac output of the right ventricle passes through the pulmonary circulation. Because the pressures in the pulmonary circulation are much lower than the systemic circulation, there are differences in blood flow between the apex and base of the lung. Apical alveoli are relatively poorly perfused, giving rise to dead space (see earlier). Conversely, basal alveoli are over-perfused and this leads to some blood not having the chance to eliminate its carbon dioxide and take up oxygen. This blood is termed 'shunted' blood. In the healthy patient, this effect is minimized by hypoxic pulmonary vasoconstriction, which has the effect of diverting blood from poorly ventilated (hypoxic) areas to those which are better ventilated.

☐ Diffusion

Gas exchange, between the alveoli and blood across the pulmonary or respiratory membrane, occurs as a result of passive diffusion as blood passes through the pulmonary capillaries.

The rate of diffusion is determined by the factors shown in Box 3.1.

BOX 3.1   Factors affecting gas exchange between alveoli and blood

- Partial pressure gradient of the gas
- Solubility
- Barrier surface area
- Barrier thickness

Gases move from areas of high to low partial pressure. Blood entering the pulmonary capillaries has a partial pressure of oxygen (PaO_2) of 40 mmHg. In contrast the partial pressure in the alveoli (PaO_2) is 100 mmHg. Consequently oxygen rapidly diffuses from the alveoli into the blood. If the gradient is reduced, for example when breathing a hypoxic mixture, the PaO_2 falls and diffusion is reduced.

The partial pressure of carbon dioxide in pulmonary capillary blood is 45 mmHg and in the alveoli it is 40 mmHg. This is a much smaller difference than the oxygen gradient, but the rate of diffusion is made up for by carbon dioxide being twenty times more soluble than oxygen. The overall effect of this is that it takes approximately the same time for the exchange of oxygen and carbon dioxide to occur in the healthy state.

The lung is ideally suited for diffusion as the surface area of the barrier is approximately 50 m^2, and the thickness is only 0.0005 mm. A reduction in the former (e.g. in pneumothorax) or an increase in the latter (e.g. in interstitial pulmonary oedema) will reduce gas exchange.

It follows from this that alveolar ventilation, low partial pressure and pulmonary perfusion will all affect alveolar PO_2 and hence arterial PO_2. What is less obvious is that the ratio of ventilation to perfusion also has a profound effect on the PaO_2. Indeed this ratio is probably the most important factor in determining the PaO_2. The ventilation/perfusion ratio has succeeded in confusing students all over the world. Below we explain why this ratio has such a major effect on arterial oxygen content.

The ventilation/perfusion ratio

Imagine that there are three areas of the lung, each with its own capillary supply (Figure 3.7).

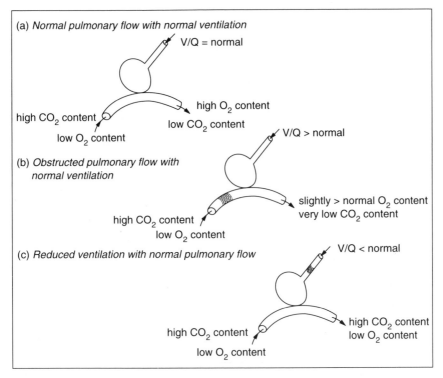

(a) *Normal pulmonary flow with normal ventilation*

V/Q = normal

high O_2 content
low CO_2 content

high CO_2 content
low O_2 content

(b) *Obstructed pulmonary flow with normal ventilation*

V/Q > normal

slightly > normal O_2 content
very low CO_2 content

high CO_2 content
low O_2 content

(c) *Reduced ventilation with normal pulmonary flow*

V/Q < normal

high CO_2 content
low O_2 content

high CO_2 content
low O_2 content

Figure 3.7   Three different V/Q ratios

In part (a), the ventilation and perfusion are matched perfectly. The oxygen in the alveoli diffuses into just the right amount of capillary blood to allow all the haemoglobin molecules to become fully saturated. A very small amount of oxygen is also dissolved in the plasma.

In part (b), there is more ventilation then there is perfusion (high V/Q ratio). Not enough blood is available to accept all the oxygen within the alveoli. This extra oxygen is 'wasted' because once haemoglobin is fully saturated the arterial content cannot be increased any further. (This is due to the flat top of the oxygen dissociation curve – see Figure 4.4.) The only effect is a small increase in the oxygen dissolved in plasma. Part (b) is equivalent to the situation described earlier, the physiological dead space.

In part (c), the alveoli are being perfused more than they are being ventilated (low V/Q ratio). All the oxygen available is taken up by the haemoglobin, but the haemoglobin is not fully saturated – there is spare oxygen-carrying capacity in the haemoglobin, and the arterial oxygen content is reduced. Part (c) has the same effect as the shunt described previously, where blood with a low oxygen content bypasses the lung and returns directly to the systemic circulation.

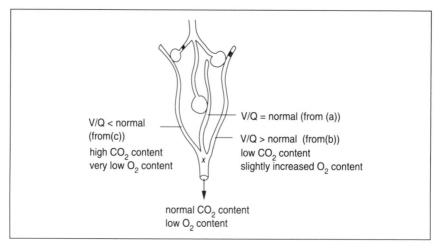

V/Q < normal
(from(c))
high CO_2 content
very low O_2 content

V/Q = normal (from (a))

V/Q > normal (from(b))
low CO_2 content
slightly increased O_2 content

x

normal CO_2 content
low O_2 content

Figure 3.8   Mixed blood returning from three sites at point *x*

Now the difficult bit! The oxygen content of the blood at point *x* in Figure 3.8 depends on the mixture of the blood coming from all three parts. It is not simply a middle point between (b) and (c) because the *small* extra amount of oxygen dissolved in plasma, from part (b), cannot offset the *massive* decrease in oxygen content produced by not fully saturating the haemoglobin molecules in part (c). Therefore the oxygen content is much lower than the half-way point between (b) and (c). In the trauma situation, an increase in the areas of V/Q mismatching is primarily responsible for the falls in PaO_2.

In summary, an area of the lung that has a high V/Q ratio cannot offset the fall in oxygen content produced by areas of the lung that have low V/Q ratios.

If the arterial oxygen content is affected by V/Q mismatching, why isn't the carbon dioxide content? The reason is that there is an almost straight-line (i.e. linear) relationship between the partial pressure of carbon dioxide and the carbon dioxide content of arterial blood. Figure 3.9 compares this with the oxygen dissociation curve. Consequently, an area of high ventilation can compensate for the failure of areas of low ventilation to eliminate carbon dioxide. Furthermore, if the $PaCO_2$ rises above a particular level, the respiratory rate is increased. This will further enhance carbon dioxide elimination by all ventilatory areas and so the $PaCO_2$ will fall back to normal levels.

An example of ventilatory, perfusional and diffusional pathology is seen in *pulmonary contusion*, which represents one of the commonest causes of death following thoracic trauma. It usually follows a blunt injury

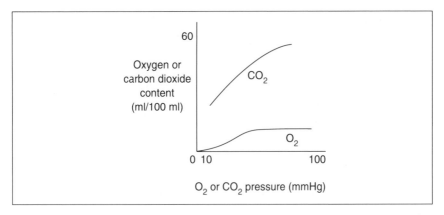

Figure 3.9 Graph showing CO_2 and O_2 content in blood against $PaCO_2$ and PaO_2. The CO_2 curve does not have a flat portion: as the $PaCO_2$ increases there is a steady increase in the carbon dioxide content of blood

which transmits its energy to the underlying lung tissue. This results in an increase in permeability of the small pulmonary capillaries leading to interstitial and alveolar oedema. The epithelial barrier is further damaged by any associated hypoxia. The affected lung area becomes more 'stiff' (i.e. less compliant), and less air is drawn into the lungs with each breath. Therefore a greater area of lung is being perfused but not ventilated (low V/Q, or shunt).

As the lungs become 'stiff', the work needed to inflate them increases. The respiratory rate increases but the tidal volume decreases, with the result that the alveoli ventilation also decreases. Further hypoxia ensues, particularly as the patient becomes exhausted and the process becomes self-perpetuating. Infection in the contused area frequently develops at a later stage if the patient survives. Trauma victims who are elderly or have coexistent lung disease are at particular risk.

■ Assessment and management

☐ Primary survey and resuscitation

The tried and tested systems of care as laid down in the ATLS/ATNC/TNCC are used to manage the problems encountered in thoracic trauma.

The initial plan of action is the same as that described in Chapter 1. Individual team members should have particular tasks allocated before the patient arrives so that the ABCs can be assessed and stabilized as quickly as possible.

The aim of the primary survey is to detect and correct any immediately life-threatening condition. With respect to thoracic trauma there are six conditions that fall into this category (Box 3.2).

BOX 3.2 Immediately life-threatening thoracic conditions

- Airway obstruction
- Tension pneumothorax
- Cardiac tamponade
- Open chest wound
- Massive haemothorax
- Flail chest

(A mnemonic for this list is: *All Trauma Clinicians Occasionally Miss Fractures*)

All of these six conditions will be covered, in the order in which they are most likely to be discovered in the primary survey.

Airway

Airway obstruction has been dealt with in detail in Chapter 2. The doctor and nurse responsible must assess, clear and secure the airway whilst maintaining cervical inline stabilization. All trauma patients have an increased oxygen demand and therefore require a high inspired oxygen concentration (see Chapter 4). The position of the trachea should be checked and any visible neck injury or venous distension noted before the cervical collar is replaced.

The patient's chest must be exposed so that it can be inspected for bruising, penetrating wounds, intercostal or supraclavicular indrawing, and abnormal chest movement. This is usually carried out by the team leader. The rate and volume of breathing should also be noted by the circulation nurse, because frequently a rapid, shallow respiratory pattern accompanies a chest injury or developing hypoxia. Both axillae are then auscultated to determine whether the air entry is equal over both sides of the thorax. If this is not the case, the chest is percussed to determine whether one side is hyper-resonant (pneumothorax) or dull (haemothorax or a ruptured diaphragm) compared to the other.

Breathing

Tension pneumothorax

Tension pneumothorax (Box 3.3) is commonly due to rupture of an emphysematous bulla, but can also result from trauma to the lung directly. Classically the patient will be tachypnoeic and tachycardic, with hyper-resonance of the hemithorax on the affected side. In the latter stages, the trachea will be deviated to the contralateral side. In a short period of time these patients become shocked as cardiac output falls and ventilation becomes progressively more difficult as the intrapleural pressure increases. This may be noticed in patients who are being ventilated, either as increasing resistance to manual ventilation or raised inflation pressures on a ventilator.

A raised jugular venous pressure (JVP) will occur only if there is sufficient blood volume. Cyanosis is a late sign (which in any situation depends on there being more than 5 g of deoxygenated (reduced) haemoglobin in circulation).

In the trauma patient a tension pneumothorax can be missed, so a high index of suspicion is required by the team leaders. It can also occur at any point in the resuscitation, especially after insertion of a central line or during manual or mechanical ventilation where there are rib fractures.

BOX 3.3 Signs of a tension pneumothorax

- Tachypnoea
- Shocked
- Hyper-resonant hemithorax
- Decreased air entry to the hemithorax
- Deviated trachea (late)
- Raised JVP (if no hypovolaemia)
- Cyanosis (very late)

The patient can die from this condition in the time it takes to obtain and process a chest x-ray. As an emergency measure, therefore, the chest must be decompressed by a needle thoracentesis.

Needle thoracentesis: procedure

The skin over the 2nd intercostal space of the affected hemithorax is cleaned. A 16 g cannula connected to a 10 ml syringe is inserted at this level in the midclavicular line (Figure 3.10), directly over the superior edge of the rib. Rapid release of air confirms the diagnosis, following which the cannula can be slid over the needle and into the pleural cavity, and the syringe and needle removed. This procedure will give the circulation nurse and doctor enough time to definitively treat the condition by inserting a chest drain (see below).

If, after insertion of the cannula, there is only a slow release of air and froth, then the diagnosis remains in doubt. There is also now a risk that a pneumothorax has been *created* as a result of the needle puncturing the lung. This creates a simple pneumothorax, but this may be transformed into a tension pneumothorax, particularly if the patient is being ventilated. An urgent chest x-ray is therefore now required. If this is not possible then the safest course is to insert a chest drain. The team leader must remember that

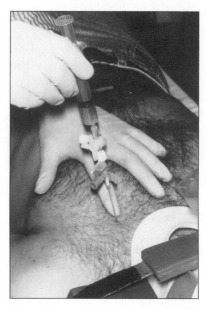

Figure 3.10   Needle thoracocentesis

the cause of shock still has to be found. A possible missed diagnosis is a cardiac tamponade.

Chest drain insertion: procedure

A chest drain should be inserted initially into the 5th intercostal space just anterior to the mid-axillary line (Figure 3.11). The equipment required is listed in Box 3.4.

BOX 3.4   Equipment required for a chest drain insertion

- Skin-preparation solution
- Swabs
- Sterile sheets
- Sterile gowns and gloves for the doctor and nurse
- Local anaesthetic (10 ml of 1% lignocaine)
- Syringe and needle
- Scalpel and blade
- Suture (at least 0 in thickness) and sterile scissors
- 36 g silastic chest drain with trocar removed
- Portex™ chest drainage bag or underwater drain with 200 ml of sterile water
- 1 large straight clamp
- 1 curved clamp

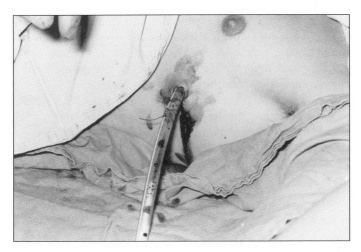

Figure 3.11 Chest drain insertion

Procedure The patient's arm is abducted and the 5th intercostal space palpated, usually at the level of the nipple in males. If there is an underlying rib fracture then an intercostal space immediately above or below is chosen.

Using an aseptic technique, the patient's chest is cleaned and draped. Local anaesthetic is injected into the skin over the area identified for insertion of the drain. The deeper structures are then infiltrated. Finally the needle is directed down onto the rib and local anaesthetic is injected onto its periosteum and over its *superior* surface into the underlying pleura. This approach is important because the intercostal vessels lie under the inferior surface of the ribs.

It is important to draw back frequently on the syringe to make sure that the needle has not entered a blood vessel. A 3 cm transverse incision is then made down to the 6th rib, through the anaesthetized area. Using the curved clamp, the pleura above the rib is breached and a track formed. The operator must now insert a finger through the incision and sweep around the intrapleural space to detect the presence of a ruptured diaphragm or lung adhesions. If adhesions prevent the passage of a finger, then a fresh incision should be made in the 4th or 6th intercostal space, just anterior to the mid-axillary line.

The straight clamp is then put across the proximal end of the chest drain and the tip inserted into the incision, directed with the curved clamp if necessary. Condensation of water vapour in air escaping from the pleural cavity causes fogging of the tube, once it is in the intrapleural space. It is then connected to the Portex™ chest drainage bag or underwater seal and the clamps are removed. If the underwater seal is used, there is initially a rush of air into the container, demonstrated by a mass of bubbles. Later, this settles and the fluid level is observed to rise and fall with the respiratory cycle.

The chest drain must then be secured: this is done with both suture and tape. The incision is now covered with gauze and waterproof tape.

Although trocars are usually supplied in chest drains, they should *never* be used as they can seriously injure the patient's lung, mediastinum and abdominal viscera due to inappropriate placement.

Once a chest drain has been inserted, the patient's chest needs to be re-examined to ensure that the lung is now ventilating, and a chest x-ray should be taken to ascertain the position of the drain and the presence of residual lung pathology.

If an underwater drainage system is used, it is important to remember three points:

1   The container must not be lifted higher than the patient, as fluid would drain back into the chest.

2   The chest drain should be clamped only when bottles are being changed.

3   Connections between the chest drain and the drainage tube are re-inforced with waterproof tape to prevent inadvertent disconnections.

Complications   The insertion of a chest drain should be carried out by trained staff because it can give rise to several complications if it is per-formed incorrectly. The main ones are these:

• bleeding;
• damage to the intercostal vessels and nerves;
• lung and mediastinal injury;
• damage to abdominal organs and vessels;
• infection;
• allergic reactions to the local anaesthetic or cleaning solution.

The circulation nurse must monitor drainage from the chest and ensure that, if an underwater seal is used, the water continues to swing with respiration. If this stops it implies that the drain is blocked and the medical team leader should be informed immediately.

Kinking of the chest drain, clogging of the chest drain with blood, or displacement of the chest drain may each cause a recurrence of the initial problem.

Open chest wound

This will automatically produce a pneumothorax on the ipsilateral side. If the wound is greater than two-thirds the diameter of the trachea then air preferentially enters the chest through this hole during inspiration. This causes failure of ventilation of the lung, which eventually collapses. A particularly dangerous situation is when air can *enter* via the hole but cannot escape (the 'sucking chest wound'). This gives rise to a tension pneumothorax, because the wound acts as a one-way valve (due to its shape) or from an inadequately applied dressing.

The immediate management of an open chest wound is to apply a sterile dressing, sealed on three sides. Air can escape via the free edge during expiration but cannot enter through the wound during inspiration, as the dressing is 'sucked' into the wound. A chest drain should then be inserted by the circulation nurse and doctor, via a freshly created hole, to drain the pneumothorax. In the acute situation of a tension pneumothorax develop-ing, any occluding dressing must be removed by the team leader, thereby opening the wound and allowing air to escape. The long-term management of the majority of these patients is by definitive surgical closure.

A flail chest

Examination of the chest wall will reveal crepitus, instability and, in the conscious patient, pain.

These patients must be managed in such a way that their hypoxia is corrected. Initially this is by high-flow, warm, humidified oxygen and adequate fluid resuscitation (see pulmonary contusion, page 90) during the primary survey. Analgesia, by intercostal or epidural block, is given during the definitive management phase. A selected group of patients (Box 3.5) require a more aggressive approach to correct their hypoxia, namely intubation and ventilation, usually early on in the resuscitation. In all cases the ABGs need to be monitored frequently.

BOX 3.5   Patients with a flail chest who require artificial ventilation

- Falling PaO_2 or < 50 mmHg on air
- PaO_2 < 80 mmHg with supplemental oxygen
- Rising $PaCO_2$ or > 45 mmHg
- Exhaustion
- Respiratory rate > 30 breaths/min
- Significant associated injuries of the abdomen and/or head

Circulation

The medical team leader must quickly assess the patient's colour and capillary return, and the presence of carotid, femoral and radial pulse. Two large (14–16 g) peripheral intravenous lines need to be inserted by the circulation nurse and doctor and 20 ml of blood should be taken at this point for laboratory investigations and possible cross-matching or typing (see Chapter 4). A poor cardiac output can result from a tension pneumo-thorax (which should already have been treated), or either of the following conditions.

Cardiac tamponade

As these patients are usually victims of penetrating trauma it is important to suspect this condition if there is a wound within an area indicated in Figure 3.12. The classic presentation of Beck's triad, pulsus paradoxus and Kussmaul's sign are only seen in a third of trauma patients (Box 3.6). Muffled heart sounds, due to blood in the pericardium, are always difficult to hear in the resuscitation room. Typically the patient is shocked, due to impaired filling of the left ventricle; but paradoxically has an elevated central venous pressure (seen clinically as distended neck veins) due to impaired venous return to the right ventricle. However, time should not be wasted inserting a central venous line during the primary survey and resus-citation phase, and in any case coexisting hypovolaemia may prevent a rise in the pressure.

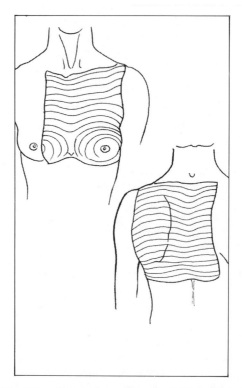

Figure 3.12 Sites of wounds associated with cardiac tamponade
Source: © Landon B, Driscoll P & Goodall J 1993. *The Atlas of Trauma Management.* Carnforth, Lancashire: Parthenon. Reproduced by kind permission.

BOX 3.6   Signs of a cardiac tamponade

- Beck's triad
  - Shocked
  - Raised JVP
  - Decrease in heart sounds
- Pulsus paradoxus of >10 mmHg
- Kussmaul's sign – raised JVP on inspiration

Pericardiocentesis

Temporary relief of the symptoms of cardiac tamponade can be gained by optimizing venous return by increasing the rate of intravenous infusions and aspiration of the pericardial sac (pericardiocentesis; Box 3.7). This latter procedure has significant risks and can be falsely negative in 25 per cent of cases, usually because the blood has clotted. If blood is aspirated then the cannula can be left in the pericardial space and allowed to drain freely. This will delay the development of any recollection, but in all cases a thoracotomy will be required for definitive care.

Pericardiocentesis: procedure

BOX 3.7   Equipment required for pericardiocentesis

- Skin-preparation solution
- Swabs
- Sterile sheets
- Sterile gowns and gloves for the doctor
- 15 cm, 16 g or 18 g cannula connected to a 10 ml syringe
- Three-way tap
- ECG monitor

The presence of any significant mediastinal shift is determined and the position of the xiphisternum noted.

If there is time, aseptic precautions are taken and the patient's subxiphoid area is cleaned, draped and anaesthetized.

The skin is then punctured, 1–2 cm inferior and to the left of the xiphochondral junction at a 45° angle. Whilst aspirating continually, the needle is advanced towards the tip of the left scapula. Simultaneously, the ECG monitor must be constantly checked for injury patterns (ST segment elevation or depression) and dysrhythmias (ventricular ectopics). Their appearance indicates that the needle has advanced too far and is now touching the myocardium. It should therefore be withdrawn slowly until a normal ECG is achieved.

Once the needle enters the pericardium as much blood as possible should be aspirated. As the cardiac tamponade is drained, ventricular filling will increase and the myocardium will move towards the needle: the ECG may change as described previously. Once again, slowly withdrawing the needle should result in a normal ECG. The cannula is left in place and connected to the three-way tap. The tap and cannula are then secured in place with gauze and tape.

Should the symptoms of a cardiac tamponade recur, the pericardium can be reaspirated.

Complications:

- Pneumothorax.
- Damage to the coronary arteries and veins.
- Damage to the myocardium.
- Damage to other mediastinal structures.
- Infection – skin; mediastinum; peritoneum.

Massive haemothorax

This is defined as greater than 1.5 litres of blood in the chest cavity (Figure 3.13) or drainage of greater than 200 ml/hour for four hours. It usually

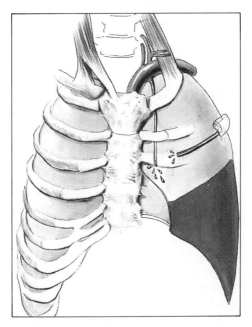

Figure 3.13 A massive haemothorax

Source: © Landon B, Driscoll P & Goodall J 1993. *The Atlas of Trauma Management.*
Carnforth, Lancashire: Parthenon. Reproduced by kind permission.

results from a laceration of either an intercostal vessel or the internal mammary artery. Bleeding from the lung parenchyma usually stops once the lung has re-expanded because of the low pulmonary perfusion pressure. However, a torrential bleed will result if the hilum is torn, and this will also require an emergency thoracotomy.

The physical signs are listed in Box 3.8. Interestingly the JVP may be high or low, depending on coexisting problems. To correct this condition some patients require a formal thoracotomy, therefore the appropriate surgeon should be informed. In the meantime the team must continue to resuscitate the patient with type-specific blood and complete the rest of the primary and secondary surveys.

BOX 3.8 Signs of a massive haemothorax

- Decreased air entry to the hemithorax
- Dull percussion note over the hemithorax
- Shock, grade 2–3 (Chapter 4)
- Raised JVP

At the end of the primary survey and resuscitation phase, the medical and nursing team leaders must ensure that the airway, ventilatory and circulatory resuscitative procedures have been started and that there has been no change requiring further intervention.

Attaching the patient to automatic blood pressure and ECG monitors enables frequent measurements to be taken. However, the former are not always reliable and so should not replace the regular, close observations of the patient by one of the circulation nurses: she must continue to record the respiratory rate, pulse, skin perfusion and conscious level.

Each of these patients will require a good-quality chest radiograph and a 12-lead ECG at the end of the secondary survey.

An arterial blood sample should be sent for analysis and the vital signs recorded. A gross estimation of the expected PaO_2 in a patient can be estimated by multiplying the inspired percentage of oxygen by 6. For example, if the inspired percentage is 60% then the expected PaO_2 would be about 360 mmHg.

Thoracotomy

Resuscitation-room thoracotomy is reserved for patients who are in electro-mechanical dissociation and have a penetrating injury to the chest. Delays in carrying out this procedure decrease the patient's chances of survival and therefore it should be carried out earlier rather than later. It must be performed by a trained clinician working with one of the circulation nurses. Both need to be familiar with the equipment (Box 3.9) and the procedure.

Thoracotomy: procedure

BOX 3.9   Equipment required for an emergency thoracotomy

- As for a chest drain insertion (page 80)
- Rib spreaders (Finocchetietto)
- Bone cutters
- Satinsky vascular clamp
- Metzenbaum scissors
- Vascular clamps
- Long forceps (toothed and non-toothed)
- Needle holder
- Felt pledgets
- 2–0 double-armed Ethibond™ suture

A prophylactic chest drain is first inserted into the contralateral hemithorax. The approach to the chest is through an anterolateral incision in the interspace immediately below the nipple. This is usually carried out on the left side, as this provides access to the heart and descending aorta. The operator should avoid the internal mammary artery by starting the incision approximately 5 cm lateral to the sternum. Further access can be achieved by extending the incision posteriorly and having the patient partially turned. The latter manoeuvre is dependent on the team leader's suspicion of a potential spinal injury.

Once this wound has been opened with the rib spreaders the clinician can deal with most emergency problems inside the chest. After a rapid inspection the emergency procedures which may be carried out are as follows:

(a) Compressing the aorta just above the diaphragm, to selectively shunt the available blood into the central circulation. It is preferable if the operator carries this out by squeezing the aorta between his hand and the thoracic vertebrae. This is safer than blindly clamping the aorta, which can result in the oesophagus being torn. Periodic assessment of the patient's volume status is needed once the aorta is compressed, to prevent ventricular distension and other problems of aortic occlusion.

(b) Opening the pericardium, to release any cardiac tamponade and allow the source of the bleeding to be controlled by direct pressure or suture. The phrenic nerve is at risk during this procedure, so the operator must identify this structure and cut anteriorly and parallel to it. The incision should extend from the apex of the heart to the base of the ascending aorta.

(c) External cardiac compression in a patient with a normal blood volume only produces 10–30 per cent of the normal cardiac output (see Chapter 4). This can be increased to 50 per cent with internal cardiac massage. This is carried out, inside or outside the pericardial sac, by compressing the heart between the operator's palms at a rate of approximately 60/minute. It is preferable to use the palms as fingertips can traumatize the heart wall. This can be an exhausting activity as the operator needs to squeeze hard and then abruptly relax to facilitate ventricular filling. Barring defibrillation, this must be continued without interruption until a spontaneous cardiac output is established or the patient is pronounced dead by the team leaders.

(d) Internal defibrillation is necessary if ventricular fibrillation develops. However the paddles should be covered with wet saline gauze to prevent burning the myocardium. One paddle needs to be placed over the base of the right atrium, the other over the cardiac apex. Lower energies are needed compared with external defibrillation (10–60 J compared with 200–360 J).

(e) Significant bleeding can usually be controlled by direct pressure using either finger compression or laparotomy pads. Occasionally a bleeding organ, such as the hilum of the lung, will require direct application of a non-crushing clamp to the vascular pedicle.

Once the emergency procedures have been accomplished the patient must be transferred to theatre, where the definitive surgery can be carried out.

☐ Secondary survey

Upon completion of the primary survey a detailed head-to-toe assessment of the patient should be carried out in the way described in Chapter 1.

The front and sides of the chest should be fully examined, with each rib being palpated for tenderness and crepitus and the thoracic cage squeezed in two planes to determine rib stability. Surgical emphysema should also be noted. Examination of the back of the chest is carried out when the patient is log-rolled onto his side.

With regard to thoracic trauma, there are six potentially life-threatening conditions which need to be ruled out during the secondary survey (Box 3.10).

BOX 3.10   Potentially life-threatening thoracic conditions

- Pulmonary contusion
- Cardiac contusion
- Ruptured diaphragm
- Dissecting aorta
- Oesophageal rupture
- Airway rupture

Unlike the thoracic problems detected during the primary survey, these conditions cannot be immediately corrected or their presence easily confirmed. Knowledge of the mechanism of the injury and a detailed physical examination are essential for their early detection.

Pulmonary contusion

On examination respiration is often rapid and shallow and there may be tenderness or marks on the chest wall due to the original injury. Overlying fractured ribs may be present, but in the young the natural elasticity of the chest wall may prevent this. Auscultation can be normal. As the disease process develops the respiratory distress increases and ventilation becomes progressively more difficult.

A plain chest radiograph and serial ABGs are essential. The former will show a hazy shadowing after a few hours (Figure 3.14). The PaO_2 gradually falls as the ventilation/perfusion mismatch develops.

These patients require a high inspired oxygen concentration, careful fluid administration and close observation, preferably in a high-dependency unit. This is particularly true if a selective approach to mechanical ventilation is instituted. The criteria for this form of treatment vary between units; one example is listed in Box 3.11.

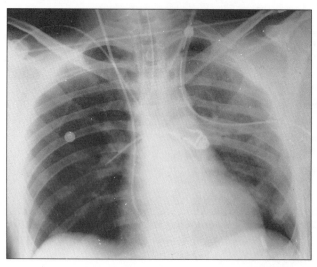

Figure 3.14   Chest radiograph showing pulmonary contusion

BOX 3.11   Patients with pulmonary contusion who require artificial ventilation

---

- Elderly
- Decreased level of consciousness
- Associated long-bone fractures
- Progressive rise in $PaCO_2$
- Progressive fall in PaO_2
- Requiring a general anaesthetic for surgery
- Requiring transfer
- Renal failure
- Pre-existing lung disease

The increase in pulmonary oedema resulting from over-transfusion is well recognized in these patients. What is less well known is the deleterious effect of *under*-transfusion. The latter leads to a fall in the cardiac output and so, in turn, a reduction in the pulmonary perfusion. Further hypoxia results, causing additional leakage through the alveolar membrane. Invasive monitoring (see Chapter 4) is the only true way of determining the appropriate fluid requirements. This is a further reason why these patients should be subsequently managed in a high-dependency unit.

Cardiac contusion

In this condition there is bleeding into the myocardium. It results from blunt trauma to the chest and it can lead to coronary artery occlusion due to spasm, neighbouring tissue oedema, or intimal tearing. These will lead to further myocardial damage due to ischaemia. Cardiac contusion has an incidence of 16–76 per cent in the reported cases of thoraco-abdominal trauma.

On examination, the patient may have sternal bruising and tenderness due to blow to the front of the chest. A common mechanism of injury is when a vehicle driver is thrown against the steering column following a head-on crash. There is an association between cardiac contusions and fractures of the sternum or wedge fractures of the thoracic vertebrae (see Chapter 8).

Should the contusion be significant then the patient may develop dysrhythmias, heart failure or hypotension which does not respond to resuscitation. The incidence of dysrhythmias increases if there is any associated hypoxia or acidosis.

Cardiac contusions can be extremely difficult to diagnose as in the majority of cases the patient is asymptomatic. The principal investigations are a 12-lead ECG and a plasma assay of the cardiac isoenzyme CPK-MB. A variety of dysrhythmias may be present, particularly premature ventricu-

lar contractions, atrial fibrillation, sinus tachycardia, and ST segment elevation or depression. A right bundle branch block pattern may also be seen.
An elevation of greater than 30 per cent in the enzyme assay is diagnostic of
myocardial damage. Unfortunately, there are few hospitals that can do this
biochemical investigation whilst the patient is in the resuscitation room: it
tends therefore to be used as a retrospective test.

Heart failure and dysrhythmias producing haemodynamic instability
should be treated by standard medical protocols. During the definitive
phase a 2D echocardiogram or isotope studies can be undertaken to gain
information on the ventricular wall motion.

Patients with confirmed cardiac contusion with dysrhythmias require
the facilities of a high-dependency unit for their long-term management.
The team leader should make sure the appropriate doctor is informed
during the definitive phase.

Ruptured diaphragm

This can result from either blunt or penetrating trauma. In the latter case
75 per cent are associated with intra-abdominal injury and there is usually
a discrete tear in the diaphragm. It should be suspected if a wound is found
lying between the 5th and 12th ribs. Blunt trauma produces irregular
multiple tears, usually on the left-hand side (79 per cent).

On examination, the patient must be checked for any wounds or marks.
Breath sounds may be decreased over the inferior aspect of the affected
hemithorax and, rarely, bowel sounds may be heard on auscultation of the
chest. Unfortunately these physical signs are not always present and the first
suspicion comes from the plain chest radiograph. The affected hemidiaphragm
is elevated and occasionally bowel is seen herniating through it into the
pleural space (see Figure 5.2, page 143). As these features are difficult to see
on a supine x-ray, an erect chest radiograph is preferable but this should be
obtained only once spinal injury has been eliminated. If a naso- or orogastric
tube has been inserted then its tip may be seen above the diaphragm in the
chest. A peritoneal lavage (see Chapter 5) can be negative if there is no intra-
abdominal injury other than a ruptured diaphragm and a chest drain has
not been inserted. Lavage fluid will leak out of a chest drain if the diaphragm is ruptured.

This condition requires early surgical advice to confirm its diagnosis
and to detect any associated intrathoracic or abdominal injury. Operative
repair of the diaphragm is needed to prevent later bowel herniation and
possible obstruction.

Dissecting thoracic aorta

About 90 per cent of these patients die at the scene of the incident. In the
remaining 10 per cent, the adventitial layer provides a tamponade effect and

only around 500 ml of blood will be lost from the systemic circulation. Consequently the patient will not demonstrate the classic signs of shock (providing there are no other sources of haemorrhage). Variable signs that may be present are hoarseness, upper-limb hypertension, and pulse differences between upper and lower limbs. An erect plain chest radiograph can demonstrate several features which should make one suspect a dissecting thoracic aorta (Box 3.12). A widened mediastinum is the most important sign (Figure 3.15). The definitive investigation is either angiography or a CT scan of the aortic arch, the choice depending on the local policy of the thoracic surgeons.

BOX 3.12   Radiological features of a dissecting aortic aneurysm

- Widened mediastinum
- Fractured first two ribs
- Trachea displaced to the right
- Oesophagus displaced to the right
- Pleural capping
- Blurring of the aortic notch
- Elevation of the right mainstem bronchus
- Depression of the left mainstem bronchus
- Decrease in space between the pulmonary artery and aorta

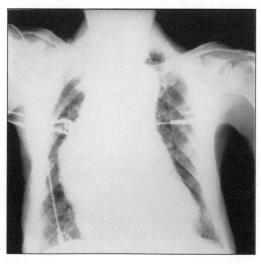

Figure 3.15   Chest radiograph showing a widened mediastinum

If these patients are to survive then the aorta needs to be surgically repaired by a thoracic surgical team before the adventitial layer ruptures. Of the 10 per cent of patients who reach hospital alive, half of the survivors will die each day if no operation is performed. The trauma team therefore needs to have a high index of suspicion of this injury and request early thoracic surgical input. If there is no thoracic surgical team in the receiving hospital, advice must be sought on where the CT scan or angiography should be performed, and how the hypertension, if present, should be managed.

Oesophageal rupture

Following a severe blow to the epigastrium, gastric contents are forced into the lower oesophagus and this may result in a linear tear. Penetrating trauma can also rupture the oesophagus at any level, and there is a high association with injuries of neighbouring structures.

On examination the patient has a degree of shock and pain greater than that due to the apparent injuries. Surgical emphysema in the neck and upper chest may develop with time. Suspicions should be further raised if a left pneumothorax or pleural effusion are seen on the chest radiograph, without there being any history of left-chest trauma or fractured ribs on the left side. Occasionally, a pneumomediastinum or a fluid level may be present behind the heart shadow on the chest x-ray. Once a chest drain has been inserted the fluid swing should be noted. Normally this is maximal during expiration, but with the air leak coming from the oesophagus the swing is equal in both stages of the ventilatory cycle. Very occasionally bowel contents are extruded through the chest drain.

These patients will require further investigations and in almost all cases a surgical repair. Therefore the appropriate surgical team should be involved in their management once the secondary survey is finished.

Airway rupture

This can occur at three different anatomical levels.

Larynx

Impacts with dashboards, steering wheels, clotheslines and fists or feet can fracture this cartilaginous structure. Penetrating trauma can also produce extensive damage.

On examination the three classic signs may be present: hoarseness, crepitus and surgical emphysema. Any tenderness, bruising around the larynx, reduced prominence of the thyroid notch or dyspnoea should also be noted.

The first priority in these patients is to ensure that they have a patent airway. In those cases where the airway has to be created, orotracheal intubation may be technically impossible. These patients will require a tracheostomy, *not* a cricothyroidotomy (see Chapter 2). Once the airway has been cleared and secured, a CT scan can be performed.

The patient will require the skills of an ENT surgeon during the definitive treatment phase.

Trachea

With regard to blunt trauma, the trachea is usually torn at the crico-tracheal junction. The mechanisms are similar to those fracturing the larynx. Penetrating trauma can occur at any level but especially in the neck, when it is frequently associated with injuries to other vital structures such as the carotid arteries, the jugular veins, the oesophagus, and the laryngeal and phrenic nerves.

If the lumen of the trachea is exposed, blood, spray and bubbles are seen escaping from the base of the wound. The airway nurse and doctor must immediately clear and secure the airway. Occasionally it may be possible to insert an endotracheal tube directly into the trachea through the wound. In cases of complete obstruction, signs of respiratory distress will be present; in the unconscious patient such distress could be the only sign of injury to the trachea. If the defect is only small then basic airway control may be all that is required until a detailed examination of the trachea can be performed.

Bronchi

The bronchi are firmly anchored anatomically and so are unable to move when the body is subjected to rapid deceleration forces. The tear usually occurs within 2–3 cm of the carina and it can be either partial or complete. This condition has a 30 per cent mortality rate, but this is due to the associated injuries that occur with this type of injury.

On examination there may be haemoptysis, surgical emphysema, a pneumothorax and overt signs of a chest injury. If oral intubation is attempted (for another reason), then it may be technically difficult or impossible to perform. A plain chest x-ray usually demonstrates a pneumothorax. After a chest drain has been inserted, suspicion should be further raised if the initial rush of air does not settle, but instead bubbles continue to be produced with each expiration.

These patients require the expertise of a thoracic surgeon for their definitive management. Some will require surgery, others will be managed conservatively, but all will require a bronchoscopy.

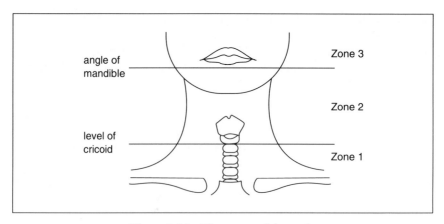

Figure 3.16   The zones of the neck

☐ Neck wounds

The neck has been divided into zones to help classify the potential severity of particular wounds (Figure 3.16).

Zone 1 extends from the level of the manubrial notch to the cricoid cartilage. It is not surprising that injury to this area has the highest incidence of mortality and morbidity because penetrating trauma to this area can involve the trachea, the oesophagus, the carotid arteries, the jugular veins and the cervical spine. In addition, haemorrhage is difficult to control and vital structures are difficult to visualize in this area.

Zone 2 lies between the cricoid cartilage and the angle of the mandible. Penetrating trauma to this area could potentially damage the same structures as mentioned in relation to zone 1. However, they are easier to visualize and haemorrhage control is simpler to apply.

Zone 3 lies above the level of the angle of the mandible and contains the pharynx and salivary glands.

No wound on the neck which has gone into the platysma should be explored in the A/E department. A detailed examination of the vascular, neurological and visceral structures needs to be made. These patients will require radiological investigations and in appropriate cases panendoscopy.

☐ Definitive care

In 15 per cent of cases of chest trauma thoracic surgical expertise is required. The medical team leader must make sure a thoracic surgeon has been called for the appropriate patients.

The management of the following conditions should be the responsibility of any trauma team.

Pneumothorax

Each traumatic pneumothorax needs to be treated with an appropriately-sized chest drain in the recommended location. If the lung becomes fully inflated and the pleural space dry, then there is a less than 1 per cent chance of complications such as infection and adhesions.

Haemothorax

Bleeding into the pleural cavity usually follows lung or vessel injury and is often self-limiting. The only treatment required is drainage of the blood through a large chest drain to stop the formation of clots which would prevent full expansion of the lung.

Occasionally, the bleeding does not stop. To ensure that this is detected one of the circulation nurses must closely monitor the amount of blood draining, as this could be a cause of hypovolaemia and might require surgical intervention to arrest the haemorrhage (see pages 87–9).

Surgical emphysema

Air in the subcutaneous tissues (surgical emphysema) does not need treating unless it is severe enough to interfere with respiration. However, a detailed examination is required to identify the cause (Box 3.13) because this will require definitive treatment.

BOX 3.13   Causes of surgical emphysema

- Laryngeal, tracheal or bronchial tears
- Oesophageal tear
- Sucking chest wound
- Blast injury
- Lung injuries

Fractured ribs

Ribs usually fracture at their point of maximum curvature, which is in the lateral thoracic position. The trauma team need to be aware that young people, especially children, have very pliable bones: this prevents them from breaking, even when subjected to considerable forces. Consequently there can be significant internal thoracic injuries *without* rib fractures. In adults the fractures are usually not visible on the initial chest x-ray unless there is significant displacement. Later, as the muscular spasm relaxes, the fractures open out and they can be clearly seen on the chest x-ray.

Fractures of the upper three ribs require great force and are usually associated with severe intrathoracic pathology and a mortality of 50 per cent. The presence of such life-threatening conditions must be identified or excluded.

Ribs 4–9 may be broken in the axillary region either from a direct blow or as a result of an antero-posterior compression force. The former will push the broken ends of the bone into the chest cavity, with an increased risk of lung damage.

The lower ribs also cover the abdominal cavity. When fractured, they may therefore be associated with intra-abdominal visceral injury. This needs to be excluded.

In all cases of multiple rib fractures, once underlying pathology has been ruled out, the patients require analgesia. This can be achieved by a variety of techniques (e.g. local or regional anaesthesia), depending upon the expertise available. Whichever method is used, it must be sufficient to allow intensive chest physiotherapy to be started. In spontaneously-breathing patients, the presence of severe pain will restrict expansion of the lungs and inhibit coughing, leading ultimately to retention of secretions, consolidation and infection.

Chest compression

If severe, this can obstruct venous return, causing raised intrathoracic and intracranial pressure. Patients are plethoric and cyanotic, with an engorged face, upper limbs and chest. They may be confused or unconscious. Other associated signs are petechial and scleral haemorrhages, and respiratory distress. Once the compression force has been relieved, the raised pressures abate: mortality is then related to any associated injuries.

■ Summary

The majority of chest injuries can be treated initially by the trauma team. However, in certain cases the expertise of the thoracic surgeon and intensive care specialist will be needed for the definitive care of the patient. If these specialists are not already members of the team, the nursing and medical team leaders must be aware of when it is appropriate to involve them.

There are six immediately life-threatening conditions which must be detected and treated during the primary survey and resuscitation phase. However, these conditions may occur spontaneously at any stage, so careful monitoring of the patient must be maintained. It is important to remember that when a patient is developing even minor signs of irritation this may indicate the development of hypoxia.

During the secondary survey, there are six potentially life-threatening conditions and several minor thoracic problems which must be detected. The management of these conditions is carried out during the definitive care phase.

■ Appendix 3.1: Partial pressures

The pressure in the airways is due to the molecules in the air colliding with the airway walls. As air is made up of several gases, including oxygen, nitrogen and water vapour, each will produce a proportion of the pressure in the airways.

The total airway pressure is the sum of all the individual gas pressures. The contribution made by an individual gas is known as its partial pressure. It can be calculated by multiplying the concentration of the specific gas, expressed as a percentage of the total, by the total pressure. For example, the partial pressure of oxygen in dry air is:

$$20.9\% \times 760 \text{ mmHg} = 159 \text{ mmHg}$$

where 20.9% is the concentration of oxygen in air and 760 mmHg is the total (atmospheric) pressure at sea level.

Pressure can also be measured in pascals (Pa). Atmospheric pressure is 101 000 Pa or 101 kPa.

$$1 \text{ kPa} \simeq 7.6 \text{ mmHg}$$

When a gas mixture is in contact with a liquid, some of the gas will dissolve in the liquid. The volume that dissolves is dependent on both the partial pressure of the individual gas, which forces molecules into the liquid, and the solubility of the individual gas in the liquid. For example, carbon dioxide is twenty times more soluble in plasma then oxygen. Therefore more carbon dioxide than oxygen will dissolve in plasma at any particular partial pressure.

Eventually, in a closed system, an equilibrium is achieved, in which the number of molecules of the gas *leaving* the liquid is equal to the number *entering* the liquid. At this point the partial pressure of each gas *within* the liquid is equal to the partial pressure of the same gas *in contact with* the liquid.

□ Symbols used

P : The partial pressure of a particular gas.
A : Alveolar (e.g. PAO_2 = partial pressure of alveolar oxygen).
a : Arterial (e.g. $PaCO_2$ = partial pressure of arterial carbon dioxide).
v : Venous.

V : The volume of gas.
Q : The volume of blood.

☐ Normal arterial blood-gas values

pH	7.35–7.45
$PaCO_2$	35–45 mmHg
PaO_2	95–100 mmHg
Bicarbonate	24–32 mmol/l
Base excess	±2 mmol/l

■ References and further reading

American College of Surgeons Committee on Trauma 1993. *Advanced Trauma Life Support Course for Physicians*. Chicago: American College of Surgeons.

Bodai B, Smith P, Ward E, *et al.* 1983. Emergency thoracotomy in the management of trauma – a review. *JAMA* **249**: 1891.

Champion H, Danne P & Finelli F 1986. Emergency thoracotomy. *Arch. Emerg. Med.* **3**: 95.

Clark G, Schecter P & Turnkey D 1988. Variables affecting outcome in blunt chest trauma: flail chest vs. pulmonary contusion. *J. Trauma* **28**: 298.

Cowley A & Dunham M 1986. *Shock Trauma/Critical Care Manual*. Maryland: Aspen Publishers.

Demetriades D, Kakoyiannis S, Parekh D, *et al.* 1988. Penetrating injuries of the diaphragm. *Br. J. Surg.* **75**: 824.

Durham L, Richardson R, Wall M, *et al.* 1992. Emergency centre thoracotomy: impact of prehospital resuscitation. *J. Trauma* **32**: 775.

Emergency Nurse Association 1988. *TNCC Course Manual*, 2nd Edn. Chicago: Award Printing Corporation.

Hammond S 1990. Chest injuries in the trauma patient. *Nurs. Clin. N. Am.* **25**(1): 35.

Hiatt J, Yeatman L & Child J 1988. The value of echocardiograph in blunt chest trauma. *J. Trauma* **28**: 914.

Hodgkinson D, O'Driscoll R, Nicholson D, *et al.* (in press). The chest. In Nicholson D & Driscoll P (eds): *ABC of Assessing Emergency Radiographs*. London: BMJ Publications.

Jones T, Barnhart G & Greenfield L 1987. Cardiopulmonary arrest following penetrating trauma: guidelines for emergency hospital management of presumed exsanguination. *J. Trauma* **27**: 24.

Jordan K 1990. Chest trauma. How to detect – and react to – serious trouble. *Nursing* **20**(9): 34.

Kaulesar Sukul D, Kats E & Johannes E 1991. Sixty-three cases of traumatic injury of the diaphragm. *Injury* **22**: 303.

Lorenz H, Steinmetz B, Lieberman J, *et al.* 1992. Emergency thoracotomy: survival correlates with physiologic status. *J. Trauma* **32**: 780.

Macnaughton P & Evans T 1992. Management of adult respiratory distress syndrome. *Lancet* **339**: 469.

Maddox P, Mansel R & Butchart E 1991. Traumatic rupture of the diaphragm: a difficult diagnosis. *Injury* **22**: 299.

Menaopace M 1989. Instituting the six-hour protocol for patients with asymptomatic thoracic stab wounds: a nursing perspective. *Trauma Quarterly* **6**: 33.

Murphy R & Jones J 1991. Acute lung injury. *Br. J. Int. Care* **3**: 110.

Myers E & Iko B 1987. The management of acute laryngeal trauma. *J. Trauma* **27**: 448.

Ordog G 1987. Penetrating neck trauma. *J. Trauma* **27**: 543.

Repine J 1992. Scientific perspectives on adult respiratory distress syndrome. *Lancet* **339**: 466.

Ross S 1990. Epidemiology of thoracic injuries: mechanisms of injury and pathophysiology. *Top. Emerg. Med.* **12**: 1.

Sheehy S 1992. Chest trauma. In Sheehy S, Marvin J & Jimmerson C (eds): *Emergency Nursing, Principles and Practice*, 3rd Edn. St. Louis: C V Mosby.

Sinkinson C (ed.) 1991. The continuing saga of penetrating neck injuries. *Em. Med. Repts* **12**: 135.

Treasure T & Raphael M J 1991. Investigation of suspected dissection of the thoracic aorta. *Lancet* **338**: 490.

West J 1987. *Pulmonary Pathophysiology – the essentials*. Baltimore: Williams & Wilkins.

West J 1990. *Respiratory Physiology – the essentials*. Baltimore: Williams & Wilkins.

Chapter 4

Shock

Peter Driscoll, Carl Gwinnutt, Terry Brown and Olive Goodall

Objectives

The objectives of this chapter are that members of the trauma team should understand:

- the definition of shock;
- the normal cardiovascular response to hypovolaemia;
- the importance of oxygen delivery and consumption;
- the initial management of the shocked patient.

■ Introduction

Shock is a term used frequently, but inexactly, by the media and lay people. Medically, the term should be reserved to define *inadequate oxygen delivery to vital organs*. It is in this restricted sense that the word is used throughout this book.

■ Cardiovascular pathophysiology

To comprehend the pathophysiology of shock it is important to understand the regulatory factors responsible for maintaining the circulation and oxygen delivery in the healthy state.

For the reader who is particularly interested, the formulae for calculating the various parameters discussed are listed in Appendix 4.1 (page 131).

□ Circulatory control

The amount of blood reaching a particular organ is dependent on several factors:

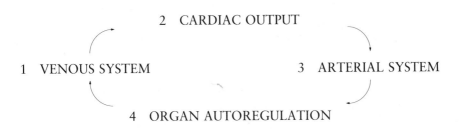

2   CARDIAC OUTPUT

1   VENOUS SYSTEM   3   ARTERIAL SYSTEM

4   ORGAN AUTOREGULATION

Venous system

The venous system is capable of acting as a reservoir for over 50 per cent of the circulating blood volume and is therefore often referred to as a capacitance system. The amount of blood stored at any one time is dependent on the size of the vessel lumen. This is controlled by sympathetic innervation and local factors (see later) which can alter the tone of the vessel walls. If the veins dilate, more blood remains in the venous system and less returns to the heart. Should there be a requirement to increase venous return, sympathetic stimulation increases, reducing the diameter of the veins and the capacity of the venous system. A change from minimal to maximal tone can increase the venous return by approximately 1 litre.

Cardiac output

Cardiac output (CO) is defined as the volume of blood ejected by each ventricle per minute. Clearly, over a period of time the output of the two ventricles must be the same, or the circulating volume would eventually end up in either the systemic or pulmonary circulation.

It follows from the definition that the cardiac output is the product of the volume of blood ejected with each beat (stroke volume) and the heart rate (beats per minute) and is expressed in litres/minute:

cardiac output = stroke volume × heart rate   (Eqn 4.1)

To allow a comparison between patients of different sizes, the *cardiac index* (CI) is used. This is the cardiac output divided by the surface area of the person and hence is measured in litres/square metre:

CI = CO/body surface area   (Eqn 4.2)

The cardiac output can be affected by various factors, as described below.

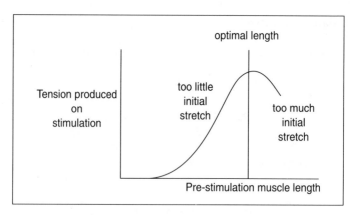

Figure 4.1 Starling's curve – single muscle

Preload

A feature of any muscle is that the magnitude of the contraction increases if the muscle is stretched before it is stimulated to contract (Figure 4.1). However, this phenomenon has an upper limit due to the internal molecular structure of the muscle cell. If the muscle is stretched beyond this point, a *smaller* contraction is produced.

This principle also applies to the heart. The cardiac muscles are stretched during diastole because this is when the heart is being filled with returning blood. Therefore, 'The more the myocardial fibres are stretched during diastole, the more forcibly they contract during systole and therefore more blood will be expelled' (Starling's law).

This venous filling of the heart is termed the *preload*. Up to a certain point, the greater the preload, the greater the stroke volume.

Unfortunately it is not possible to measure the length of each of the hundreds of myocardial cells in the ventricle in order to determine the degree of stretching produced by the blood in the chamber at the end of diastole. Instead, a clinical estimate is obtained by measuring the ventricular pressure at the end of diastole. This is known as the *end diastolic pressure* (EDP). As the left ventricular EDP (LVEDP) increases, so does the stroke volume; but as with the individual muscle cell, if the EDP exceeds a critical level the myocardium in the left ventricle begins to produce smaller contractions (Figure 4.2) and eventually left ventricular failure results.

An increase in the venous filling (preload) will only lead to an increase in the cardiac output if it is kept below a critical level.

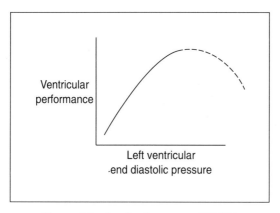

Figure 4.2   Starling's curve – LVEDP

Afterload

As the left and right ventricles contract, pressures within the chambers increase until they exceed those in the aorta and pulmonary artery respectively. The aortic and pulmonary valves open and the blood is ejected. The resistance faced by the ventricular myocardium during ejection is termed the *afterload*. In the left ventricle this is a combination of the resistance offered by the aortic valve and the arterial blood vessels. This latter component is the most important and is termed the *systemic vascular resistance* (SVR). Clinically afterload is frequently approximated to SVR, as this is more easily measured.

When afterload is reduced (whilst maintaining preload), the ventricular muscle shortens more quickly and extensively, thereby increasing the stroke volume.

Myocardial contractility

This is the rate at which the myocardial fibres contract for a given degree of stretch. Substances affecting myocardial contractility are termed *inotropes*. They can be positive or negative in their actions. A positive inotrope produces a greater contraction for a given length (or EDP, clinically), the equivalent of shifting the curve in Figure 4.2 to the left (Figure 4.3). Adrenaline, noradrenaline and dopamine are naturally-produced substances which have this effect. Dobutamine and isoprenaline are synthetic catecholamines with positive inotropic activity. Along with dopamine, they are frequently administered in the management of cardiogenic and septic shock (see later).

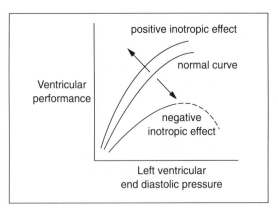

Figure 4.3 Starling's curve – LVEDP
with positive/negative inotropic effects

Negative inotropes result in a reduced contractility for a given muscle length. These substances are often drugs being taken by the patient (e.g. anti-arrhythmics) or administered acutely (e.g. anaesthetic agents). Many of the physiological states produced by shock will also depress contractility (e.g. hypoxia and acidosis).

Heart rate

Increases in heart rate are mediated by the sympathetic nervous system directly, or indirectly by the release of catecholamines from the adrenal medulla. This is termed a *positive chronotropic effect*. Conversely, the release of acetylcholine from the vagus nerve near the sino-atrial node and atrio-ventricular node result in a decrease in heart rate, a *negative chronotropic effect*.

An increase in the heart rate can lead to an increase in cardiac output (see Equation 4.1). However, ventricular filling occurs during diastole and it is this phase of the cardiac cycle that is predominantly shortened at fast heart rates. As the rate rises above 160 bt/min in the young adult, very little time is left for the heart to fill. This leads to a progressively smaller stroke volume and a fall in cardiac output. The critical heart rate when this occurs is also dependent on the age of the patient and the condition of the heart – for example, in the elderly rates over 120 bt/min may cause inadequate filling.

An increase in the heart rate will only lead to an increase in the cardiac output if it is kept below a critical level.

In summary, the main factors affecting the cardiac output of the left ventricle are listed in Box 4.1.

BOX 4.1 Factors that affect the left ventricular cardiac output

- Preload (or LVEDP)
- Afterload (or SVR)
- Myocardial contractility
- Heart rate

The arterial system

If there were a total loss of arterial tone (SVR), the capacity of the circulatory system would be increased so much that the total blood volume (Box 4.2) would be insufficient to fill it, blood pressure would fall, and flow through organs would be dependent upon their resistance.

BOX 4.2 Blood volumes

- Adult: 70 ml per kilogram ideal body weight
- Child: 80 ml per kilogram ideal body weight

Some organs would receive more than the normal amounts of oxygenated blood (e.g. the skin), at the expense of others which would receive less (e.g. the brain). To prevent this, the arterial system is under constant control by sympathetic innervation and local factors to ensure that blood goes where it is needed most.

This is exemplified in the shocked patient where differential vasoconstriction maintains supply to the vital organs (e.g. the heart) at the expense of others (e.g. the skin). Hence the skin is cold and pale.

Systemic arterial blood pressure

This is the pressure exerted on the walls of the arterial blood vessels. *Systolic pressure* is the maximal pressure generated in the large arteries and *diastolic pressure* is the minimum during each cardiac cycle. The difference between them is the *pulse pressure*. The *mean arterial pressure* is the average pressure during the cardiac cycle and is approximately equal to diastolic pressure plus one-third the pulse pressure.

The mean arterial pressure is the product of the cardiac output and the systemic vascular resistance (and is therefore affected by all the factors already discussed). Should either of these fall, then compensatory changes occur in an attempt to maintain the mean pressure. For the trauma team, the commonest cause for this fall in blood pressure is hypovolaemia reducing cardiac output. Initially blood pressure will be maintained by vasoconstriction (increasing SVR) and a tachycardia. A fall in blood pressure will take place only when no further compensation is possible, and is therefore a *late* sign in shock.

Autoregulation

Organs also have a limited ability to regulate their own blood supply so that perfusion is maintained as blood pressure varies. This process is known as *autoregulation*. This is bought about by the presence of smooth muscle in the arteriolar walls which alters the calibre of the vessels to maintain flow. Furthermore, other local factors such as products of anaerobic metabolism, acidosis and a rise in temperature all cause the local vascular tree to dilate. This enables active tissues to receive increased quantities of nutrients and oxygenated blood.

□ Oxygen delivery

The delivery of oxygen (DO_2) to the tissues is dependent on its transfer from alveoli into blood flowing through the pulmonary capillaries, its transport to the tissues and, finally, its release to the cells of the tissues.

Transfer from alveoli to blood

The factors affecting this – namely ventilation, perfusion diffusion and V/Q ratios – are discussed on pages 72–7.

Transport to the tissues

The amount of oxygen transported from the lungs to the tissues in arterial blood (CaO_2) is dependent on the saturation of haemoglobin with oxygen, the haemoglobin concentration and the cardiac output.

The vast majority of oxygen carried in the blood is taken up by the haem molecule, with only a small amount dissolving in the plasma. The relationship between the PO_2 and oxygen uptake by haemoglobin is not linear, because each oxygen molecule added facilitates the uptake of the next oxygen molecule. This produces a sigmoid curve (Figure 4.4). Furthermore, because haemoglobin is virtually fully saturated at a PO_2 of 100 mmHg (i.e. that found in the normal healthy state), increasing the PO_2 further has little effect on oxygen transport.

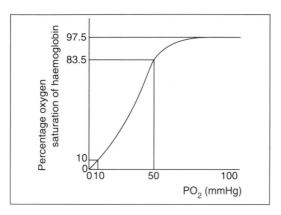

Figure 4.4 Oxygen association curve

The affinity of haemoglobin for oxygen at a particular PO_2 (commonly known as the O_2–Hb association) is also affected by other factors. It is increased (i.e. shifting the curve to the left) by an alkaline environment, low PCO_2, low concentrations of 2,3-diphosphoglycerate (2,3-DPG) in the red cells, carbon monoxide, and a fall in temperature. (The opposite of these factors *reduces* the affinity – see later.)

At first sight, it would seem logical that a greater haemoglobin concentration would allow more oxygen to be carried. Unfortunately, however, increasing the haemoglobin concentration leads to an increase in blood viscosity, which impedes blood flow and so offsets this advantage. The normal haemoglobin concentration (as measured by haematocrit) is usually just above the point at which the oxygen transportation is optimal. A slight fall in haemoglobin concentration (and hence viscosity) will actually *increase* oxygen transportation.

The factors affecting cardiac output are described on pages 103–7.

Oxygen release to tissue

At the tissue level, the partial-pressure gradient is opposite to that found at the alveolar/capillary interface (see Chapter 3). The capillary PaO_2 is approximately 20 mmHg and cellular PO_2 only 2–3 mmHg. Local factors also decrease the affinity of haemoglobin for oxygen (shifting the curve to the right), allowing oxygen to be released more readily. This occurs with an increase in $PaCO_2$, increased temperature and acidosis, and with an increase in 2,3-DPG.

To help remember these effects, think of the athlete during a race. The active muscles require more oxygen than when they are at rest. Due to the increased metabolism they generate lactic acid, carbon dioxide and heat, all of which will assist in the release of oxygen by haemoglobin. Finally, local autoregulatory mechanisms will affect oxygen release.

☐ Tissue oxygen consumption

In the normal subject, total consumption of oxygen per minute (VO_2) is constant throughout a wide range of oxygen delivery (DO_2; Figure 4.5). The normal VO_2 for a resting male is 100–160 ml/min/m², and the normal value of DO_2 in the same person is 500–720 ml/min/m². Therefore tissues are taking up only 20–25 per cent of the oxygen brought to them. This is known as the *oxygen extraction ratio* (OER) and demonstrates that normally there is great potential for the tissues of the body to extract more oxygen from the circulating blood.

Following trauma both oxygen delivery and consumption can be affected. Tissue damage results in an early increase in consumption, despite the fact that the delivery of oxygen falls because of the reduced blood volume. The increase in consumption is achieved by increasing the extraction of oxygen from the blood. This compensatory response only works if the delivery of oxygen is greater than 300 ml/min/m². With levels below this the tissues cannot increase oxygen extraction any further – oxygen extraction is at its maximum. Oxygen consumption therefore progressively falls because it is now directly dependent on the rate of delivery to the tissues.

It is important to remember that pain has an adverse effect on the patient's tolerance of shock, as it increases the tissue's oxygen requirements. Therefore every effort should be made to reduce the level of pain for both humanitarian and physiological reasons.

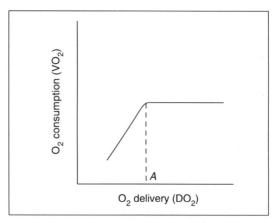

Figure 4.5 Graph showing the relationship between oxygen delivery and consumption. *A* is the critical level for DO_2: below this, VO_2 is dependent on DO_2; above *A*, VO_2 is maintained by an increase in the oxygen extraction ratio. *A* is elevated in the critically ill patient

■ Cellular and tissue effects due to shock

Patients cannot remain permanently in a state of shock: they either improve or die. Indeed shock could be looked upon as a momentary pause on the way to death. This pause gives the trauma team time to prevent further deterioration and, ultimately, death.

If the shock persists, tissue oxygenation becomes markedly compromised and the cells revert to anaerobic metabolism. This results in the formation of lactic acid which eventually leads to intracellular and systemic acidosis. Eventually autolysis occurs and the toxins released can lead to the development of multiple organ failure. This condition is one of the commonest causes of late death after trauma. The chances of this happening increase if there is inadequate early resuscitation and correction of the shock state.

In the later stages of shock there are microcirculatory changes leading to stagnation of blood flow, sludging of red cells, and a further impairment of tissue perfusion. In addition, the hydrostatic pressure within the capillaries increases because blood can still perfuse the capillaries but cannot escape; as a consequence, further intravascular fluid is lost as it diffuses through the capillary wall into the interstitial space.

■ Compensatory mechanisms

When a sufficient cell mass has been damaged, the shocked state becomes irreversible and the death of the patient is inevitable. Fortunately the body has several compensatory mechanisms which attempt to maintain adequate oxygen delivery to the essential organs of the body and help prevent this stage being reached.

□ Circulatory control

Pressure receptors in the heart and baroreceptors in the carotid sinus and aortic arch trigger a reflex sympathetic response via control centres in the brain stem in response to hypovolaemia.

The sympathetic discharge stimulates many tissues in the body, including the adrenal medulla which leads to an increased release of systemic catecholamines, enhancing the effects of direct sympathetic discharge, particularly on the heart. This has the effect of preventing or limiting the fall in cardiac output by positive inotropic and chronotropic effects on the heart and by increasing venous return as a result of venoconstriction. Furthermore, selective arteriolar and pre-capillary sphincter constriction of non-essential organs (e.g. the skin and the gut) maintains perfusion of vital organs (e.g. the brain and the heart).

Selective perfusion also leads to a lowering of the hydrostatic pressure in those capillaries serving non-essential organs. This reduces the diffusion of fluid across the capillary membrane into the interstitial space, thereby decreasing any further loss of intravascular volume.

Any reduction in renal blood flow is detected by the juxtaglomerular apparatus in the kidney, which releases renin. This leads to the formation of angiotensin II and aldosterone which, together with antidiuretic hormone released from the pituitary, increase the reabsorption of sodium and water by the kidney (thereby reducing urine volume), which helps maintain the circulating volume. Renin, angiotensin II and ADH can also produce generalized vasoconstriction and so help increase the venous return.

In addition to these hormones, insulin and glucagon are also released to assist the supply and utilization of glucose by the cells. Furthermore, the body attempts to enhance the circulating volume by releasing osmotically-active substances from the liver. These increase plasma osmotic pressure, and so cause interstitial fluid to be drawn into the intravascular space.

☐ **Oxygen delivery**

Unfortunately, although the sympathetically induced tachypnoea occurs, this does not produce any increase in oxygen uptake because the haemoglobin in blood passing ventilated alveoli is already fully saturated.

In summary, therefore, shock can result from vascular, cardiac and tissue pathology, acting separately or in combination to cause an inadequate delivery of oxygen to vital structures of the body. Each of these elements has a finite capacity to maintain adequate oxygen delivery. This enables the patient to compensate, to a limited extent, when one or more of the elements are defective.

■ **Causes of shock**

Each of the four components on page 113 can be responsible alone or in combination as the cause of shock:

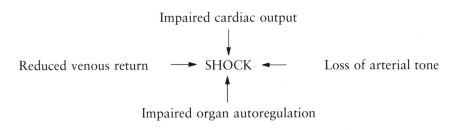

Impaired cardiac output

Reduced venous return ⟶ SHOCK ⟵ Loss of arterial tone

Impaired organ autoregulation

For example, following a car crash a patient may have both cardiac con-tusion, reducing cardiac output by a negative inotropic effect, and hypovolaemia, reducing venous return. However after trauma, shock usu-ally has a hypovolaemic component. Fortunately, this is the causative factor most easily corrected and it should be treated before the other causes are assessed and managed.

☐ Reduced venous return

The most common cause of shock in the trauma patient is haemorrhage. This may be occult, as the thorax, abdomen and pelvis have large potential spaces in which blood may collect. Significant haematomas can also develop in potential spaces in the body (e.g. the intrapleural and retroperitoneal spaces), as well as in muscles and tissues around long-bone fractures. Intravascular volume may also be reduced by fractures as a result of leakage of plasma into the interstitial spaces. This may account for up to 25 per cent of the volume of tissue swelling following blunt trauma.

The rate of blood returning to the heart is dependent on the pressure gradient created by the high hydrostatic pressure in the peripheral veins and the low hydrostatic pressure in the right atrium of the heart. Any reduction in this gradient (e.g. tension pneumothorax or cardiac tamponade increas-ing right atrial pressure) will lead to a fall in the venous return to the heart. External compression on the thorax or abdomen can have a similar action in obstructing the venous return.

☐ Impaired cardiac output

Both ischaemic heart disease and cardiac contusions have negative inotropic effects, but do not produce cardiogenic shock in the trauma victim unless more than 40 per cent of the left ventricular myocardium has died or has been severely damaged. Cardiac tamponade, in addition to its effect on venous return, also impedes ventricular filling. It is important to remember that anti-arrhythmic drugs – being taken by the patient, or administered acutely – may have a significant negative inotropic effect.

In cardiogenic shock the compensatory sympathetic and catecholamine responses only serve to increase the myocardial oxygen demand and further increase the degree of ischaemia.

☐ Loss of arterial tone

Neurogenic shock

A spinal injury above T6 will impair the sympathetic nervous system outflow from the spinal cord below this level. As a consequence both the reflex tachycardia and vasoconstriction responses to hypovolaemia are eliminated. The result is generalized vasodilatation, bradycardia and loss of temperature control. This is known as *neurogenic shock*, and it leads to a reduction in blood supply to the spinal column and so additional nervous-tissue damage ensues. Any associated haemorrhage from the injury will aggravate this situation, further reducing spinal blood flow (see Chapter 8).

Septic shock

Circulating endotoxins, from sepsis or bacteraemia, also produce vasodilatation and impair energy utilization at a cellular level. The source is usually gram-negative bacteria.

In this type of shock, tissue hypoxia can occur even with normal or high oxygen delivery rates because the tissue oxygen demand is extremely high. In addition, the capillary walls at the site of the infection become leaky due to the endotoxin. Later on this becomes more generalized, allowing sodium and water to move from the interstitial space to the intracellular space. With time, this leads to hypovolaemia and the condition becomes indistinguishable from hypovolaemic shock.

Further cellular damage by endotoxins causes the release of proteolytic enzymes. These paralyse pre-capillary sphincters, enhance capillary leakage, and increase hypovolaemia. The situation is aggravated by the endotoxin acting on the myocardium as a negative inotrope. Therefore in the late stage of sepsis there are several causes for the shock state.

(Further details on the pathophysiology of septic shock is beyond the scope of this book. For the interested reader, several references are listed in the 'Further reading' section.)

■ Estimating volume loss and grading shock

The compensatory mechanisms produce signs and symptoms dependent on the severity of the shock. It follows that by monitoring the decline in function of the various organs, a grading of the degree of shock can be made (see below). Capillary refill (see below), conscious level, heart rate, blood pressure and urine output can be readily measured and so are important indicators of the grade of shock, and also allow assessment of the response to treatment.

A *positive capillary refill* is defined as the return of blood within 2 seconds to the base of the thumb following digital pressure.

These physiological changes can be used to divide hypovolaemic shock into four categories, dependent on the percentage blood loss (Table 4.1 and Figures 4.6a–d) and so enable the team leader to estimate the loss of circulating volume.

In Grade 2 shock (Figure 4.6b), diastolic blood pressure rises, without any fall in the systolic component, leading to a narrowed pulse pressure. This is due to the compensatory vasoconstriction that occurs. Consequently, a narrow pulse pressure with a normal systolic blood pressure is an early sign of shock.

☐ Limitations to estimations of hypovolaemia

For some patients, blindly following the signs in Table 4.1 could lead to a gross over- or underestimation of the blood loss (Box 4.3). It is therefore important that management is based on the overall condition of the patient and not on isolated physiological parameters.

Table 4.1 Categories of hypovolaemic shock

Grade	1	2	3	4
Blood loss (litres)	< 0.75	0.75–1.5	1.5–2.0	> 2.0
Blood loss (% BV)	< 15 %	15–30 %	30–40 %	> 40 %
Heart rate	< 100	> 100	> 120	140 or low
Systolic BP	normal	normal	decreased	decreased ++
Diastolic BP	normal	raised	decreased	decreased ++
Pulse pressure	normal	decreased	decreased	decreased
Capillary refill	normal	delayed	delayed	delayed
Skin	normal	pale	pale	pale/cold
Respiratory rate	14–20	20–30	30–40	> 35 or low
Urine output (ml/hr)	> 30	20–30	5–15	negligible
Mental state	normal	anxious	anxious/ confused	confused/ drowsy
Fluid replacement	colloid	colloid	blood	blood

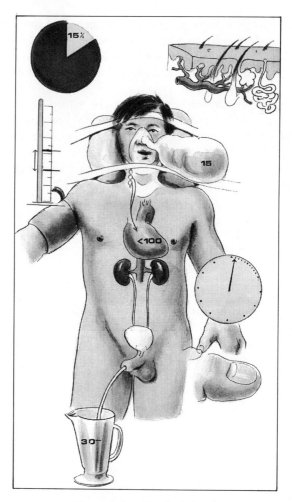

Figure 4.6a   Grade 1 shock
Source: © Landon B, Driscoll P & Goodall J 1993. *The Atlas of Trauma Management.*
Carnforth, Lancashire: Parthenon. Reproduced by kind permission.

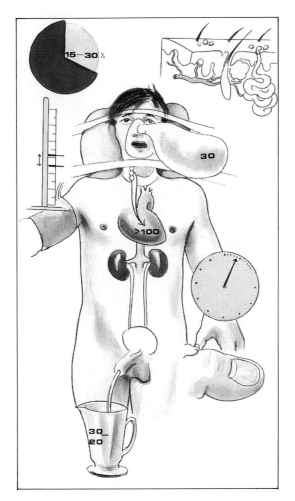

Figure 4.6b   Grade 2 shock
Source: © Landon B, Driscoll P & Goodall J 1993. *The Atlas of Trauma Management.*
Carnforth, Lancashire: Parthenon. Reproduced by kind permission.

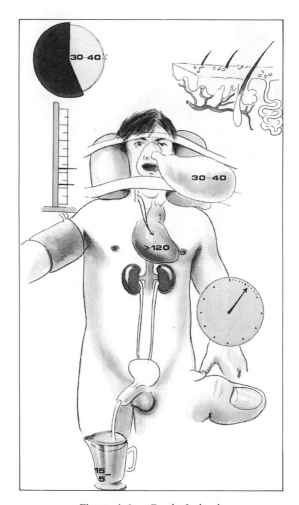

Figure 4.6c Grade 3 shock
Source: © Landon B, Driscoll P & Goodall J 1993. *The Atlas of Trauma Management*.
Carnforth, Lancashire: Parthenon. Reproduced by kind permission.

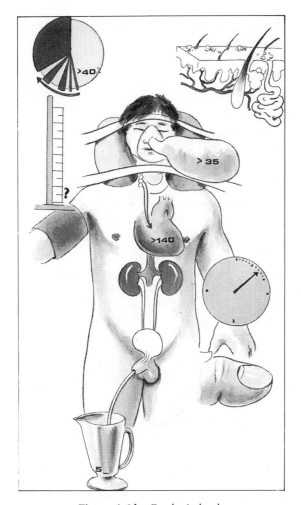

Figure 4.6d Grade 4 shock
Source: © Landon B, Driscoll P & Goodall J 1993. *The Atlas of Trauma Management.*
Carnforth, Lancashire: Parthenon. Reproduced by kind permission.

BOX 4.3   Patients with a risk of over- or underestimation of blood loss

---

- Type of patient
  - elderly
  - drugs/pacemaker
  - athlete/pregnancy
- Environment/pre-hospital
  - hypothermia
  - time
  - type of injury

The elderly patient

This type of patient is less able to compensate for acute hypovolaemia than the young trauma victim. Consequently the loss of smaller volumes can produce a fall in blood pressure. Reliance only on the blood pressure could therefore lead to an overestimation of the blood loss.

The patient taking drugs or fitted with a pacemaker

Various drugs which are commonly taken can alter the physiological response to blood loss. The best example of this is beta-blockers. These drugs will prevent tachycardia and also inhibit the normal sympathetic positive inotropic response. Therefore, a patient taking a beta-blocker who has lost over 15 per cent of his blood volume may not have the compensatory tachycardia. This could lead to an underestimation of the blood loss. It is also important to remember that the blood pressure falls at lower volumes of blood loss in these patients by the same mechanisms.

An increasing number of patients each year have pacemakers fitted. These devices may allow the heart to beat only at a particular rate, irrespective of the volume loss. They will therefore give rise to the same errors in estimation as beta-blockers.

The athletic or pregnant patient

These patients have already undergone various physiological changes before the accident. Both have larger blood volumes (and the athlete, a lower heart rate) than normal (Box 4.4).

BOX 4.4   Heart rate, blood pressure and blood volume in the athlete or the pregnant woman

---

Pregnancy
Heart rate increases through pregnancy. By the third trimester it is 15–20 beats faster than normal. Blood pressure falls by 5–15 mmHg in the second trimester and returns to normal during the third trimester. The blood volume has increased by 40–50 per cent by the third trimester.

Athlete
The resting heart rate in a moderate athlete is 50 beats per minute. Therefore a compensatory tachycardia, in a trained athlete, can be less than 100 bt/min. A further source of possible underestimation of blood loss comes from the increase in normal blood volume by 15–20 per cent as a consequence of training.

The patient with hypothermia

Hypothermia will reduce the blood pressure, pulse and respiratory rate in its own right, irrespective of any blood loss. If this is ignored then there would be an overestimation of any hypovolaemia. It has also been found that hypothermic patients who are bleeding are resistant to appropriate fluid replacement. The estimation of the fluid requirements of these patients can therefore be very difficult and often invasive monitoring is required (see Chapter 13).

Compensation

The longer the time the patient spends without resuscitation (especially in the young), the longer the normal compensatory mechanisms will have to work. This will lead to improvements in blood pressure, respiratory rate and heart rate. An underestimation of the blood loss could then occur.

■ Management of the shocked patient

As previously stated, the state of shock is defined as *inadequate delivery of oxygen to vital organs*. It therefore follows that the detection of this condition is dependent on certain physical signs that are produced as a result of poor oxygen delivery. Similarly, the treatment of shock consists of the restoration of an adequate delivery of oxygen, and not simply the restoration of a normal blood pressure.

☐ **Primary survey and resuscitation**

The same plan is used as is described in Chapter 1, with members of the team carrying out their tasks simultaneously.

It is essential that the airway nurse and doctor clear and secure the patient's airway and administer oxygen at 15 l/min (see Chapter 2). Adequate ventilation with a high inspired oxygen concentration is required for optimizing oxygen uptake and delivery. Unconscious patients with grade 4 shock should be intubated and ventilated with 100% oxygen. At the same time the spinal column in general, and the cervical spine in particular, should be immobilized.

The remaining five immediately life-threatening respiratory problems need to be excluded or treated if they are present (see Chapter 3).

A patient presenting in a state of shock is presumed to be suffering from hypovolaemia until this has been excluded. The primary aims of treatment of this type of shock are to stop any further loss and to replace the circulating volume. Red-cell replacement is secondary, becoming more important with progressively larger blood losses. (Remember the advantages effect of a reduced haematocrit on blood flow.)

Any overt bleeding is stemmed by direct pressure. Two large-bore peripheral IV lines (14 g or 16 g) should be inserted by the team members allocated to be responsible for 'circulation'. The antecubital fossa is the site of choice, provided that there is no proximal arm injury. If the latter is the case, any available site, other than the arm, should be used. It is important that fluid is infused quickly, therefore short, wide cannulae should be used because the flow of a liquid in a tube is inversely proportional to the length and directly related to its diameter (Box 4.5).

BOX 4.5 Relationship between cannula diameter and flow rate

Catheter	Rate of flow (ml/min)
14 g short	175–200
14 g long	150
16 g short	100–150
16 g long	50–100

The intraosseous route can be used in children if it is not possible to cannulate a peripheral vein. This technique is described in Appendix 4.2 (page 134).

In adults, there are two alternatives if a peripheral site is not available: central line and cutdown.

Central line

An appropriate cannula of similar diameter should be inserted into a central vein (usually the subclavian vein) using a Seldinger technique. This technique involves threading a guide wire through a needle which has been inserted into the central vein. This procedure should be carried out only by experienced staff because it has potential for damaging the vein and neighbouring structures. One of the circulation nurses should prepare the equipment listed in Box 4.6 and assist in the procedure (Figure 4.7).

Central venous cannulation: procedure

BOX 4.6   Equipment required for central venous cannulation

- Skin-preparation solution
- Swabs
- Sterile sheets
- Sterile gowns and gloves for the nurse and doctor
- Local anaesthetic
- Syringe and needle for administering the anaesthetic
- Scalpel and blade
- Suture and sterile scissors
- Central line pack:
  - Syringe
  - Large-bore needle
  - Guide wire
  - Dilators
  - Cannula
- Three-way tap
- Giving set, attached to intravenous fluid for infusion
- Opsite™
- Monitor and appropriate tubing

The patient is placed supine with his arms at his side. The operator, standing on the same side as that to be punctured (usually the right), identifies the midclavicular point and the suprasternal notch.

Under sterile conditions, the needle is inserted 1 cm below the midclavicular point and advanced along the posterior surface of the clavicle towards a finger in the suprasternal notch (Figure 4.7). The syringe and needle must be kept horizontal during the insertion, aspirating at all times.

When the needle enters the subclavian vein blood flows easily into the syringe. The syringe is then removed and the end of the cannula blocked by a thumb to prevent air entering the central vein. The floppy end of the guide wire is then inserted into the needle and advanced 4–5 cm into the vein. The

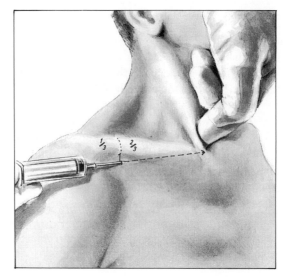

Figure 4.7   Procedure for central line insertion
Source: © Landon B, Driscoll P & Goodall J 1993. *The Atlas of Trauma Management.*
Carnforth, Lancashire: Parthenon. Reproduced by kind permission.

needle is then removed over the wire, taking care not to accidentally extract the wire along with the needle.

A dilator is then loaded onto the wire, ensuring that the proximal end of the latter protrudes from the dilator. While holding onto the proximal end of the wire, the dilator is slid along the wire, into the vein. Occasionally it is necessary to make a small incision in the skin to allow this to happen. Next, a wide, short catheter is loaded onto the guide wire and slid into the vein. The wire is then removed whilst holding the catheter in position.

A syringe is now reattached and blood aspirated to confirm the correct placement of the catheter. If difficulty is encountered during insertion, the needle and wire must be removed together so that the wire is not damaged on the tip of the needle. After 3 minutes of gentle pressure, a fresh attempt can be made.

A chest x-ray should be taken as soon as possible to exclude complications such as a pneumothorax and to confirm correct positioning of the catheter.

Complications

- Pneumothorax.
- Haemothorax.
- Brachial plexus injury.
- Tracheal puncture.
- Infection – skin, mediastinum.

Cutdown

An alternative method is to cut down onto the long saphenous or medial basilic vein. The same circulating nurse mentioned above will need to be familiar with the equipment described in Box 4.7.

Venous cutdown: procedure

BOX 4.7 Equipment required for a venous cutdown

- Skin-preparation solution
- Swabs
- Sterile sheets
- Sterile gowns for the nurse and doctor
- Local anaesthetic
- Syringe and needle for administering the anaesthetic
- Scalpel and blade
- Suture and sterile scissors
- Small haemostats
- Cannula
- Giving set, attached to intravenous fluid for infusion
- Opsite™

The operator should identify the important landmark. In the case of the long saphenous vein, this is the medial malleolus; with the medial basilic vein, it is the medial epicondyle of the humerus.

Following routine skin preparation and local anaesthesia, a 3 cm transverse incision is made either 2 cm anterior and superior to the medial malleolus or 2–3 cm lateral to the medial epicondyle at the flexion crease of the elbow.

Using blunt dissection, the 2–3 cm of vein is then freed from neighbouring tissue. The distal end is tied off, with the suture being kept in place to allow traction on the vein. Proximally, however, a loop of suture is placed around the vein but the knot is not tied.

Using the scissors or scalpel, a small transverse hole is then made in the side of the vein and a wide-bore cannula inserted. The proximal loop is tied off so that the cannula is secured in place.

Blood should now be aspirated from the cannula. If placement in the vein is confirmed, the intravenous tubing can be connected and the skin closed with interrupted sutures. Finally a sterile dressing is placed over the operation site.

Complications

- Infection – skin, vein.
- Haematoma.
- Venous thrombosis.
- Nerve, vein and artery transection.

Immediately following successful venous cannulation, 20 ml of blood is taken for estimation of serum electrolytes, full blood count, and grouping and crossmatching (if required). By the time the cannulae are in place, the medical team leader should quickly have assessed the patient with regard to the grade of shock. If this is estimated to be grade 2 or higher, 1 litre of colloid is then infused with each giving set connected to a 0.5 litre bag. Where there has been over 30 minutes' delay in starting the infusion, 2 litres of Hartmann's solution should be used instead, to compensate for the interstitial fluid volume loss. This can then be followed with colloid or blood, depending on the response. The aim should be to maintain the haematocrit (packed cell volume) at 30–35 per cent so that oxygen delivery is optimized. In grade 1 shock, 0.5 litres of colloid is infused and the response monitored. The arguments for and against crystalloid and colloid infusions are described in Appendix 4.3 (page 134).

All fluids given to trauma patients need to be warmed before administration, to prevent iatrogenically-induced hypothermia. A simple way of achieving this is to store a supply of colloids and crystalloids in a warming cupboard. This eliminates the need for warming coils during this phase of resuscitation, which increase resistance to flow and thereby slow the rate of fluid administration.

In those trauma victims with ischaemic heart disease, the increase in cardiac work and oxygen demand may be critical. Therefore the need for high inspired levels of oxygen and accurate monitoring is extremely important in these patients.

Simultaneously with the stemming of any overt blood loss and gaining intravenous access, the team leader should rapidly inspect the patient for gross signs of shock. Consequently, the presence of pale, cold and clammy peripheries must be noted. Other signs which should be quickly checked are an altered conscious level, tachypnoea, tachycardia and loss of palpable main pulses. Using Table 4.1, an estimation can then be made of the degree of intravascular volume loss.

As these tasks are being carried out the second circulation nurse should begin monitoring the patient and measuring the vital signs (Box 4.8).

BOX 4.8   Vital signs that must be monitored in trauma patients

---

- Heart rate, blood pressure, pulse pressure
- Respiratory rate
- Capillary refill
- Urinary output
- Glasgow Coma Scale
- Chest leads (ECG rhythm and waveform)
- Peripheral oxygen saturation
- Temperature (core and peripheral)

Accurate measurement of urinary volume will obviously require the insertion of a urinary catheter which should be connected to a system permitting accurate volume measurement. The volume is then recorded whenever the other vital signs are measured. However, this will have to wait if a urethral injury is suspected (see Chapter 1). Consequently, catheterization is usually carried out at the end of the secondary survey.

As described in Table 4.1, if there is a reduced blood pressure, then the trauma patient will require blood, because he will have already lost at least 30 per cent of his intravascular volume. A decision to transfuse the patient may also be made if there is a poor or transient response to the initial colloid challenge (see later). In the majority of trauma cases typed blood is required – that is, blood checked only for ABO and Rhesus compatibility. Most laboratories can provide typed blood within 10 minutes. If there is no recordable BP then the patient will require uncrossmatched blood initially, because he will have lost over 40 per cent of his intravascular volume and so will require blood urgently. Once the uncrossmethod blood has been given, the typed blood should be available.

Coagulation abnormalities can occur after massive blood loss because of dilution of clotting factors by administered fluids, the release of tissue factors which inhibit clotting, and the low concentration of clotting factors in stored blood. The coagulation abnormality needs to be treated precisely, using information gained by a regular assessment of the patient's clotting status. This approach is preferable to the practice of blindly treating any bleeding problem with platelets and fresh frozen plasma.

The rest of the primary survey is completed as previously described in Chapter 1. At the end, the nursing and medical team leaders must ensure that the required tasks have been, or are being, carried out. An arterial blood sample can be sent at this stage. Acidosis should be treated with increased ventilation and fluid administration because it is invariably a result of anaerobic metabolism in poorly perfused tissues. Sodium bicarbonate is reserved for cases where the pH is less than 7.2.

The goal of the team at the end of this stage in the resuscitation is for the patient to achieve an adequate organ perfusion, demonstrated by a urine flow greater than 50 ml/hr, a normal conscious level and an adequate blood pressure with no tachycardia. The team leader must reassess the ABCs if these targets have not been reached to make sure that a correctable life-threatening condition has not been missed.

☐ **Secondary survey**

After the detailed head-to-toe assessment of the patient has been carried out, the team should have a reasonable estimation of the blood loss and its source. They should also know the patient's allergic history, current medication, past medical history, time of last meal and the mechanism of the injury (remember 'AMPLE' in Chapter 1).

Pain relief will usually be required, in order to relieve the suffering, to increase the patient's ability to compensate for any hypovolaemia, and also to reduce the catecholamine secretion. It is achieved by diluting 10 mg of morphine to 10 ml in saline and administering it intravenously in 1 ml increments, until analgesia is achieved. An appropriate dose of an antiemetic (e.g. metoclopramide 5–10 mg) should be administered at the same time. Analgesia should never be given by the intramuscular route because of the erratic uptake in the shocked patient. Initially there is only limited systemic distribution due to the poor perfusion of the patient's muscles. However after resuscitation, when perfusion has improved, a large bolus of narcotics can be released into the bloodstream.

In the time it takes an efficient trauma team to reach this stage in the resuscitation, the first litre of colloid will have been given to the patient. The original estimated blood loss can therefore be compared with the patient's response to the fluid volume provided. There are only three options available with regard to the change in the patient's state after reassessment:

The patient is improving

This implies that the intravascular volume loss is less than 20 per cent and that the rate of fluid supply is greater than the rate of fluid loss. Such a patient may require blood later but one can afford to wait for a full crossmatch. He still requires close monitoring because he may suddenly deteriorate (see below).

The patient initially improves, then deteriorates

In these cases the rate of bleeding has suddenly increased. This may be due to a new source or a loss of haemostasis at the original source. The majority of these patients will require an operation, and so they all require early involvement from the appropriate surgical team. Blood is required, the choice being between typed or uncrossmatched unless fully crossmatched blood had been previously prepared. The decision will depend on the clinical state of the patient (as above).

The patient does not improve

These patients are either bleeding faster then blood is being supplied or not suffering primarily from hypovolaemic shock. In the former group the patient will have lost over 40 per cent of his blood volume and therefore will require surgery and blood.

Alternatively, the shock may be due to a cardiogenic, neurogenic or septic cause. Aspects of the history, examination and physiological recordings are essential to distinguish between these possibilities.

Cardiogenic shock

Signs, symptoms and treatment of both cardiac tamponade and tension pneumothorax are described in Chapter 3. Their presence should be rapidly excluded because these conditions can quickly kill the patient.

Shock resulting from failure of the heart itself is not common in trauma victims. If heart failure is suspected, it is essential to discover the past medical history and current medication. Clinically, there may be evidence of chest trauma, dysrhythmia and a raised central venous pressure (CVP) as displayed by engorged jugular veins, in addition to the more usual signs of shock. These patients are also less able to compensate for hypovolaemia should that coexist.

Measurement of the CVP does not provide an accurate estimate of the LVEDP in those patients with heart failure (Box 4.9). These patients are best managed using a pulmonary artery (Swann-Ganz) catheter which enables both the filling pressure of the left side of the heart and the cardiac output to be estimated. It has been demonstrated that the first management priority is correction of hypoxaemia, even if this requires intubating and ventilating the patient with supplemental oxygen. The filling pressures, which may be high in heart failure, can be reduced in a controlled fashion with intravenous nitrates, which will lower the systemic vascular resistance. Dopamine and dobutamine may also be required to provide inotropic support and improve the cardiac output. Any dysrhythmia causing haemodynamic compromise has to be treated.

BOX 4.9   Disadvantages of a central venous pressure measurement in heart failure

- Poor estimate of LVEDP
- CVP is often raised due to lung pathology
- CVP is affected by positive pressure ventilation
- Malpositions of the central line may cause false elevations

---

It is not unusual to find that a combination of mechanical ventilation, vasodilators, inotropes and expansion of the circulating volume is required to increase the cardiac index and DO_2. Clearly these are not procedures to be undertaken in A/E, but require the facilities available in the ITU.

Neurogenic shock

Patients with neurogenic shock will have the history and physical findings of spinal damage (see Chapter 8). It is important that these patients are neither under- nor over-transfused: the former leads to further spinal injury, the latter to pulmonary oedema. Over-transfusion was a leading cause of death in spinally-injured service personnel in the Vietnam war. When this injury occurs in people with no previous heart or lung disease, the CVP and the LVEDP have a close correlation. In the early stages, therefore, a CVP will be of help in estimating the fluid requirements, but later the patient will require much more intensive and accurate fluid monitoring.

Septic shock

It takes time to develop septic shock, so these patients are usually transfers from other hospitals or the victims of bowel perforation some hours previously.

Early signs are a wide pulse pressure and warm skin due to the dilated peripheral vessels. The cardiac output may also be raised. The patient is frequently agitated and pyrexial, and has an increased respiratory rate due to the hypoxia. Later on the classic features of hypovolaemic shock are manifested. There may also be evidence of problems with coagulation, for example disseminated intravascular coagulation. This abnormality often manifests as blood oozing around wounds and cannula sites.

In the late stages, septic shock will affect all four parts of the circulatory system: the venous return is reduced; there is a negative inotropic effect due to the circulating endotoxins; the arterial system is dilated; and the tissue autoregulation system is disrupted. In addition to all these changes, the oxygen demand of the tissues increases and there is a decrease in the tissues' ability to take oxygen up. It will not therefore be surprising to find that, in its late stages, septic shock has an extremely high mortality rate.

If these patients are to survive, the source of the infection needs to removed. Repeated blood cultures are required to determine the causative organism. The patient will require cardiovascular and respiratory support, as well as intensive monitoring of his fluid and antibiotic regimes.

Treatment is aimed at maintaining high cardiac index (over 4.5 l/min/m^2), a high DO_2 (above 600 ml/min/m^2), and a high tissue perfusion pressure. This usually entails intubation and ventilation of the patient with supplemental oxygen, correction of hypovolaemia with colloid, and the use of inotropes. Noradrenaline is frequently needed for its alpha-agonist activity which helps counteract some of the profound vasodilatation.

■ Summary

The trauma team leaders and the circulation nurses must recognize and treat as early as possible all shocked patients. They should also constantly reassess and monitor the appropriate physiological parameters. Any deterioration must be detected quickly and treated appropriately. As the patient improves, other problems may become apparent.

■ Appendix 4.1: Invasive monitoring

In the case of the critically ill patient it is now recognized that manipulating the patient's haemodynamic status and oxygen transportation, such that they achieve optimal goals (Box 4.10), markedly reduces the mortality rate.

BOX 4.10   Optimal goals in securing adequate oxygen transportation

- Cardiac index (CI) > 4.5 l/min/m²
- Oxygen delivery (DO_2) > 600 ml/min/m²
- Oxygen consumption (VO_2) > 170 ml/min/m²

The routine recordings therefore need to be augmented, during the definitive care phase, by more sophisticated monitoring devices. Other than CVP measurements, these invasive techniques are usually reserved for the intensive care unit. The normal ranges of values for these parameters are listed in Box 4.11.

BOX 4.11   Normal ranges of values for cardiorespiratory variables

- CI   = 2.8–3.6 l/min/m²
- DO_2 = 500–720 ml/min/m²
- VO_2 = 100–160 ml/min/m²
- Mixed venous oxyhaemoglobin saturation (SvO_2) = 75%
- Oxygen extraction ratio (OER) = 22–30%
- Whole-blood lactate concentration = <2 mmol/l

A Swann-Ganz pulmonary artery catheter (PAC) is a device commonly used to enable these parameters to be measured or calculated.

☐ Cardiac output

The CO can be measured directly by a thermodilution technique using the PAC.

☐ Left ventricular end diastolic pressure

The LVEDP cannot be measured directly. Instead it is estimated from the pulmonary artery occlusion (wedge) pressure (POWP). This is again measured by the PAC when its tip has been advanced into a pulmonary capillary. An inflatable balloon at the end of the catheter enables it to be wedged into place for the reading. Normal values range through 4.5–13 mmHg.

☐ Systemic vascular resistance

The SVR is another parameter that cannot be measured directly, but it can be calculated from the mean arterial pressure (MAP), the central venous pressure (CVP) and the cardiac output (CO; Box 4.12).

BOX 4.12   Calculating the systemic vascular resistance

MAP = diastolic pressure + $\frac{1}{3}$ (systolic pressure – diastolic pressure)

SVR = (MAP – CVP) 80/CO

Normal values are 800–1400 dynes s^{-1} cm^{-5}

☐ Oxygen content of arterial blood

An accurate measurement of haemoglobin oxygen saturation (SaO_2), PaO_2 and haemoglobin concentration is needed to calculate the oxygen content of arterial blood (CaO_2):

CaO_2 (in ml/dl) = amount carried by haemoglobin + amount carried by plasma where:

the amount carried by Hb = concentration of Hb (in g/dl) $\times$ SaO$_2$ $\times$ 1.34

(when fully saturated, 1 g of Hb carries 1.34 ml of O$_2$), and:

the amount carried by plasma = PaO$_2$ $\times$ 0.003

(each mmHg of PO$_2$ represents 0.003 ml of oxygen dissolved in plasma). Therefore:

CaO$_2$ (in ml/dl) = [Hb (in g/dl) $\times$ SaO$_2$ $\times$ 1.34] + [PaO$_2$ $\times$ 0.003]

☐ Delivery of oxygen

The delivery of oxygen to the body (DO$_2$) is dependent on the amount of oxygen in the blood and the amount of blood reaching the tissues. It is possible to calculate the DO$_2$ from the cardiac index and the oxygen content of arterial blood (CaO$_2$):

DO$_2$ (in ml/min/m^2) = CI $\times$ CaO$_2$ $\times$ 10

Normal values are 500–720 ml/min/m^2. (The 10 is to change the content of oxygen per decilitre to the content per litre.)

The important feature of this equation is that DO$_2$ is produced by *multiplying* the cardiac index by the oxygen content. Therefore if either or, more importantly, if both of these parameters change, the DO$_2$ will be altered considerably – much more so than if DO$_2$ were calculated by simply adding the parameters together.

☐ Consumption of oxygen

In order to assess the oxygen consumption for the whole body (VO$_2$), the amount of oxygen in the blood which has left the tissues has to be measured. If this is low, then this indicates that the tissues are extracting large amounts of oxygen from the blood as it passes through them (i.e. the oxygen extraction ratio is high).

A sample of blood is therefore taken from the distal lumen of the PAC. This represents blood which has crossed every point in the body where oxygen would be released, and it is called the *mixed venous sample.*

The oxygen content of the mixed venous blood sample (CvO$_2$) is measured using a similar formula to that used to calculate the CaO$_2$:

CvO$_2$ (in ml/dl) = [Hb (in g/dl) $\times$ SvO$_2$ $\times$ 1.34] + [PvO$_2$ $\times$ 0.003]

SvO$_2$ and PvO$_2$ represent the oxygen saturation and the oxygen partial pressure of the mixed venous sample.

The VO$_2$ can now be calculated from this equation:

VO$_2$ (in ml/min/m²) = CI × [CaO$_2$–CvO$_2$] × 10

■ Appendix 4.2: Intraosseous infusion

This technique is carried out when it is not possible to cannulate a peripheral vein in a child. It is simple to learn and has a low incidence of complications. Osteomyelitis and local soft-tissue infection usually occur only when the needle has to be in place for several days or when a hypertonic solution has been infused.

Ideally an intraosseous infusion needle should be used, but spinal and bone-marrow needles can be used instead. No matter which is chosen, the needle must have a trocar to prevent it being obstructed when it traverses the cortex. The commonest site used for inserting the needle is 2–3 fingerbreadths below the tibial tuberosity on the anterior tibial surface.

A leg without a fracture proximal to the insertion site is chosen and the site cleaned. The needle is then pushed into the bone at 90° to the skin's surface. Steady pressure is maintained until there is a sudden fall in resistance, indicating that the needle is in the bone marrow. This position must be checked firstly by removing the trocar and aspirating marrow, and secondly by noting a free flow of fluid into the bone without there being any subcutaneous leakage.

The aspirated marrow must not be discarded; instead it should be sent for blood-typing. The choice and quantity of fluid needed to resuscitate children is described in Chapter 11.

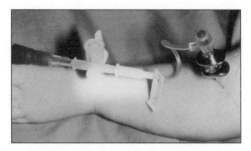

Figure 4.8   Intraosseous infusion

■ Appendix 4.3: Colloids versus crystalloids

Much has been written about which fluid is the most appropriate in treating shocked patients. Advocates for colloids state that the rapid replacement of intravascular volume is of primary importance. Those supporting crystalloids consider that a fluid is required to restore the loss in the entire extracellular space.

☐ **Colloids**

Colloid solutions are usually isotonic and can be used to replace intravascular loss up to 1 litre, on a 1:1 basis. Greater degrees of blood loss require packed cells to be added such that the haematocrit remains at around 30 per cent. A variety of colloid solutions exists. They are either plasma derivatives (5% albumin and human plasma protein fraction (HPPF)) or plasma substitute (gelatins, dextrans, Hetastarch™). Plasma derivatives are expensive and have a limited availability. The two common types of gelatins are Haemaccel™ and Gelofusine™. They have a half-life of 2–4 hours, after which the gelatin has been removed and only normal saline remains. These fluids do not adequately replace the interstitial loss but they produce less tissue oedema then crystalloids. However cardiac failure has been reported more often in patients receiving inappropriately large volumes of colloids. Haemaccel™ has a higher calcium concentration and a lower sodium concentration then Gelofusine™. It can also produce flocculation (clumping) of red cells if Haemaccel™ and blood are administered via the same giving set.

Dextrans are hydrolytic products of starch, fractionated to produce solutions with a limited range of molecular weight. A number, representing this weight in daltons, is used to describe the solution. Dextran 70 is the only type used for trauma resuscitation. Its intravascular half-life can be measured in days, but it interferes with coagulation due to its effect on platelet function and fibrin formation. Dextran-diluted blood can still be used for crossmatching purposes but it is more time-consuming for the laboratory. As a consequence of all these features, 1 litre is the maximum that can be used, and only when a better type of resuscitation fluid is unavailable.

Another type of colloid solution is Hetastarch™ (6% hydroxyethyl starch in isotonic saline). This has a longer half-life than polygelatins (12–14 hours), so care must be taken to avoid fluid overload when blood is added later to restore the haematocrit. Both these classes of colloids have a low incidence of allergic reaction.

☐ **Crystalloids**

The most commonly used crystalloid solutions are Hartmann's solution (Ringer's lactate) and 0.9%N saline. The former is preferred because it contains a lower concentration of sodium and chloride ions. There is, therefore, less chance of producing hyperchloraemic acidosis in the shocked patient. There is a risk that lactate may accumulate in shocked patients when Hartmann's solution is administered. This results from the decreased liver perfusion inhibiting the metabolism of lactate to bicarbonate. This is unlikely to be a problem during the initial resuscitation.

Both types of crystalloid have an intravascular life of 30–60 minutes before they diffuse to all fluid compartments of the body, especially the interstitial spaces. Over 60 per cent is taken up by the latter in normal conditions, and up to 90 per cent in the shocked patient. Consequently three times the estimated intravascular loss has to be infused as crystalloid to maintain the intravascular volume. This becomes a major problem when there is large volume loss (grade 3 or 4 shock). It is difficult to infuse such large volumes of crystalloid (>4.5 litres) quickly, and tissue oedema can result. This is of particular importance in brain and lung injury, when further cerebral swelling or reduced lung compliance can be produced. The latter would add to the tissue hypoxia. Renal complications probably also occur, more often in elderly patients receiving large volumes of crystalloids. The advantages of using crystalloids are that they restore intracellular and interstitial fluid loss, they are cheap and convenient, and they have a low incidence of infection or allergic reactions, and a long shelf-life. Fluid resuscitation using only Ringer's lactate and blood is a technique commonly used in the United States.

Recently hypertonic-hyperosmotic crystalloid solutions have been advocated for the initial resuscitation. It is suggested that this may be superior to either crystalloid or colloid separately.

There should no longer be a crystalloid versus colloid controversy. Instead the most appropriate fluid for the affected body spaces should be chosen. Blood should be given as early as possible for patients in grade 3 or 4 shock. For lesser grades there is mainly an intravascular loss initially, so in this situation the primary fluid is colloid. (Crystalloid, in adequate volumes, can be given as a substitute). Later on crystalloids will be needed to replace the interstitial loss.

■ References and further reading

Baskett P & Small D 1989. Blood substitutes: a review. *Int. Ther.* 10: 283.

Brenner M & Welliver J 1990. Pulmonary and acid-base assessment. *Nurs. Clin. N. Am.* 25(4): 761.

Bressack M & Raffin T 1987. Importance of venous return, venous resistance and mean circulatory pressure in the physiology and management of shock. *Chest* 92: 906.

Buckley R 1992. The management of hypovalaemic shock. *Nursing Standard* 6: 25.

Cohen J & Glauser M 1991. Septic shock: treatment. *Lancet* **338**: 736.

Cullen S 1992. Intravenous therapy. In Sheehy S, Marvin J & Jimmerson C (eds): *Emergency Nursing, Principles and Practice*, 3rd Edn. St. Louis: C V Mosby.

Edwards J 1990. Practical application of oxygen transport principles. *Crit. Care Med.* **18**: S45.

Edwards J, Nightingale P, Wilkins R, *et al.* 1989. Haemodynamic and oxygen transport response to modified gelatin in critically ill patients. *Crit. Care Med.* **17**: 996.

Frayn K 1987. Fuel metabolism during sepsis and injury. *Int. Ther.* **8**: 174.

George R & Winter R 1985. The clinical value of measuring cardiac output. *Br. J. Hosp. Med.* August: **89**.

Glauser M, Zanetti G, Baumgartner J, *et al.* 1991. Septic shock: pathogenesis. *Lancet* **338**: 732.

Hardy G 1992. Blood, fluids and electrolytes. *Br. J. Int. Care* **194**.

Hurley J 1993. Reappraisal of the role of endotoxin in the sepsis syndrome. *Lancet* **341**: 1133.

Kirkman E & Little R (in press). The bradycardic phase in hypovolaemic shock; cardiovascular regulation during hypovolaemic shock and central integration.

Little R 1989. Heart rate changes after haemorrhage and injury – a reappraisal. *J. Trauma* **29**: 903.

Little R, Randall P, Redfern W, *et al.* 1984. Components of injury (haemorrhage and tissue ischaemia) affecting cardiovascular reflexes in man and rat. *Q. J. Exp. Physiol.* **69**(4): 753.

Neugebauer E & Lorenz W 1988. Causality in circulatory shock: strategies for integrating mediators, mechanisms and therapies. *Perspec. in Shock Res.* **295**. Alan Liss, Inc.

Nimmo G & Grant I 1990a. Oxygen transportation in the critically ill, Part I. *Int. Ther.* **11**: 88.

Nimmo G & Grant I 1990b. Oxygen transportation in the critically ill, Part II. *Int. Ther.* **11**: 126.

Nimmo G & Grant I 1990c. Oxygen transportation in the critically ill, Part III. *Int. Ther.* **11**: 219.

Scalea T, Simon H, Duncan A, *et al.* 1990. Geriatric blunt multiple trauma: improved survival with early invasive monitoring. *J. Trauma* **30**: 129.

Secher N, Jensen K, Werner C, *et al.* 1984. Bradycardia during severe but reversible hypovolaemic shock in man. *Cir. Shock* **14**(4): 267.

Sheehy S 1992. Shock. In Sheehy S, Marvin J & Jimmerson C (eds): *Emergency Nursing, Principles and Practice*, 3rd Edn. St. Louis: C V Mosby.

Shoemaker W 1985. Critical care. *Surg. Clin. N. Am.* **4**: 65.

Shoemaker W & Czer L 1979. Evaluation of the biologic importance of various haemodynamic and oxygen transport variables: which variables should be monitored in postoperative shock? *Crit. Care Med.* **7**: 424.

Shoemaker W & Fleming A 1986. Resuscitation of the trauma patient: restoration of haemodynamic functions using clinical algorithms. *Ann. Emerg. Med.* **15**: 1437.

Sinkinson C A (ed.) 1990. Septic shock: where we are now? *Em. Med. Repts* **11**: 177.

Stoner H 1993. Responses to trauma: fifty years of ebb and flow. *Cir. Shock* **39**: 316.

Sutcliffe A 1990. Resuscitation. *Injury* **21**: 317.

Thompson D, Adams S & Barrett J 1990. Relative bradycardia in patients with isolated penetrating abdominal trauma and isolated extremity trauma. *Ann. Emerg. Med.* **19**: 268.

Topley E 1987. The contribution of Ruscoe Clarke and his team to knowledge relevant to blood loss after injury. *Injury* **18**: 373.

Van der Poll T 1991. Tumour necrosis factor and septic shock. *Int. Ther.* **12**: 20.

Wilson R 1988. Fluid and electrolyte problems. In Tintinalli J, Krome R & Ruiz E (eds): *Emergency Medicine: a comprehensive study guide*. New York: McGraw-Hill.

Yates D & Magill P J (eds) 1984. Plasma volume replacement. *Arch. Emerg. Med.* Suppl. 1.

Chapter 5

Abdominal and pelvic trauma

Terry Brown, Abigail Hamilton
and Peter Driscoll

Objectives

The objectives of this chapter are for members of the trauma team to understand:

- the importance of abdominal trauma;

- relevant abdominal anatomy;

- how the abdomen can be injured;

- the management of a patient with abdominal trauma.

■ Introduction

Injury to the abdomen is relatively uncommon in this country as compared with injury to other body regions. Nevertheless it accounts for a high proportion of deaths following trauma. There are several reasons for this apparent anomaly:

1   The symptoms and signs of abdominal trauma are subtle, and may be overshadowed by more obvious injuries to other body regions.

2   The presence of associated head injury, or the effects of various intoxicants, alter the patient's perception of any abdominal injury.

3   The abdomen is particularly vulnerable to trauma, both because of its position in the centre of the body and because it is largely unprotected by any bony covering.

As a result of the difficulty encountered in diagnosing abdominal injury, it is not surprising that many deaths that occur following abdominal trauma do so as a result of missed diagnoses, or inadequate treatment, or both. These deaths may be prevented if those concerned with the management of trauma victims have a high index of suspicion and an aggressive approach to the management of such injuries.

The nurse's role in this is of prime importance. The patient who arrives as a 'standby' from a major accident poses no difficulties in triage. Often, however, patients present to the emergency department with apparently minor injuries. It is the responsibility of the nurse to decide which patients need to be seen immediately, and by whom. Similarly, the nurse is intensively involved in the assessment and management of these patients.

This chapter will outline the principles involved in the management of abdominal trauma. The anatomy of the region, the mechanism of injury, and the team's role in the assessment and management of the patient will all be considered.

■ Applied anatomy and pathophysiology

In order to appreciate the nature of the problems faced when dealing with the patient who may have suffered an injury to his abdomen, it is essential to have a good working knowledge of the anatomy of this region.

The borders of the abdomen are the diaphragm above, the pelvis below, the abdominal musculature in front, and the vertebral column behind. As we shall see later on, this concept needs to be modified slightly when we consider the mechanism of injury, but it will serve as a useful model for most of our purposes.

The abdomen may be divided into regions based either on the contents of each region or on the surface anatomy of the region. In this section we will divide the abdomen into three regions, based on the contents of each. Later on, when we address the concept of mechanism of injury, the abdomen will be considered in terms of its surface anatomy.

The contents of the abdomen occupy the following three regions:

- the peritoneal cavity;
- the retroperitoneum;
- the pelvis.

The peritoneum is an extensive serous membrane which covers certain organs in the abdomen. It consists of a closed sac and has two layers:

- the parietal layer, which lines the abdominal wall;
- the visceral layer, which covers the surface of the organs.

The two layers of peritoneum are actually in contact, so the peritoneal cavity is only a *potential* cavity. If the organs that are lined by the peritoneum are damaged, haemorrhage occurs into this potential space, con-

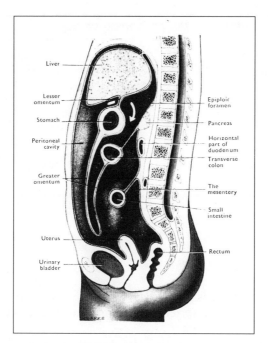

Figure 5.1 Contents of the peritoneal cavity and retroperitoneum
Source: © Romanes G J (ed.) 1969. *Cunningham's Manual of Practical Anatomy*, Vol. 2,
13th edn. Oxford: Oxford University Press. By permission of Oxford University Press.

verting it into an actual cavity. This becomes important when we come to consider the diagnosis of concealed intra-abdominal haemorrhage (see later).

Those organs that are not contained by the peritoneum lie in the posterior part of the abdomen and are thus referred to as retroperitoneal (Figure 5.1).

For the purposes of this chapter the contents of the pelvis will be considered as being intra-abdominal.

☐ The peritoneal cavity

This region can be further subdivided into intrathoracic and abdominal (Box 5.1). It is important to remember that, on expiration, the diaphragm rises to the level of the 4th intercostal space (the nipple line). As a result, several of the 'abdominal' organs actually lie within the bony thorax and are therefore at risk of injury if the patient suffers trauma to the lower chest.

BOX 5.1   Contents of the peritoneal cavity

Intrathoracic:
- Diaphragm
- Liver
- Spleen
- Stomach

Abdominal:
- Small intestines
- Large intestines

Intrathoracic

The diaphragm

This muscular structure is dome-shaped and is attached posteriorly to the 1st, 2nd and 3rd lumbar vertebrae, anteriorly to the lower sternum, and laterally to the costal margins.

Injury to the diaphragm is uncommon, and may occur as a result of either blunt or penetrating trauma. The former tends to occur with greater force than the latter, and usually leads to larger tears in the diaphragm through which abdominal contents may enter the thorax.

Both types of injury are commoner on the left, because the right side of the diaphragm is protected by the liver (which will also act to plug any tears on that side). In addition, as most assailants are right-handed, stab wounds are usually inflicted on the left side of the victim's body.

Injuries to the diaphragm may be so slight that the patient is asymptomatic and the damage may not be discovered until weeks, months or even years later. When the tear in the diaphragm is large, the abdominal contents may herniate into the thoracic cavity, compromising the patient's respiration.

The diagnosis of significant diaphragmatic injury relies on the team having a high index of suspicion. The patient may complain of chest pain or difficulty breathing. Physical examination may reveal absent breath sounds on the left, dullness to percussion, mediastinal shift, and the presence of bowel sounds in the chest. Anybody who has been in a crowded resuscitation room during a trauma resuscitation will appreciate the difficulties involved in listening for these subtle signs!

X-rays may be helpful, either by demonstrating the presence of bowel in the thorax (Figure 5.2), or by revealing the position of the nasogastric tube coiled above the diaphragm. More commonly, however, the abnormalities on the x-ray are non-specific.

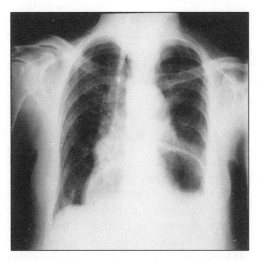

Figure 5.2   Radiograph of a diaphragmatic hernia

The treatment of a patient with a tear in his diaphragm is by surgical repair of the defect. How rapidly this operation is undertaken will depend on the condition of the patient. While the patient is awaiting surgery a nasogastric tube should be passed in order to decompress the stomach and relieve any respiratory embarrassment.

A special situation which deserves mention is the use of the pneumatic anti-shock garment (PASG – see Figure 5.8). One of the complications of this device is the creation or exacerbation of a diaphragmatic hernia. For this reason, any patient who develops respiratory problems whilst the device is in operation should have it deflated, following the procedure explained in Chapter 4.

The liver

The liver is situated in the right upper quadrant of the abdomen. It is covered over a large part of its surface by the ribcage, which affords it some protection from injury. In terms of function, all that needs to be remembered about the liver is that it is extremely vascular, and therefore can bleed torrentially when injured.

Unrecognized liver injury is an important cause of preventable death. Although numerically less common than splenic injury, liver injuries are reported as causing more deaths because of unsuspected intra-abdominal haemorrhage. A high index of suspicion is essential, therefore, when assessing trauma victims. Any injury to the right lower chest or upper abdomen should alert the team to the possibility of underlying liver damage. The presence of hypovolaemic shock in the trauma patient, in the absence of any obvious cause, should be assumed to be secondary to hepatic or splenic injury until proven otherwise.

Major injuries to the liver which cause severe haemorrhage require immediate surgical repair. Less severe injuries may be managed conservatively, depending on the patient's condition.

The gall bladder and extrahepatic biliary tract

These organs are located under the right lobe of the liver and are therefore usually damaged in association with other viscera. Liver trauma is the most common coexisting pathology (50 per cent of cases), but there is a significant chance of the pancreas being injured also (17 per cent of cases). As a consequence of this, the clinical presentation of trauma to the gall bladder and biliary tree is usually masked by symptoms resulting from damage to the surrounding viscera. The overall mortality of 16 per cent in this condition is also due to the coexisting organ injuries.

Blunt trauma is the usual cause of gall bladder damage and rupture is more likely when the gall bladder is distended. This happens after a meal and during alcohol intoxication.

These patients require surgical exploration, intra-operative cholangiography to check the biliary tree and, usually, cholecystectomy if there is damage to the gall bladder.

The spleen

The spleen is situated in the left upper quadrant of the abdomen. It lies at the level of the 7th–11th ribs, which protect it from injury.

Like the liver, the most important aspect of the spleen is its highly vascular nature. It is the most commonly injured solid organ in the abdomen following blunt trauma, and as such is a frequent cause of shock in patients with abdominal injury. Any injury to the left lower chest or upper abdomen may lead to splenic injury. This may range from small tears to complete shattering of the organ.

The diagnosis of severe splenic injury is suggested by the combination of left upper quadrant or shoulder-tip pain and hypotension. X-rays may show lower-rib fractures, a raised left hemidiaphragm, or displacement of the gastric air bubble.

As with liver injury, the management of splenic injury revolves around resuscitation of the shocked patient and deciding on the need for immediate life-saving surgery. The trend at the moment amongst surgeons is to try to conserve the spleen wherever possible, especially in children, because splenectomy renders the patient at risk from severe infection (especially pneumococcal).

Both the liver and the spleen are susceptible to delayed rupture following trauma. Patients in whom hepatic or splenic injury is suspected should therefore be admitted for observation, even if there are no physical signs. Similarly, a patient who presents some days after trauma with shoulder-tip pain (indicating diaphragmatic irritation) or signs of effusion or consolidation in the lower lobes of the lungs should be carefully assessed to exclude the possibility of delayed rupture.

The stomach

The stomach occupies the epigastric region of the abdomen. Injury to the stomach following blunt trauma is rare; it is however sometimes injured as a result of penetrating trauma.

Injury to the stomach usually presents as peritonitis. The diagnosis is made on the basis of the history and physical signs. There may be blood in the nasogastric tube or free gas visible on plain x-ray.

The treatment of gastric injuries usually necessitates surgical repair.

Abdominal

The contents of the abdominal section of the peritoneal cavity are the small and large intestines. For practical purposes these may be considered together.

Damage to the bowel may result from either blunt or penetrating trauma as well as from blast injuries (see Chapter 10). Blunt trauma and blasts commonly cause bowel injury in one of two ways:

1 The bowel may rupture as a result of a sudden increase in pressure within the lumen, such as may occur when the abdomen is compressed (the closed-loop phenomenon).

2 The bowel may become ischaemic because of damage to the mesentery and its arteries. This usually arises when the abdomen is subjected to deceleration or shearing forces.

Penetrating injury to the bowel usually results in small tears in the bowel wall. Occasionally, the bowel may become completely transected.

Unlike injuries to the liver and spleen, trauma to the bowel is rarely immediately life-threatening. The major problem is peritonitis, which occurs as a result of leakage of bowel contents into the peritoneum. This usually arises several hours after injury, and is therefore common in patients who have suffered a delay in transport to the hospital. Obviously, it is also a problem in those patients whose bowel injury has gone unrecognized.

The treatment of bowel injury is surgical exploration and repair. In view of the dangers of peritonitis, the patient should receive prophylactic antibiotics whilst in the resuscitation room.

☐ The retroperitoneum

The most important point to remember about the contents of this region is that it is much more difficult to diagnose injury to these organs than injury to those in the peritoneal cavity. The main reasons for this are that the viscera contained within this region are less accessible to physical examination, and any bleeding from these structures will be contained within the retroperitoneum. As a result of the latter, the degree of hypotension may be deceptively slight, and a diagnostic peritoneal lavage will be negative (see later).

The organs that lie within the retroperitoneal space are listed in Box 5.2.

BOX 5.2 Contents of the retroperitoneum

- Pancreas
- Duodenum (excluding the first part)
- Colon
- Aorta
- Inferior vena cava
- Genito-urinary tract

For the sake of clarity, injuries to the kidneys and ureters will be dealt with along with injuries to the bladder and urethra, in the section on genito-urinary trauma.

The pancreas

This organ lies at the level of the first lumbar vertebra and extends from the curve of the duodenum to the spleen.

The pancreas may be injured as a result of both blunt and penetrating trauma – for the purposes of this chapter, they may be considered to produce the same effect. The commonest mechanism of injury resulting in pancreatic damage is that of the unrestrained driver impacting with the steering wheel.

Unfortunately, the signs of pancreatic damage are non-specific. The patient may have epigastric tenderness or a paralytic ileus. The serum amylase may be high, but it should be remembered that injuries to other abdominal organs may also produce this effect. Similarly, a normal serum amylase does not exclude pancreatic damage.

If pancreatic injury is suspected, ultrasound and CT scans may help confirm the diagnosis. Close observation and frequent estimations of the serum amylase are required. If the presence of injury is confirmed the treatment may be surgery or observation, depending on the nature of the damage and the patient's condition.

The duodenum

The first part of the duodenum lies within the abdominal peritoneal cavity. The remainder is attached to the posterior abdominal wall and is retroperitoneal.

Like the pancreas, the duodenum may be injured following either blunt or penetrating trauma, but the commonest mode of injury is a steering-wheel impact.

As with all the retroperitoneal structures, the diagnosis of injury is difficult. The patient may complain of abdominal or testicular pain, and x-rays may show free gas in the abdomen. The presence of blood in the nasogastric tube should make one suspicious that duodenal injury may have occurred.

If in doubt (which is usually the case!), CT scanning or contrast studies will confirm the diagnosis. The treatment of duodenal injury is usually surgical repair.

The colon

All of the caecum and ascending colon, as well as one-third to two-thirds of the circumference of the descending colon, lie within the retroperitoneal space. The remainder of this organ is located within the peritoneal cavity.

Blunt or penetrating trauma is capable of damaging any part of the colon and causing leakage of bowel contents. However, in cases of retroperitoneal perforation, the symptoms are usually ill-defined and slow in onset. This often leads to delays in diagnosis and increases the chances of abscess formation.

In view of this nondescript presentation it is important that the team leader considers the possibility in all cases of abdominal trauma. Water-soluble contrast radiology, with or without computerized tomography, can help confirm the diagnosis. Occasionally plain abdominal radiography will show loss of the psoas shadow and air bubbles in the retroperitoneal space.

If colonic injury is confirmed, then treatment is by surgical intervention.

The aorta

The abdominal aorta lies in front and slightly to the left of the vertebral column. It is rarely injured as a result of blunt trauma, but is susceptible to damage as a result of penetrating injury. As would be expected, injury to the aorta produces two types of symptoms: those secondary to blood loss and those secondary to ischaemia distal to the injury.

Severe trauma is almost invariably lethal, but lesser degrees of injury will manifest as hypotension or symptoms of ischaemia, or both. The latter will depend on at what level the injury is, and may include abdominal pain, poor renal function and cold, pale lower limbs.

If the haemorrhage is contained within the retroperitoneum then the hypotension may be mild and respond to fluid resuscitation. A retroperitoneal haematoma may be visible as bruising in the flank or back (Grey Turner's sign).

If the diagnosis is in doubt and the patient's condition allows, CT and ultrasound scans may provide useful information. The treatment of injury to the aorta is by surgery.

The inferior vena cava

The inferior vena cava (IVC) lies to the right of the aorta and it is susceptible to the same types of injury. Trauma to the IVC can result in significant blood loss, however this is usually less than that from an equivalent injury to the aorta. This is because of the lower pressure within the vessel, and the relatively high pressure in the surrounding tissues. However, if this pressure is lost, as occurs in the presence of a large wound, the blood loss from the IVC is severe and may be life-threatening.

Not surprisingly, the symptoms of damage to the IVC will depend upon the severity of the blood loss. If the damage is relatively minor, the patient may simply complain of back pain. Physical examination may reveal bruising or swelling of the back.

CT scans or an ultrasound investigation may reveal the extent of the damage, but they should only be carried out in the haemodynamically stable patient. Surgical repair is the usual treatment.

The genito-urinary tract

This consists of the kidneys, the ureters, the bladder and the urethra.

The kidneys

The kidneys lie on the posterior abdominal wall at the level of T12-L3. The right kidney is slightly lower than the left, but both are well protected by soft tissue in front and bone and muscle behind. As a result, isolated injury to the kidneys is uncommon. They are injured, however, in association with other organs as a result of either blunt or penetrating trauma.

Renal injury may occur following a penetrating wound to the back or flank. Similarly, a blow to the renal angle may result in renal damage. The latter injury often arises following a blow from an opponent's shoulder during a rugby match.

Injury to the kidneys is rarely immediately life-threatening. The exception is when the kidney is avulsed from its blood supply, which can lead to severe haemorrhage. More commonly, it is the parenchyma of the kidney that is damaged. This will lead to long-term problems if not diagnosed at the time of injury.

Haematuria is an indicator of urinary tract damage. However, it is neither sensitive nor specific: microscopic haematuria is seldom associated with significant urinary tract damage, whereas 70 per cent of potentially lethal injuries to the renal pedicle do not produce gross haematuria.

If renal damage is suspected a one-shot intravenous urogram may be performed in the emergency room. This investigation requires the presence of an adequate blood pressure in order to transport the dye to the kidneys. Ultrasound and CT are useful adjuncts in the diagnosis of renal damage.

Most renal trauma is managed conservatively, with surgical intervention reserved for those patients in whom the damage is life-threatening.

As with the liver and spleen, the kidney is susceptible to delayed injury. This usually takes the form of secondary haemorrhage as a result of the lytic action of urinary enzymes released at the time of trauma.

The ureters

The ureters connect the kidneys to the bladder. They lie behind the peritoneum and in front of the psoas muscle. Injury to the ureters, as a result of either blunt or penetrating injury, is uncommon.

The bladder

The bladder lies within the pelvis, but it should be remembered that, when full, it may extend as high as the umbilicus. This means that it is susceptible to injury following trauma to the lower abdomen. An important factor, therefore, which will determine the risk of bladder injury, is how full it is at the time of injury. It is useful to ask the patient the time that he or she last micturated.

Injury to the bladder may follow compression of the abdomen, thus increasing intravesical pressure. More commonly, it is damaged as a result of penetrating injury from fragments of bone produced when the pelvis is fractured.

When the bladder is ruptured, the urine leaks into the surrounding tissues. This may occur in one of two ways:

1   The urine leaks into the peritoneal cavity, causing peritonitis.

2   The urine leaks into the perineum and surrounding structures. This usually produces a less dramatic picture than intraperitoneal leakage, but it is important to diagnose this condition early as necrosis of the tissues will follow if it is missed.

Clinically, the presence of bladder rupture is suspected if the bladder is found to be completely empty, if the patient has signs of peritonitis, and if there is a boggy swelling noted in the perineal region.

Cystography will show extravasation of urine from the bladder, and peritoneal lavage fluid may be observed to drain from the urinary catheter.

The initial treatment of bladder injury is to pass a urinary catheter, thus reducing the leakage of urine. If the damage is not severe, the patient may be managed conservatively with an indwelling catheter and antibiotics for 10 days. If the injury is severe, surgical repair is undertaken.

The urethra

The urethra is rarely injured in women, due to its being short. In men, injuries are divided into those above the urogenital diaphragm (posterior) and those below (anterior). This level is indicated by the sphincter urethrae in Figure 5.3.

Posterior urethral injury usually arises as a result of pelvic fracture, and is therefore often associated with injuries to other body regions. Anterior urethral injury occurs as a result of blunt trauma to the perineum (e.g. falling astride a beam) and is therefore usually an isolated injury.

The diagnosis of urethral injury is suspected from the history, and from the presence of a desire to micturate coupled with an inability to do so. Important physical signs include a palpable bladder, blood at the urinary meatus and a high-riding prostate on rectal examination.

If the diagnosis of urethral injury is suspected, and the patient's condition permits, urethrography may be performed to confirm the diagnosis. Similarly, a one-shot urogram may show a high-riding bladder if the urethra is completely disrupted.

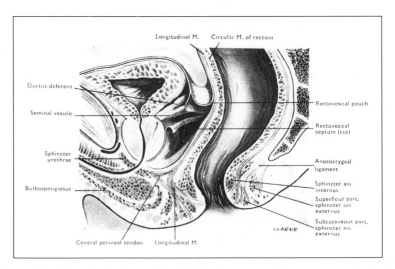

Figure 5.3   The relationship of the bladder to surrounding structures, including the urogenital diaphragm

Source: © Romanes G J (ed.) 1969. *Cunningham's Manual of Practical Anatomy*, Vol. 2, 13th edn. Oxford: Oxford University Press. By permission of Oxford University Press.

A urethral catheter should not be passed on any patient in whom the diagnosis of urethral injury is suspected, as it may cause further damage. A suprapubic catheter should be passed to relieve any retention. As a temporary measure, needle aspiration of the bladder may be performed.

If the urethral damage is slight, treatment is conservative, involving a suprapubic catheter and antibiotics. When more major damage has occurred, surgical repair is the treatment of choice.

☐ **The pelvis**

The pelvic contents

The pelvis contains the rectum, the bladder, and, in women, the female reproductive organs. Injuries to the rectum are dealt with along the lines described in the section on injuries to the intestine (page 145). Injuries to the uterus are uncommon and will not be considered here. Injuries to the bladder have been described along with injuries to the rest of the genitourinary tract, in the previous section.

The bony pelvis

The pelvis is composed of three bones: the sacrum and two innominate bones. They are held together by several extremely strong ligaments which are crucial for maintaining pelvic stability. The bones of the pelvis can only be separated if these ligaments are torn. When this occurs, structures that run close to the ligaments – that is, vessels and nerves – can be damaged. The bleeding which results is usually venous and extraperitoneal, and can be life-threatening. An open pelvic fracture is associated with a 50 per cent mortality rate, however some tamponading effect can be achieved if bones fracture whilst the ligaments remain intact. In these cases the degree of haemorrhage is less severe, and the mortality rate is reduced.

The sciatic nerve lies close to the sacral wing. It is therefore not surprising that with 30 per cent of the fractures to this bone there is associated sciatic nerve damage. Similarly, the urethra and bladder are damaged in 20 per cent of cases where there is disruption of the pubic symphysis.

Plain x-rays of the pelvis can reveal some fractures, but special views may be needed.

As with injury to the liver and spleen, management of severe pelvic fracture revolves around the restoration of an adequate circulating blood volume. However, unlike these organs, bleeding from the pelvis may be temporarily reduced in the emergency department (see later).

■ Mechanisms of injury

One of the most important concepts in trauma management is that of the mechanism of injury. A knowledge of the pattern of injury associated with particular types of trauma is essential if we are to avoid missed diagnoses and preventable deaths.

For the purposes of trauma management, damage is considered to occur as a result of either blunt or penetrating trauma or a blast injury. Obviously, this classification is not comprehensive and does not cover injury occurring following deceleration and shearing forces (so-called indirect injury). However, it is useful for professionals involved in the management of victims of trauma because it heightens awareness as to what sort of injuries to expect following a given type of trauma.

When we consider certain abdominal structures it is apparent that the effects produced by trauma are the same irrespective of the mechanism of injury. For example, injury to the spleen will produce haemorrhage whatever the nature of the insult. Some structures, however, manifest different responses to injury depending on the nature of the forces involved. The diaphragm is a good example of this: a penetrating injury may be so innocuous as to be asymptomatic, whereas a blunt injury can lead to severe respiratory embarrassment as a result of a diaphragmatic hernia.

☐ Blunt trauma and blast injuries

Blunt trauma is by far the commonest type of abdominal trauma seen in the UK, and usually occurs as a result of motor vehicle accidents. The abdomen is subjected to rapid changes in speed which result in visceral damage, whether from a direct blow, shearing or rotational forces, or closed-loop phenomena. The last of these arises when the pressure within the bowel lumen suddenly increases following compression of the abdomen.

Other types of blunt trauma include blows to the renal angle from an assailant (producing kidney damage), falls from a bicycle (a commonly overlooked cause of a ruptured spleen in children and young adults), and blast injuries (see Chapter 10).

The liver, the kidneys and the spleen are the organs commonly injured as a result of blunt trauma. In addition, the bowel can burst and the mesentery may tear if they are subjected to sufficient energy. Occasionally this occurs following incorrect seatbelt usage (along with bladder rupture). Blast injuries can also lead to multiple intestinal perforations and areas of infarction (Figure 5.4).

The diagnosis of visceral damage following blunt abdominal trauma is fraught with difficulties. Physical examination has been shown to be accurate in only 50–80 per cent of patients. In addition, blunt abdominal trauma

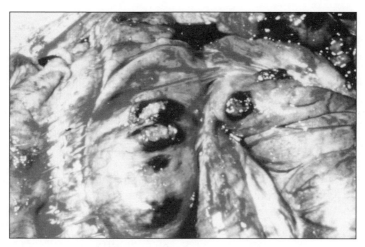

Figure 5.4 Bowel damaged by a blast injury
Source: © Prof. J Ryan. Reproduced by kind permission.

rarely occurs in isolation from other body regions, which makes the diagnosis of injury even more difficult. The presence of tenderness, guarding and hypotension are all indicators that visceral injury has occurred. A diagnostic peritoneal lavage (see later) will confirm the diagnosis with an accuracy of 98 per cent.

The bony pelvis is usually injured as a result of road traffic accidents or falls from a height. These mechanisms give rise to three forces (Box 5.3), which can act on the pelvis either singularly or in combination. They are all capable of producing pelvic instability and haemorrhage because of the vascular and bony damage. However, antero-posterior compression and vertical shearing have a greater chance of causing significant vascular damage and pelvic instability due to disruption of the sacroiliac joint and the closely aligned major blood vessels.

It follows that a patient with pelvic fractures may present *in extremis* due to profound hypotension. Conversely if the injury is less severe, he may simply complain of lower abdominal pain or a desire to micturate.

BOX 5.3   Forces resulting from blunt trauma which may lead to pelvic damage

---

- Antero-posterior compression
- Lateral compression
- Vertical shear
- Combinations of the above forces

☐ **Penetrating trauma**

Penetrating trauma to the abdomen is relatively uncommon in this country, unlike the situation in parts of South Africa and North America. It usually follows stab or gunshot wounds, although almost any sharp implement can be (and has been!) used to inflict damage to the viscera.

As would be expected, the incidence of injury to viscera following penetrating trauma depends on the size of the organ and its proximity to the entrance wound. Not surprisingly, therefore, the organs commonly injured are the liver, the small bowel, the colon and the stomach.

Stab injuries damage structures that are adjacent to one another, because the path of the blade is straight. Bullets, however, may ricochet within the abdomen and travel in several different directions, thereby injuring structures which are distant from one another. Because of this phenomenon, it is wise to consider the abdomen as extending from the nipples to midthigh. A seemingly innocuous buttock wound may hide extensive damage to the abdominal viscera.

Furthermore, a missile entering the body at speed produces an effect known as cavitation. This phenomenon occurs as a result of the pressure wave which spreads radially from the missile as it passes through the tissues, and causes extensive damage. Thus, the track left by a bullet as it passes through the body is several times wider than the diameter of the bullet. Usually also it is contaminated by debris that has been sucked into the wound as a result of the temporary vacuum caused by the bullet's passage. For this reason, bullet wounds require extensive débridement in order to prevent infection (see Chapter 10).

When considering the structures which are at risk from penetrating trauma, it is useful to divide the abdomen into regions based on surface anatomy, as follows:

The lower chest

This is the area bounded by the nipples anteriorly, the costal margins laterally, and the tips of the scapulae posteriorly.

The anterior abdominal wall

This region lies between the anterior axillary lines laterally, the costal margin above, and the groin below.

The posterior abdominal wall

This is the area medial and posterior to the posterior axillary lines.

The flank

This is the region at the side of the abdomen, bounded by the anterior and posterior axillary lines.

Considerations in treatment of these regions

Each of the regions discussed poses different problems in terms of incidence of visceral injury, diagnosis, investigation and management.

The lower chest

Some 15 per cent of stab wounds to this region will be associated with significant visceral damage. Surgical exploration of this region is difficult and most cases can be successfully managed conservatively.

By contrast, up to 50 per cent of gunshot wounds will cause visceral injury and in the vast majority of these cases most surgeons will explore the wound.

The anterior abdominal wall

About 60 per cent of stab wounds to this region penetrate the peritoneum. Of these, 40–50 per cent cause significant visceral injury. Physical examination is only accurate in diagnosing 65–75 per cent of visceral injuries in this situation, therefore most wounds are explored either locally or at laparotomy.

Visceral damage results from 96 per cent of gunshot wounds to this region. All such injuries are explored at laparotomy.

The posterior abdominal wall

Both stab wounds and gunshot wounds to this region will be associated with visceral injury in 10 per cent of cases. However, not only is physical examination unreliable but DPL will be falsely negative in up to 25 per cent of cases.

The consequences of missing a visceral injury in this area (most notably colonic perforation) are so severe that most surgeons will explore the region at laparotomy. However, the use of triple-contrast abdominal CT scans may increase the selectivity and specificity of this operation.

The flank

Around 30 per cent of injuries to this region result in visceral damage, whether the trauma is blunt or penetrating. This region suffers the same problems as the posterior abdominal wall with respect to examination, DPL and organs injured. It is no surprise, therefore, that most injuries in this area are explored surgically.

Note Although not covered by our classification of abdominal regions, remember that both stab and gunshot wounds to the perineum may result in visceral injury.

■ Assessment and management

As mentioned elsewhere in this book, assessment of the victims of trauma follows the protocol of primary survey, resuscitation, secondary survey, and definitive management.

Assessment of the patient begins while he is still in the ambulance. The medical team leader should take a detailed history from the ambulance crew, which must include the mechanism of injury, the patient's condition at the scene, and any change in this condition while in transit. The gathering of this information should in no way delay the transfer of the patient to the emergency room.

☐ The primary survey

The function of the primary survey is to identify *and treat* any condition that is immediately life-threatening. When we apply this concept to abdominal trauma, only hypovolaemic shock, arising as a result of visceral or pelvic injury, falls into this category.

After the airway and breathing have been assessed and stabilized, the condition of the circulation is assessed. With abdominal trauma there are only two questions which need to be answered at this stage:

- Is the patient shocked?
- Does the patient require immediate surgery to stop the bleeding?

Shocked patients should be managed by the doctor and nurses assigned to circulation, along the lines discussed in Chapter 4. If there is no response to fluid therapy, and there is evidence of abdominal trauma, the patient should go to theatre immediately. In cases of significant pelvic damage, the rapid application of a pelvic external fixator may enable the team to gain temporary haemostasis. This can be put on either in the resuscitation room or in the operating theatre, depending on the local policy. As a temporary measure, the PASG may be used to control haemorrhage whilst awaiting the arrival of the orthopaedic surgeon.

If the patient is stable, or becomes so after treatment with fluids, then the assessment can proceed to the rest of the primary and secondary survey.

☐ The secondary survey

The abdomen

The abdomen is assessed using the following sequence: *look, feel and listen.*

Look

The patient must be completely exposed and the surface of the abdomen thoroughly inspected for signs of injury such as bruising, seatbelt and tyre marks, entry and exit wounds, and evisceration (Figure 5.5). The team leader should not forget to turn the patient and inspect the back, flank, perineum and scrotum. The urethral meatus should also be inspected for blood.

Feel

The abdomen should be gently palpated to assess the presence of tenderness, swelling or distension. Any guarding is recorded, but injuries to the chest and pelvis may also produce guarding and so can mimic abdominal injury.

On examination the pelvis may be obviously deformed and there could be scrotal or perineal bruising. The practice of 'springing' the pelvis in order

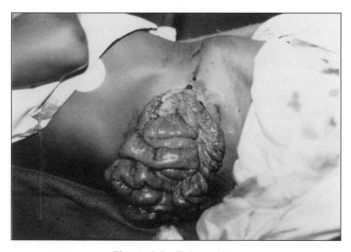

Figure 5.5 Evisceration

to discover the presence of a fracture is to be deplored. This manouevre is painful and can exacerbate bleeding. It is also not helpful in diagnosis unless the disruption is gross. Instead, a plane pelvic radiograph should be taken as soon as possible as this provides the team with invaluable information with regard to the degree of pelvic damage (see below).

Percussion of the abdomen is a useful (and humane!) method of demonstrating peritonism. Peritonitis is a relatively late development and initial signs may be equivocal. It is necessary, therefore, continually to re-evaluate the abdominal findings as the resuscitation progresses.

Listen

Using a stethoscope, each quadrant of the abdomen should be auscultated, with the presence or absence of bowel sounds recorded. This information is of little use when considered on its own, but may help if viewed in the light of other findings.

The rectum

A rectal examination should now be performed to assess the presence of blood, the integrity of the bowel wall, the presence of bony fragments from a pelvic fracture, and the position of the prostate.

The vagina

Similarly, a vaginal examination should also be performed.

Passing a nasogastric tube

At this stage, and in the absence of major facial injuries, a nasogastric tube should be passed. This may reveal blood, suggesting injury to the stomach or duodenum. It will also decompress the stomach, which is very important if the patient is shocked or has a diaphragmatic hernia, stomach injuries or an ileus following a high spinal lesion (see Chapter 8).

Passing a urethral catheter

Similarly, a urethral catheter should be passed if injury to the urethra has been ruled out. This will demonstrate any haematuria, relieve retention and reduce leakage from a ruptured bladder. It will also prevent inadvertent damage to the bladder as a result of DPL.

Blood tests

Blood will have been taken during the primary survey. This should be sent to the laboratory for estimation of the usual baseline values, but also for estimation of the serum amylase.

☐ Further investigations

X-rays

A chest x-ray, taken at the end of the primary survey, may show a diaphragmatic hernia or the presence of lower-rib fractures. Gas under the diaphragm is best seen in erect chest radiographs.

Pelvic radiograph

It is important that there is a disciplined 'ABCs' approach to interpreting the pelvic radiograph once the adequacy of the film has been determined (cf. cervical radiographs, Chapter 8):

- *A* – Alignment;
- *B* – Bones;
- *C* – Cartilage and joints;
- *s* – Soft tissue.

In 94 per cent of cases a correct diagnosis can be made using only an antero-posterior radiograph of the pelvis (Figure 5.6).

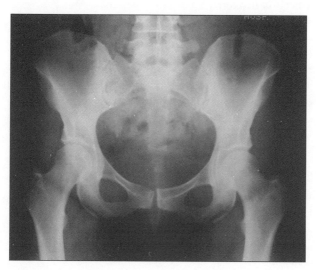

Figure 5.6 AP pelvic radiograph showing the pelvic brim, the two obturator foramina and Shenton's line

Check the adequacy and quality of the film

The medical team leader must ensure that the whole of the pelvis can be seen, including the iliac crests, both hips, and femurs distal to the lesser trochanters. The penetration should also be assessed.

(A) Alignment

The pelvic radiograph can be considered to enclose three circles (Figure 5.6):

- one large circle, formed by the sacrum and pelvic brim;
- two small circles, formed by the inner margins of the obturator foramina.

The large circle of the pelvic brim should have a smooth edge. This is not disrupted by the sacroiliac joints or pubic symphysis unless the patient is very old, when osteophytes may disrupt the line. It is important to note that if this circle is broken, this invariably occurs in two places. The breaks can take the form of bone fractures or opening of the joints (sacroiliac or pubic symphysis).

A similar inspection of the inner margins of both obturator foramina should be carried out. These should have smooth edges when seen on the x-ray. Again, if a disruption is present, it is rarely due to damage at just one point.

Examination of the obturator foramina is completed by tracing along its superior border and continuing along the inferior surface of the neck of the femur (Figure 5.6). This is called Shenton's line and it is disrupted when the femoral neck is broken.

(B) Bones

The outer edges of the pelvis and its bony structure can now be inspected for fractures. These can present as areas of increased density or lucency or alteration of the internal trabecular pattern. Unlike the situation discussed previously, fractures not involving the three bony circles can occur in isolation.

(C) Cartilage and joints

The right and left sacroiliac joints must be checked for widening, an intact cortical surface, overlapping of bone, and congruity of the joint margin.

The cortical margins of the acetabulum should be inspected for fractures. These can easily be missed because they are covered by the shadow of the femoral head.

(s) Soft tissue

Haematoma or tissue oedema, sufficient to produce bladder displacement, can be detected on the plane radiographs by asymmetry of the fat planes (dark-grey lines) around this organ. This appearance may be the only indication that a fracture of the superior pubic ramus has occurred.

Abdominal radiographs

At the end of the secondary survey, a plain film of the abdomen may be taken, looking for free gas or foreign bodies. If injury to the bowel or genitourinary tract is suspected, contrast studies may be performed. If available, ultrasound and CT scans can provide useful information – especially in cases of blunt trauma. However, these investigations should only be carried out if the patient is haemodynamically stable.

Diagnostic peritoneal lavage

This investigation is of prime importance when assessing the victims of trauma. If performed properly it is accurate in up to 98 per cent of cases.

Diagnostic peritoneal lavage (DPL) is carried out when the diagnosis of visceral injury is in doubt (Box 5.4). It is *not* performed if the patient obviously has a visceral injury and will be going to theatre anyway.

BOX 5.4   Indications for diagnostic peritoneal lavage

- Unexplained hypotension
- Clinical examination is
  - equivocal
  - unreliable
  - impractical

DPL is useful when clinical examination is unreliable, for example if the patient has an altered level of consciousness or if there are injuries to the chest or pelvis. Similarly, if the patient has suffered injury to his spinal cord then examination may not reveal tenderness or guarding.

One area where DPL is less accurate is when the patient has suffered injury to retroperitoneal structures. In this situation, any bleeding will be contained within the retroperitoneal space and will therefore not appear in the lavage fluid. Similarly, if the patient has a pelvic fracture the presence of an associated haematoma may cause the lavage fluid to contain blood, even if no visceral injury has occurred.

DPL is a commonly performed procedure and nurses involved in the management of trauma victims should become familiar with the equipment used and the protocol followed (Box 5.5).

Diagnostic peritoneal lavage: procedure

BOX 5.5 Equipment required for a diagnostic peritoneal lavage

- Naso-/orogastric tube
- Urinary catheter
- Skin-preparation solution
- Lignocaine *with adrenaline*
- Scalpel
- Sterile gauze swabs
- Small retractors
- Sterile forceps
- 10 ml syringe
- Peritoneal dialysis catheter
- IV giving set
- 1 litre warmed saline/Hartmann's
- Sterile specimen pot
- Suture material
- Dressing

Explain the procedure to the patient. He will feel bloated after the fluid is instilled into the abdomen. Written consent is not required for this investigation, however verbal consent should be obtained, witnessed and documented. If the patient is unable to give consent – for example due to unconsciousness or being under the influence of alcohol – and a potentially life-threatening condition is suspected, then consent is not necessary (see Chapter 17).

A nasogastric tube and urinary catheter should be passed to decompress the stomach and empty the bladder.

A point is chosen in the midline of the abdomen, one-third of the distance between the umbilicus and the pubic symphysis. A supra-umbilical approach is used if the patient is pregnant or has a pelvic fracture. This area is infiltrated with lignocaine and adrenaline (the latter is to reduce bleeding from the incision which might cause a false positive result).

The operator then makes a small longitudinal incision and dissects down to the fascia. The fascia is grasped with the forceps and put under gentle traction while a small incision is made in it. (This procedure is safer and more accurate than the practice of 'blind' peritoneal lavage. In the latter technique, a hole is made in the peritoneum by pushing a trocar through an

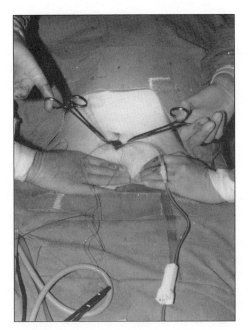

Figure 5.7   Diagnostic peritoneal lavage

incision made in the abdominal wall. Without direct vision of – and traction upon – the peritoneum, there is potential for injury to the underlying abdominal viscera.)

The catheter is then inserted into the abdomen, aiming towards the pelvis (Figure 5.7). An attempt is made to aspirate any free intraperitoneal blood. If more than 5 ml is obtained, this is considered to be a positive result.

If this is unsuccessful, 1 litre of warmed saline or Hartmann's is slowly infused into the abdomen and allowed to distribute. If necessary, the patient can be gently rolled from side to side.

The saline bottle is then lowered and the lavage fluid is drained by gravity. A sample of this fluid is sent to the laboratory for analysis. A positive lavage is one that contains more than 100 000 red blood cells/millilitre. The presence of food debris or bowel contents is also a positive result.

If the fluid instilled into the abdomen is not recovered then the diagnosis of diaphragmatic or bladder rupture should be considered. Similarly, the presence of lavage fluid in the chest drain or urinary catheter indicates damage to these structures.

DPL can be performed on any patient except those for whom surgery is already inevitable. Care should be taken when performing it on patients who are very obese or pregnant, those who have cirrhosis or have clotting disorders, and those who have had previous abdominal surgery.

☐ Definitive care

Further information needs to be gathered from the patient or a relative at this stage. Whether the patient has any allergies, whether he is on any medication, whether he has any previous medical problems, the time he last ate, and the 'environment' of the injury is all information that needs to be recorded. This can be easily remembered using the mnemonic AMPLE (see Chapter 1).

After the examination, resuscitation and investigation have been completed, the team leaders and surgeon must make a decision on the disposal of the patient. This will depend on the presence of pelvic and visceral injuries and their management. If there is evidence of a significant intra-abdominal haemorrhage or a ruptured viscus then a laparotomy is carried out. Conversely, if the surgeon does not consider there are any immediate indications for an operation, a policy of 'active observation' is followed. In these cases, surgery is carried out if signs of abdominal pathology develop.

The management of pelvic fractures and disruption revolves around the restoration of an adequate circulating blood volume. This is achieved by intravenous fluid resuscitation, as outlined in Chapter 4. At the same time an attempt can be made to control the haemorrhage temporarily in the resuscitation room by the application of an external fixator device or the PASG. Ultimately more definitive fixation can be carried out in theatre when the patient is haemodynamically stable. Minor fractures can be managed conservatively.

The patient may therefore be transferred straight to theatre or sent to the ward for observation. More complex radiological investigations may be performed en route, depending on the haemodynamic stability of the patient.

■ Summary

Injuries to the abdomen and pelvis range from the trivial to the lethal. In order to distinguish the former from the latter the trauma team must constantly be aware of the possibility of significant injury in patients presenting to the A/E department following trauma.

In order to do this a knowledge of anatomy and mechanisms of injury, coupled with a high index of suspicion and an aggressive approach to management are needed.

By increasing awareness of the principles involved in trauma management, we can reduce the number of unnecessary deaths that occur each year as a result of abdominal and pelvic trauma.

■ References and further reading

Anon 1989. What's your first choice for detecting abdominal injury? *Top. Emerg. Med.* **21**: 45.

Burgess A, Eastridge B, Young J, *et al*. Pelvic ring disruptions: effective classification system and treatment protocols. *J. Trauma* **30**: 848.

Burgess P & Fulton˙R 1992. Gallbladder and extrahepatic biliary duct injury following abdominal trauma. *Injury* **23**(6): 413.

Cope A & Stebbings W 1991. Abdominal trauma. In Skinner D, Driscoll P & Earlam R (eds): *ABC of Major Trauma*. London: BMJ Publications.

Cryer H, Miller F, Evers B, *et al*. 1988. Pelvic fracture classification: correlation with haemorrhage. *J. Trauma* **28**(7): 973.

Dalal S, Burgess A, Siegel J, *et al*. 1989. Pelvic fracture in multiple trauma: classification by mechanism is key to pattern of organ injury, resuscitative requirements and outcome. *J. Trauma* **29**: 981.

Deane A 1991. Trauma of the lower urinary tract. In Skinner D, Driscoll P & Earlam R (eds): *ABC of Major Trauma*. London: BMJ Publications.

Demetriades D, Rabinowitz B, Sofianos C, *et al*. 1985. Haematuria after blunt trauma: the role of pyelography. *Br. J. Surg.* **72**(9): 745.

Demetriades D, Rabinowitz B, Sofianos C, *et al*. 1988. The management of penetrating injuries to the back. A prospective study of 230 patients. *Ann. Surg.* **207**(1): 72.

Driscoll P, Hodgkinson D & Nicholson D 1992. Diagnostic peritoneal lavage. It's red but is it positive? *Injury* **23**: 111.

Driscoll P, Ross E & Nicholson D (in press). The pelvis. In Nicholson D & Driscoll P (eds): *ABC of Assessing Emergency Radiographs*. London: BMJ Publications.

Duus B, Damm P, Jensen F, *et al*. 1987. Conservative treatment of abdominal stab wounds with omental protrusion. *Injury* **18**(2): 87.

Feliciano D, Burch J, Spjut-Patrinely V, *et al*. 1988. Abdominal gunshot wounds. An urban trauma center's experience with 300 consecutive patients. *Ann. Surg.* **208**(3): 362.

Jalleh R, Greco L & Habib N 1992. Liver injury after trivial trauma: need for awareness. *Hospital Update* **18**: 872.

Leppaniemi A, Haapiainen R, Kiviluoto T, *et al*. 1988. Pancreatic trauma: acute and later manifestations. *Br. J. Surg.* **75**(2): 165.

Mariadason J, Parsa M, Ayuyao A, *et al*. 1988. Management of stab wounds to the thoracoabdominal region: a clinical approach. *Ann. Surg.* **207**(3): 335.

Merrill C 1990. Current thoughts on blunt abdominal trauma. *Top. Emerg. Med.* **12**: 21.

Nallathambi M, Ferreiro J, Ivatury R, *et al*. 1987. The use of peritoneal lavage and urological studies in major fractures of the pelvis – a reassessment. *Injury* **18**: 379.

Nicholson D & Driscoll P (in press). The abdomen. In Nicholson D & Driscoll P (eds): *ABC of Assessing Emergency Radiographs*. London: BMJ Publications.

Smith S R 1988. Traumatic retroperitoneal venous haemorrhage. *Br. J. Surg.* **75**(7): 632.

Stokes M & Jones D T 1992. Colorectal trauma. *Br. Med. J.* **305**: 303.

Terry T 1991. Trauma of the upper urinary tract. In Skinner D, Driscoll P & Earlam R (eds): *ABC of Major Trauma*. London: BMJ Publications.

Visvanathan R & Low H. Blunt abdominal trauma – injury assessment in relation to early surgery. *J. R. Coll. Surg. Edinb.* **38**: 19.

Wagner M M. 1990. The patient with abdominal injuries. *Nurs. Clin. N. Am.* **25**(1): 45.

Wilson R & Moorehead R 1992. Management of splenic trauma. *Injury* **23**(1): 5.

Young J, Burgess A, Brumback R, *et al.* 1986. Pelvic fractures: value of plain radiography in early assessment and management. *Radiology* **160**(2): 445.

Chapter 6

Head trauma

Peter Driscoll, Carl Gwinnutt
and David Hodgkinson

Objectives

The objectives of this chapter are that members of the trauma team should understand:

- basic pathophysiological changes following a head injury;

- the importance of primary and secondary brain damage;

- signs and symptoms of diffuse and focal brain damage;

- the cause and effect of an acute intracranial haematoma;

- how to assess a head-injured patient;

- the management of a head-injured patient;

- what the neurosurgeon needs to know from the trauma team.

■ Introduction

Head injuries are common. Over 10 million people per year present to A/E departments in the USA after sustaining a head injury. In the UK the figure is approximately 1.4 million, or 11 per cent of all A/E attendances. Around 50 per cent of all trauma deaths are associated with this type of injury, with 4000 children dying each year in the USA alone, due to the resulting brain damage.

■ Applied anatomy

☐ Neurocranium

This is the part of the skull which encloses the brain. Inside, it is divided into two levels by a fold of the dura mater (see later) called the *tentorium cerebelli*, or tent (Figure 6.1). This separates the cerebellum from the cerebral hemispheres. The midbrain passes through the opening in the anterior aspect of the tentorium and continues as the pons. Inferiorly the pons is continuous with the medulla, which gradually merges into the spinal cord at the cranio-cervical junction. At the level of the tent, the midbrain is partially covered on its antero-lateral aspects by the cortico-spinal tract. These are motor fibres descending from their origin in the motor cortex. They cross over to the opposite side at the lower end of the medulla (Figure 6.2).

The oculomotor (III) nerve leaves the anterior aspect of the midbrain and runs forward, lying between the free and attached edges of the tent. It eventually enters the orbit to supply most of the extrinsic eye muscles as well as conveying the pre-ganglionic parasympathetic fibres which cause constriction of the pupil.

These anatomical details are important in understanding some of the clinical signs seen after a head injury. Following head trauma, the development of a mass lesion above the tent (e.g. from a haematoma or cerebral oedema), can cause a pressure gradient to develop. If this is unrelieved it can result in one or both medial surfaces of the temporal lobes herniating

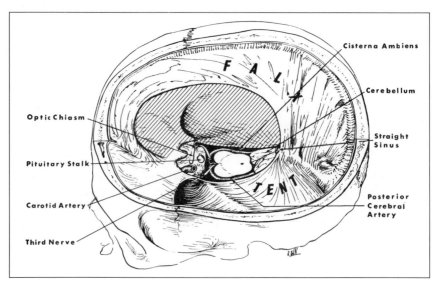

Figure 6.1 View of the neurocranium divided by the tentorium
Source: © Jennett B 1977. *Introduction to Neurosurgery*, 3rd edn. Oxford: Heinemann.
Reproduced by kind permission.

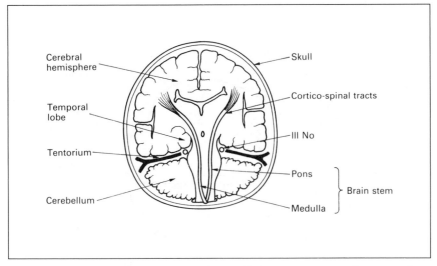

Figure 6.2 Coronal section of the brain, showing cortico-spinal tracts and III nerve

through the opening in the tent. In so doing, this brain tissue presses on, and damages, structures in this region, namely the oculomotor nerve and motor fibres in the cortico-spinal tract. This is called *tentorial herniation* and results in a fixed dilated pupil and weakness in the limb (see 'Signs following head injury', page 178). If the pressure increases further, the medulla and the cerebellum are forced downwards into the foramen magnum, a process known as *coning*. This leads to compression of the vital centres with disturbances of the cardiovascular and respiratory function (see later).

☐ **Base of the neurocranium**

This is commonly known as the 'base of the skull'. It is irregular, with two large, sharp pieces of bone projecting from its surface. These are the sphenoid wings and the petrous processes.

Following acceleration and deceleration forces, the brain moves over the base of the skull. Consequently its inferior surface can be damaged by colliding with these two large projections.

☐ **Meninges**

The internal surface of the neurocranium is lined with a thick, hard, fibrous cover called the *dura mater* (Figure 6.3). Its blood supply comes from arteries running between the dura and neurocranium. These vessels are closely adherent to the bone surface and even groove it in places. Con-

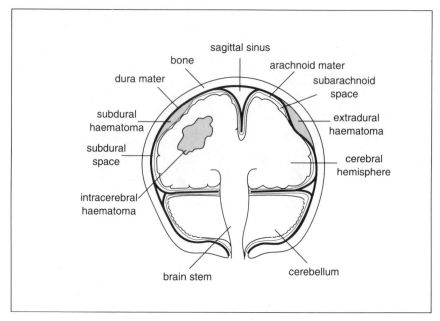

Figure 6.3 An extradural haematoma, a subdural haematoma and an intracerebral haematoma

sequently they can be torn when forces are applied to the overlying bone. The resulting haematoma collects between the bone and dura. This is therefore known as an *extradural haematoma* and 90 per cent of such injuries are associated with a fractured skull. The blood vessel most prone to this type of injury is the middle meningeal artery which lies beneath the thin, temporo-parietal area of the skull.

The brain has a complete fibro-vascular covering called the *pia mater*. In between this and the dura mater is the *arachnoid mater* (Figure 6.3), which consists of an impermeable but delicate membrane. The arachnoid mater is connected to the pia mater, across the CSF-filled subarachnoid space, by thin fibrous strands. Running between these strands are bridging veins which carry blood from the brain to the venous sinuses. With age, the brain atrophies and the subarachnoid space increases. This stretches the bridging veins and makes them more likely to tear following a head injury. The bleeding which results will collect in the subdural and subarachnoid spaces.

☐ Cerebrospinal fluid (CSF)

This is secreted by the choroid plexus in the lateral ventricles. It then passes through a series of channels inside the brain, before draining into the subarachnoid space from foramina on the surface of the midbrain.

In the intact state, there is free communication above and below the tentorium as well as between the intracranial and the spinal subarachnoid spaces. Most of the CSF is absorbed by arachnoid villi located in the dural walls of the sagittal sinus.

□ Scalp

Five layers go to make up the scalp (Box 6.1). The subcutaneous layer is very vascular and is divided into loculi by fibrous bands. The areolar layer is much looser and therefore has a greater capacity for expansion. This is the layer where the scalp haematomas usually collect. Scalp wounds tend to pout open if the aponeurosis is breached.

BOX 6.1   The layers of the scalp

- *S*kin
- sub*C*utaneous layer
- *A*poneurosis
- *L*oose (areolar) layer
- *P*eriosteum

A useful mnemonic to help remember these layers is *SCALP*.

■ Pathophysiology

□ Intracranial pressure (ICP)

As the neurocranium is a rigid box in the adult, the pressure generated inside it – the ICP – is dependent on the relationship between its volume and its contents. In the normal state the latter consist of the brain, the CSF, the blood and the blood vessels. Together, these produce an ICP of 5.8–13 mmHg in the horizontal position at the external auditory meatus.

If the ICP is to be kept at normal levels, any increase in the volume of one component must be accompanied by a decrease in one or more of the other components. CSF can be displaced into the spinal system and its absorption increased. The volume of cerebral venous blood within the dural sinuses can also decrease. Furthermore, the brain is a compliant organ, so it can mould to accommodate changes. Once the limit of these compensatory mechanisms is reached, the ICP will rise.

Head trauma results not only in mass lesions but also in an increase in the permeability of the intracerebral capillaries. This leads to interstitial oedema and cerebral swelling, making the brain relatively 'stiff'. This in turn reduces the ability of the brain to adapt to changes in the intracranial contents. This situation is worsened if ventilation is impaired, as hypoxia will produce additional cerebral swelling. Hypercapnia will result in vasodilatation of the blood vessels in the uninjured parts of the brain (see later), thereby increasing the cerebral blood volume.

The changes to the brain, the CSF and the blood vessels not only produce an elevation in the ICP, but also make each component less adaptable to any further additions in the intracranial contents. In this situation, even a small rise in volume of the intracranial contents will cause a steep rise in the ICP.

☐ Cerebral perfusion

To supply the brain with oxygenated blood, there need to be both adequate ventilation (see Chapter 3) and adequate cerebral perfusion. The latter depends on the mean arterial pressure (MAP), the resistance to blood flow due to the ICP and, to a lesser extent, the central venous pressure (CVP).

The MAP has already been defined in Chapter 4 as follows:

$$\text{MAP} = \text{diastolic pressure} + \tfrac{1}{3}(\text{systolic pressure} - \text{diastolic pressure})$$

The cerebral perfusion pressure (CPP) can be calculated from this equation:

$$\text{CPP} = \text{MAP} - \text{ICP}$$

In the multiply injured patient, not only is the ICP rising due to the head injury but the MAP may be falling because of blood loss from an extracranial trauma. In these situations, therefore, the CPP is markedly reduced.

If the CPP is 50 mmHg or less, then cerebral ischaemia will develop. As has been described above, this will lead to additional brain swelling and further rises in ICP as the cycle perpetuates itself. A CPP of less than 30 mmHg will cause death.

☐ Consciousness

This is dependent on the function of two structures: first, a network of neurons in the midbrain and brain stem known as the reticular formation, and second, both cerebral cortices. If either or both of these structures are damaged, then consciousness is lost. Hypercapnia, from any cause, can lead to a reduction in the level of consciousness. Mild hypoxia tends to make the patient restless; only when it is profound does a fall in consciousness result.

Other causes of an alteration in the conscious level, given in Box 2.2 (page 45), can be remembered from the mnemonic 'Tipps on the vowels'.

■ Pathological terms

Brain injuries are produced either by direct contact between a hard object and the neurocranium or by indirect inertial forces. These forces may act in isolation or combination.

If the object hitting the neurocranium has sufficient energy, penetration will occur. The degree of damage resulting is mainly proportional to the amount of energy delivered to the brain by the missile. This depends primarily on its velocity *on impact* unless it is very heavy (see Chapter 10). A high-energy transfer injury to the head will produce devastating damage to the brain and neurocranium (Figure 6.4).

Rapid acceleration or deceleration subjects the head to inertial forces with little of the energy being absorbed by the skull. Examples of this are shaking a child's shoulders, or when the head hits the padded interior of a car in a high-speed impact. Inertial forces are capable of producing a greater degree of neurological damage than contact forces.

☐ Primary and secondary brain injury

Primary brain injury is the neurological damage produced by the causative event, for example the blow to the head. Secondary brain injury is the neurological damage produced by subsequent insults such as hypoxia, ischaemia, hypovolaemia, metabolic imbalance, infection, and elevations in the ICP.

☐ Fractures

These usually result from a contact force and they can be associated with underlying brain injury. They are classified as being linear, depressed or compound.

Base-of-skull fractures and open fractures are particular types of compound fractures. 'Open fracture' is a term used when there is direct communication between the scalp laceration or mucous membranes and the brain substance. This diagnosis is made from inspection of the scalp wound or detection of a CSF leak from the nose or ear.

☐ Concussion

When the head is subjected to inertial forces, a spectrum of injury results, ranging from concussion as the most mild form to diffuse axonal injury as the most severe.

Concussion occurs when the head has been subjected to minor inertial

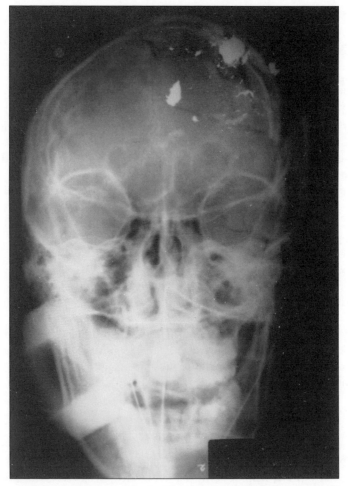

Figure 6.4 Radiograph of a skull, demonstrating the damage caused by the impact of a rifle bullet

forces. The patient is always amnesic of the event and there may be post- and antigrade amnesia as well. A transient loss of consciousness (usually less than 5 minutes) may occur. On examination, these patients do not have any localizing signs but there may be nausea, vomiting and headaches. Originally it was thought that no organic brain damage occurred in this condition. This has been found not to be the case: microscopic changes are produced. The net effect after one episode is minor, but it can be cumulative.

☐ Diffuse axonal injury (DAI)

This results in a widespread, mainly microscopic disruption of the brain consisting of axonal damage, microscopic haemorrhages, tears in the brain tissue, and interstitial oedema.

As a consequence of the widespread neuronal disruption, DAI can cause prolonged periods of coma (days or weeks) and has an overall mortality rate of 33–50 per cent. Autonomic dysfunction giving rise to high fever, hypertension and sweating are also seen in this condition.

☐ Contusion

The brain, lying under the impact point of a contact force, is subjected to a series of strains. It results from the inward deformation of bone and the shock waves spreading out from the impact. It can also occur as the base of the brain impinges on projections on the base of the skull. These produce gross neurological damage, with haemorrhages, neuronal death and brain swelling. The patient therefore invariably loses consciousness at the time of the incident and, by the time he is examined in the A/E department, has usually developed neurological signs. The most common signs are an altered conscious level, hemiparesis, ataxia and seizures.

☐ Contra coup injuries

The brain is not fixed inside the neurocranium, but instead floats in a bath of CSF, tethered by the arachnoid fibres and blood vessels. If the head moves due to an accelerating or decelerating force, the skull, and then the brain, will move in the direction of the force. As a consequence, strains develop in the brain tissue and small blood vessels opposite the impact point. This gives rise to the contusional changes described previously. Another factor giving rise to injury is that the brain will continue to move until it collides with the opposite side of the skull or its base. The result is that the brain can be injured in two places, with the site furthest from the impact being the most severe. An example of this is an occipital blow that produces temporal and frontal damage.

☐ Acute intracranial haematomas

Acute extradural haematoma (EDH)

In the majority of cases the EDH develops in the temporo-parietal area following a tear in the middle meningeal artery (Figure 6.5). However, a

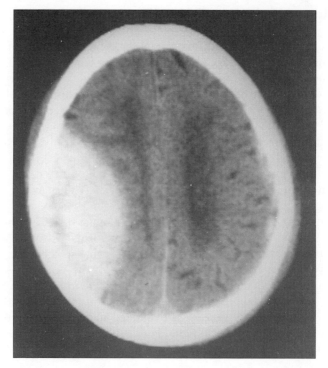

Figure 6.5 CT scan showing an extradural haematoma

small number are due to tears in one of the venous sinuses inside the neurocranium. As the source of the haematoma is usually arterial, the EDH develops quickly and so produces a rapid rise in the intracranial pressure.

The 'classic' presentation of an EDH (Box 6.2) only occurs in approximately one-third of patients. The rest either are unconscious from the time of the impact, or do not lose consciousness at the scene of the injury but go on to develop neurological signs. The most common clinical signs are a deterioration in the conscious level and pupil size changes.

BOX 6.2   The classic history of an extradural haematoma

- Transient loss of consciousness at the time of the injury from a momentary disruption of the reticular formation
- Patient then regains consciousness for several hours, the lucid period
- Localizing signs develop, with neurological deficits, headaches and eventually unconsciousness from the developing EDH, which causes the ICP to rise

Early evacuation is the treatment of choice for EDH because it will reduce the secondary brain damage. Early surgery results in a 9–36 per cent mortality, with 40 per cent making a good recovery. However, the death rate rises steeply if the patient is allowed to deteriorate from a rise in intracranial pressure before the operation.

Acute intradural haematomas (IDH)

This is a collective term used for both subdural (SDH) and intracerebral (ICH) haematomas. They frequently coexist, and are three to four times more common than extradural haematomas (Figure 6.6).

SDHs commonly develop in the temporal lobe and can be bilateral. Following an inertial force, some of the bridging veins tear and blood collects in the subdural space. Occasionally an SDH develops without there being an accompanying ICH. Rarer still is the solitary presence of an ICH; when this occurs it is often found in the frontal lobes.

Small ICHs can also be produced by inertial forces and their volume can increase over time. Depending on their location, they may cause localizing signs or a rise in the intracranial pressure and a deterioration in the clinical state of the patient.

The forces needed to produce an IDH are greater than those needed to produce an EDH, and an IDH is usually associated with cerebral contusion and cortical lacerations. Consequently the patient commonly loses consciousness at the time of the injury. Fits, which are commonly focal, a deteriorating conscious level, contralateral hemiparesis and unilateral pupil

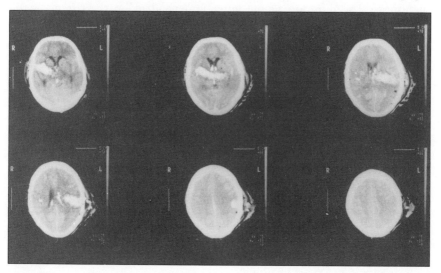

Figure 6.6 CT scan for a patient who has been shot in the head with a hand gun; the CT scan shows both a subdural and an intracerebral haematoma developing in the bullet tract

dilatation are the usual signs. If a solitary SDH occurs, the patient may have a lucid period followed by a gradual deterioration in the neurological state. This takes longer to develop than in the case of EDH, because the source of the bleeding is venous rather than arterial. If there are only a few bridging veins torn and there is plenty of intracranial space, due to brain atrophy, then it can take several days for symptoms to develop.

In view of the amount of primary brain damage, the mortality rate for an IDH is 36–74 per cent in those requiring an operation within 48 hours of the injury. Only 12 per cent will make a good recovery.

Subarachnoid haemorrhage (SAH)

This can occasionally follow a head injury. The patient often develops severe headaches and photophobia, but other signs of meningism can occur. No test for neck stiffness should be done until injury to the cervical spine has been ruled out both radiologically and clinically.

■ Signs following a head injury

☐ Signs due to a diffuse injury

If a sufficient force is sent through the brain, enough of the synapses in the reticular formation and cerebral cortices are disrupted to produce unconsciousness. The duration of the latter is dependent on the extent of the primary, and subsequent secondary, brain damage.

Diffuse brain injury can also be produced by hypoxia, hypovolaemia and hypoglycaemia. It is very important to rule out these treatable extracranial causes of unconsciousness before diagnosing an intracranial pathology.

If there is a generalized increase in brain bulk (i.e. from blood and oedema) the intracranial pressure will rise once the compensatory mechanisms have been exhausted. Eventually tentorial herniation occurs causing pupillary dilatation (III N compression) and motor weakness (cortico-spinal tract compression). With a further rise in ICP, coning occurs and the vital centres are compressed. This gives rise to the signs known as Cushing's response (Box 6.3).

BOX 6.3   Cushing's response

- Decrease in the respiratory rate
- Decrease in the the heart rate
- Increase in the systolic blood pressure
- Increase in the pulse pressure

Without treatment pontine compression gives rise to a further deterioration in motor function and bilateral pupillary constriction. In the preterminal situation, pupillary dilatation returns, the heart rate increases, the respiratory rate becomes very slow and irregular, and the blood pressure falls. Finally there is a respiratory arrest from haemorrhage or infarction of the brain stem.

☐ Signs due to a focal injury

A purely focal injury can follow a contact force. However, there is usually sufficient associated diffuse brain injury to produce an altered level of consciousness from a temporary disruption of the reticular formation.

The presenting signs and symptoms will depend on the site injured, as different parts of the brain carry out different functions. A focal lesion above the tentorium can produce ipsilateral, unilateral herniation of the medial part of the temporal lobes (diffuse brain injuries tend to be bilateral). In 90 per cent of cases, this produces an ipsilateral fixed dilated pupil and contralateral hemiplegia. With further rises in the ICP, the brain stem begins to be compressed and the patient develops the signs described previously (Figure 6.7).

Selective herniation of the cerebellum through the foramen magnum can be produced by an expanding posterior-fossa intracranial haematoma. This can lead to a whole collection of presenting signs, the most common being pupil dilatation, respiratory abnormalities, bradycardia, head tilt and cranial nerve palsies. Most alarming is the sudden respiratory arrest due to low brain-stem compression. This is the only cerebral haematoma to produce this without a preceding deterioration in conscious level.

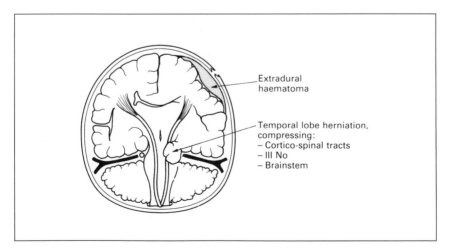

Figure 6.7 Coronal section of the brain showing herniation of medial temporal lobe (compare Figure 6.2)

Focal signs can sometimes mislead – for example, the fixed dilated pupil could be a result of direct eye trauma, and the weak upper limb could be due to a brachial plexus injury.

☐ **Signs due to both diffuse and specific injuries**

The trauma patient invariably has diffuse and specific neurological injuries. A space-occupying lesion is often accompanied by a swollen brain due to primary and secondary brain damage. This accelerates the rise in intracranial pressure and the development of further brain damage.

As there is still no method of regenerating neurons once they have died, the management of the head-injured patient concentrates on preventing those factors which would produce secondary brain damage. These patients are therefore dealt with using the same sequence as in all other circumstances.

■ Assessment and management

☐ **Primary survey and resuscitation**

When the patient arrives, the ambulance crew should inform the medical team leader about the mechanism of injury, the neurological state of the patient at the scene, subsequent changes, and the presence of associated injuries. If since the injury the trauma victim has replied logically to any question, then the primary brain damage cannot have been severe. Any subsequent deterioration will be due to secondary brain damage.

As this discussion is under way, the rest of the team will be carrying out their tasks concerned with the primary survey and resuscitation of the patient.

In many cases the head-injured patient also has serious injuries to other areas of his body. This increases the chance of secondary brain damage and complicates the resuscitation. It is therefore important that the patient is managed by the same team approach as is described in Chapter 1. **The temptation to examine and treat an obvious injury should be resisted because it may not be the problem that could kill the patient.**

It is recommended that the head-injured patient is resuscitated on a trolley capable of a 15° head-up tilt, to help reduce the ICP, once cardiovascularly stable.

Continuous communication with all trauma victims, especially those with head injuries, is very important. It is best that this is the responsibility of only a single nurse and a single doctor (usually the airway nurse and doctor) as this will enable a relationship to be built up and will also prevent the patient being confused by several people asking him questions.

Airway and cervical spine

The airway nurse and doctor must clear and secure the airway in the manner described in Chapter 2. They must also ensure that the trauma victim is adequately ventilated. Those head-injured patients who need to be intubated and ventilated are listed in Box 6.4.

BOX 6.4 Head-injured patients who require intubation and ventilation

---

- Inability to maintain the airway
- Risk of aspiration
- $PaO_2 < 100$ mmHg or $PaCO_2 > 40$ mmHg
- Hyperventilation is required to reduce the $PaCO_2$
- Chest injuries
- GCS < 9
- Neurogenic pulmonary oedema
- Protracted or recurrent seizures
- Hyperthermia
- Protection during transportation

Endotracheal intubation carries risks (see Chapter 2). Furthermore, any patient who is not deeply comatosed will respond with reflex increases in blood pressure and ICP when laryngoscopy and intubation are attempted. The airway personnel must therefore have the skills to minimize these reflexes and reduce the chances of secondary brain damage.

A method of temporarily reducing the ICP is to utilize the reactivity of normal cerebral arterioles to the $PaCO_2$. Hyperventilating the patient and reducing the $PaCO_2$ will cause vasoconstriction and thereby reduce the volume of blood in the neurocranium. However, this technique can produce cerebral ischaemia in the remaining uninjured brain due to extreme vasoconstriction if the $PaCO_2$ falls below 25 mmHg. Therefore the patient must be carefully monitored, using arterial blood analysis, whilst this procedure is carried out. In view of the potential complications with this technique, it is preferable that the neurosurgeons are contacted before it is started.

Some 5–10 per cent of patients who are unconscious following a road traffic accident or a fall have an associated neck injury. Therefore care should be taken at all times to stabilize the cervical spine in the midline with a rigid collar, sandbags and tape (or a commercially available head restraint – see Figure 1.5). Positioning the head in neutral also helps prevent obstruction of neck veins which could cause cerebral venous congestion and an increase in ICP.

Breathing

Any thoracic problems should be corrected by the medical team leader working with one of the circulation nurses (see Chapter 3). The respiratory rate and pattern should also be noted as these can indicate both intra- and extracranial pathology.

Circulation

With the exception of infants, hypovolaemia is not produced by bleeding inside the neurocranium. In a young child it can, however, be caused by a scalp haematoma.

Patients require vigorous fluid replacement if they are in a shocked state (see Chapter 4). In contrast, if there is no evidence of hypovolaemia in the head-injured patient, then only maintenance fluids should be administered as brain swelling can be exacerbated by over-transfusion. It is therefore important that the amount of fluid administered to the patient is known by both the nursing and the medical team leaders.

Dysfunction

Even though the head-injured patient may have sustained several injuries, the airway nurse should not forget the tenets of basic nursing care of the unconscious patient. Talking and listening to the patient will enable her to decide whether he is speaking spontaneously, following commands, only responding to pain, or totally unconscious. The pupillary response must also be recorded. With this information, in addition to that from the ambulance crew, the nursing and medical team leaders will now know whether the patient is deteriorating neurologically.

Changes in the neurological state will no longer be detectable if the trauma victim has received drugs to facilitate intubation and ventilation. Consequently this type of patient must have a CT scan of his head at the earliest appropriate time (see later).

Exposure

By the end of the primary survey, all the patient's clothes should have been removed. Occasionally the head-injured patient can become hyperthermic. This increases the metabolic demands of the already damaged brain and causes a further deterioration in the neurological state. Blankets should be removed from the patient if his temperature begins to rise. Ice bags in sheets should be put over the patient if the temperature rise continues.

Upon completion of the primary survey, the nursing and medical team leaders must check that all the resuscitative procedures have been started and that all the monitoring systems have been connected to the patient (see Chapter 1). By monitoring the head-injured trauma victim, the team should be able to detect:

- changes in the neurological state of the patient;
- factors which give rise to secondary brain damage.

The clinical diagnosis of intracranial pathology is unreliable if the patient is hypovolaemic or hypoxic, because these conditions can reproduce similar neurological signs. They are also the main factors giving rise to secondary brain damage in the trauma patient. Consequently, the blood pressure, the heart rate, the respiratory rate and the arterial blood gas need to be measured frequently. Each of these parameters should be reassessed if there is any change in the neurological state of the patient. This will enable the extracranial causes for the neurological deterioration to be ruled out.

☐ Secondary survey

Once the immediate life-threatening conditions have been corrected, the detailed head-to-toe assessment can commence. This has already been covered in Chapter 1, but those features pertinent to the head-injured patient will be described now in greater detail.

Scalp

The medical team leader should examine the scalp for any lacerations, bruising and swellings, and digitally explore all cuts for depressed skull fractures. Fingers are quite good at detecting these deformities, but haematomas in the loose (areolar) layer can imitate this type of fracture. If the wound goes down to the skull, it can be inspected to determine whether there is a linear, non-depressed fracture at its base. Open fractures with brain exposed should not be probed.

Major scalp bleeding must be controlled either by direct pressure or by gripping the aponeurosis with haemostats, which can then folded back on themselves.

Any foreign matter protruding from the skull following an impalement injury needs to be left for the neurosurgeon to remove in theatre.

Neurological assessment

This involves an assessment of the consciousness using the Glasgow Coma Scale, the pupillary response, and the presence or absence of lateralizing signs. Occasionally a short-term memory test is also carried out.

The Glasgow Coma Scale (GCS, Box 6.5) is the most commonly used neurological test for the trauma patient in the resuscitation room:

BOX 6.5   Glasgow Coma Scale

Eye

Opens spontaneously	4
Opens to speech	3
Opens to pain	2
None	1

Verbal

Orientated	5
Confused	4
Inappropriate words	3
Incomprehensible sounds	2
None	1

Motor

Obeys commands	6
Localizes to pain	5
Flexion (withdraws) to pain	4
Abnormal flexion to pain (decorticate)	3
Extension to pain (decerebrate)	2
None	1

A variation of this scale is used for assessing children (see Chapter 11).

The GCS records the *best* verbal and eye-opening response and the *best* motor response to standard painful stimuli. The latter are produced by pressure on the supratrochlea nerve or fingernail bed. The GCS does have a limited sensitivity in detecting focal injuries and in distinguishing between different degrees of diffuse brain injuries. However there is no universally accepted alternative.

Problems can also arise in assessing the verbal response in intubated patients, and the eye-opening response in those who have bilateral periorbital oedema. If this is the case, then appropriate records must be made rather than not carrying out the assessment.

Lateralizing signs have a strong association with intracranial pathology. Therefore a detailed neurological examination must be carried out to determine whether there is any asymmetry of motor and pupillary response. These signs may be subtle, such as a 4th cranial nerve palsy, or gross, such as a hemiplegia. A sensitive test for partial hemiplegia, in the conscious patient, is to monitor the upper-arm drift. The arms are held perpendicular to the body, palms supinated and eyes closed. The earliest sign is pronation of the palm. It is important to remember that congenital unilateral pupil dilatation is present in 10 per cent of the population. However, these pupils respond to light.

Short-term memory for three objects at 3 minutes is a sensitive test for diffuse brain injury in those patients who have a GCS of 15.

The airway nurse must continue to check the patient's GCS and pupillary size and reactivity every 15 minutes. These findings can then be compared with previous recordings to determine whether there is any *change* in the neurological state of the patient. Changes are much more important than any individual reading. Consistency of measuring the GCS is facilitated by having the same nurse taking the GCS each time.

A poor neurological response or a deterioration should never be attributed to alcohol. In all situations, the team must rule out an intracranial pathology or secondary brain damage from hypoxia, hypovolaemia or hypoglycaemia.

Agitation

This is common in head-injured patients. Though it can indicate intracranial pathology, it can also result from cerebral hypoxia and pain. The primary cause needs to be found and corrected because the agitated patient is at risk of injuring himself further, especially if there is a cervical injury. Sedation alone should never be used as these patients may prove difficult to ventilate using the bag-valve-mask technique described in Chapter 2.

If it is not possible to correct the agitation, these patients should be anaesthetized, intubated and ventilated by an experienced anaesthetist.

Convulsions

These are not uncommon after head injuries. They can result from primary brain damage, hypoxia or a raised ICP, or they can occur spontaneously in those trauma victims who have a history of epilepsy. These patients can develop further brain damage due to the hypoxia and hypercapnia which occur during the fit. Therefore, convulsions should be treated promptly. The adult patient should receive 5–10 mg of diazepam (depending on age and size) as a slow IV bolus, and the respiration and blood pressure should be monitored. This can be repeated once if the convulsion recurs or continues, or an IV dose of phenytoin (17 mg/kg) can be given. During the administration of phenytoin, the pulse and blood pressure must be monitored and the drug never given faster than 50 mg/min. If the convulsions continue, intravenous barbiturates will be needed. This almost always means the patient will have to be intubated and ventilated. Patients should *never* just be paralysed as the fits will continue.

The base of the skull

This lies at an angle to the horizontal plane (see Figure 1.7). The surface landmarks of this diagonal line are:

- mastoid process;
- tympanic membrane;
- orbits.

The medical team leader should inspect this line because the clinical features of a fracture to the base of the skull also lie on it (Box 6.6).

BOX 6.6   Signs of a fracture to the base of the skull

- Bruising over the mastoid (Battle's sign)
- Haemotympanum
- CSF with blood from the ear or nose
- Orbital bruising ('panda' or 'raccoon' eyes)
- Scleral haemorrhages with no posterior margin

Battle's sign and the orbital bruising can take 12–24 hours to develop and so are of limited use in the acute situation. The presence of CSF in the blood dripping from the nose or ear can be detected by dropping some of the fluid onto an absorbent sheet and seeing a double-ring pattern developing. Another method is to note the delay in the clotting of the bloody discharge.

A CSF leak indicates the presence of a compound fracture. Most units would recommend that these patients receive prophylactic antibiotic cover to prevent meningitis. The type of antibiotic used will depend on the local policy, and this should be known by the team leaders.

A nasogastric tube should not be used if there is a fracture of the base of the skull, because it might be pushed into the neurocranium during its insertion. The oral route must be used instead.

Eyes

The orbits must be examined for penetrating injury. Sharp objects can perforate the roof of the orbit and enter the anterior cranial fossa (see Chapter 7). The eyes should then be inspected for damage, haemorrhage, acuity and pupil size, and reactivity. If the patient is unconscious the corneal reflex should be tested. Its absence indicates a profound neurological deficit.

The rest of the secondary survey is carried out as described previously in Chapter 1. If the patient is unconscious or if there is a sensory defect then peritoneal lavage may be required to rule out an intraperitoneal bleed. This is especially important if the patient is being transferred away from General Surgical supervision.

By the time the patient has been fully examined, a complete history should have been taken (remember AMPLE in Chapter 1). Consequently, upon completion of the secondary survey both the nursing and medical team leaders should know:

- the neurological state of the patient following the injury;
- any subsequent changes in the neurological state;
- whether there are factors producing secondary brain damage;
- whether there are neck injuries;
- whether there are any associated injuries.

Narcotics seldom mask neurological changes and they may be required for analgesia. If the medical team leader decides to use them, they should be administered slowly by the intravenous route until pain relief is achieved (see Chapter 4), and a note made of the dose given and the time of admission.

☐ Definitive care

Investigation

Further investigations of the head-injured patient are dependent on the presence of any remaining respiratory or hypovolaemic problems, because these must be corrected first. In certain situations this may require an operation. For example, the hypovolaemic patient may require a laparotomy to remove a ruptured spleen, before he is sufficiently haemodynamically stable to have a CT scan of his head.

If the patient's respiratory and cardiovascular systems are stable then further investigations are warranted, the definitive test being a CT scan. An increasing number of hospitals have this facility but no neurosurgical presence on-site. In such a setting, the team should carry out a CT scan on patients in any of the following circumstances:

- if the patient has a skull fracture;
- if he has a reduced level of consciousness;
- if he displays neurological signs;
- if he has been paralysed and ventilated.

The results of the scan can then be transmitted to the neurosurgeon by a telephone link.

If a CT scan is not available, two skull x-rays should be taken (PA and lateral) in the situations listed in Box 6.7. A Towne's view is permitted only, if the cervical spine has been cleared of any abnormality, both clinically and radiologically.

BOX 6.7   Indications that a skull radiograph is required

- Loss of consciousness or amnesia at any time since the injury
- Neurological signs or symptoms
- A CSF leak or blood loss from the ear or nose
- Suspicion of a penetrating injury
- Scalp bruising, swelling or significant lacerations
- Alcohol or drug intoxication making assessment of the patient difficult

---

These plain radiographs only give information about the position of foreign matter and the presence of fractures (Figure 6.8). Base-of-skull fractures are not seen on these routine skull films but may be suspected if there is intracranial air, if the sphenoid sinus is opaque or if there is a fluid level in the sphenoid or ethmoid sinuses.

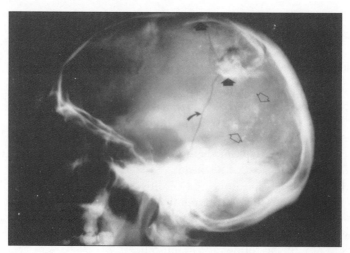

Figure 6.8   Skull radiograph showing a linear fracture and depressed fractures

The presence or absence of fractures and neurological signs significantly affects the incidence of intracranial haematomas (Box 6.8). Consequently, in the absence of a CT scan these two features are used in deciding the treatment of the head-injured patient.

BOX 6.8   Incidence of operable intracranial haematomas

- No skull fracture and no neurological signs: 1 : 6000
- No skull fracture but a GCS <15:   1 : 120
- A skull fracture but no neurological signs: 1 : 32
- A skull fracture and a GCS <15:   1 : 4

Further management

Minor head injuries

This term is applied to those patients who are fully orientated, have amnesia of less than 10 minutes, have no neurological signs or symptoms at the time of the examination in the resuscitation room, and have no skull fractures. These trauma victims still require a further 24 hours of observation by a sensible adult who has been given head-injury instructions (Figure 6.9). Observations need to be made hourly for the first 12 hours and two-hourly thereafter. Post-traumatic amnesia for a short period of time, or unconsciousness with full recovery, is not necessarily an indication for admission.

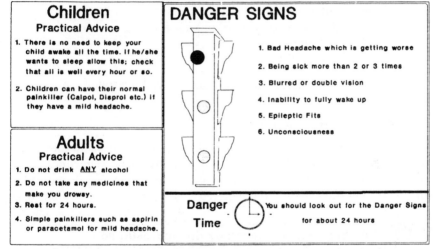

ADVICE FOLLOWING A MILD HEAD INJURY

Hope Hospital — Accident and Emergency Department

Very occasionally complications can develop after slight head injury. In order to catch this very rare possibility a responsible adult should watch carefully for the DANGER SIGNS

Children
Practical Advice

1. There is no need to keep your child awake all the time. If he/she wants to sleep allow this; check that all is well every hour or so.

2. Children can have their normal painkiller (Calpol, Disprol etc.) if they have a mild headache.

Adults
Practical Advice

1. Do not drink ANY alcohol
2. Do not take any medicines that make you drowsy.
3. Rest for 24 hours.
4. Simple painkillers such as aspirin or paracetamol for mild headache.

DANGER SIGNS

1. Bad Headache which is getting worse
2. Being sick more than 2 or 3 times
3. Blurred or double vision
4. Inability to fully wake up
5. Epileptic Fits
6. Unconsciousness

Danger Time You should look out for the Danger Signs for about 24 hours

If any of the Danger signs develop come straight back to the Hospital. We are happy to see you or give advice at any time DIRECT LINE 787 4841

Figure 6.9 Head injury instructions

Moderate head injuries

This term is applied to the following patients:

1 Those who have either a simple skull fracture or neurological signs (including confusion) at the time of the examination. These patients require an early CT scan.

2 Children under 12 years of age who have no neurological signs or fractures but who have vomited more than once since the time of the injury.

3 Patients with whom there is difficulty in assessing their condition (e.g. due to alcohol or epilepsy).

4 Patients with other medical conditions (e.g. blood-clotting disorders).

5 Patients in poor social conditions or who lack a responsible adult to monitor them.

These patients should be admitted for observation and investigation.

Serious head injuries

This term is applied to patients who have:

1 Both neurological signs and a skull fracture.
2 A compound or depressed skull fracture.
3 A base-of-skull fracture.
4 Coma (GCS ∂ 8) continuing after resuscitation.
5 Post-traumatic epilepsy.
6 A deteriorating neurological state.
7 Neurological disturbance persisting after 6 hours.
8 Amnesia for greater than 10 minutes.
9 An abnormal head CT scan.

All these patients require immediate neurosurgical referral.

Communication with a neurosurgeon

Few A/E departments have the luxury of being able to have all their head-injured patients seen in the resuscitation room by a neurosurgeon. Instead, the team leader usually has to describe the situation over the telephone. It is therefore important that all the required information is relayed (Box 6.9).

BOX 6.9   Information needed by the neurosurgeon

- The name, sex and age of the patient
- The time and mechanism of injury
- The neurological state at the scene of the injury
- The initial GCS and current GCS in the A/E department
- The pupil size and reactivity
- The presence of any localizing signs or convulsions
- The blood pressure, heart rate, respiratory rate and breathing pattern
- Any associated injuries
- The arterial blood-gas levels
- The skull and cervical-spine x-ray results
- The treatment provided in the resuscitation room, and the response
- Relevant past medical history and medications

The neurosurgeon will now know whether the patient needs to be transferred. In most cases the patient is transferred for a CT scan, and should this prove normal the patient may be returned to the referring hospital. The team leader will also receive advice about treatment and transportation. It is important that the patient is stable from a respiratory and cardiovascular aspect before he is transferred.

Additional treatment

Additional treatment for the head-injured patient should be started only if the neurosurgeon is in agreement or if there is a local policy. Such treatment includes the following:

Mannitol

This is an osmotic diuretic which decreases the cerebral water content by establishing an osmotic gradient between blood and brain in areas with normal capillary permeability (i.e. the uninjured brain). The usual dose is 0.5 g/kg as a 20% solution over 10–30 minutes (175 ml for a 70 kg patient). It is usually effective in 10–15 minutes. However, there are some problems associated with its use. Initially it may cause a slight rise in the ICP due to expansion of the circulating blood volume; and repeated doses can cause hypovolaemia (thereby reducing cerebral perfusion) and electrolyte disturbances. The diuresis will invalidate the measurement of urine volume as a monitor of hypovolaemia and also require the patient to be catheterized.

Frusemide

This is an alternative preferred by some units. It is a potent loop diuretic and has the advantage of not causing an initial rise in ICP. It also helps reduce ICP by reducing the rate of CSF formation. The dose is 0.5 mg/kg. However, it still suffers from the same problems as mannitol if repeated doses are given and large urine volumes are produced.

Hyperventilation

The mechanism behind this form of treatment is discussed on page 181.

Neurosurgery

This is rarely required in the A/E department as it is preferable to transfer the patient to the neurosurgeon once he has been stabilized. If the distance is great and a trained surgeon is available, then burr holes may be placed provided the patient shows a rapid neurological deterioration and the neurosurgeon has been consulted and agrees.

Transportation of the head-injured patient

In all cases the diagnosis, initial resuscitation and treatment of the immediately life-threatening conditions in the airway, breathing and circulation take priority over the transfer of the patient to a neurosurgical unit.

Those patients who need to be transferred require as an escort a nurse and a doctor who are competent at monitor interpretation and can deal with any resuscitation problem which may develop in transit. If the patient is already intubated, the ideal team is the airway nurse and the anaesthetist. Before leaving, the patient must be as haemodynamically stable as possible and physically secured to the stretcher so that his spine and limbs cannot be moved or injured. The lines and leads also must be secured. Finally, the transport equipment, drugs, notes and x-rays must be checked (see Chapter 1).

All the vital signs and the GCS need to be recorded frequently during the journey by the accompanying nurse.

■ Summary

The objective in managing the head-injured patient is to prevent secondary brain damage. The main factors giving rise to this are hypoxia, hypovolaemia, intracranial haematomas and infection. A significant percentage of these patients have serious injuries to other body systems, which increase the chance of secondary brain damage. It is therefore important that a co-ordinated resuscitation is carried out, and the the patient is not transferred to a neurosurgical unit until he has been stabilized from a respiratory and haemodynamic point of view.

■ References and further reading

Adams J, Graham D, Murray L, *et al.* 1982. Diffuse axonal injury due to nonmissile head injury in humans: an analysis of 45 cases. *Ann. Neurol.* **12**(6): 557.

Aldrich S & Eisenberg M 1990. Pitfalls in acute emergency department evaluation of head-injured patients. *Top. Emerg. Med.* **11**: 53.

Ammons A 1990. Cerebral injuries and intracranial haemorrhages as a result of trauma. *Nurs. Clin. N. Am.* **25**(1): 23.

Bullock R & Teasdale G 1991. Head injuries. In Skinner D, Driscoll P & Earlam R (eds): *ABC of Major Trauma*. London: BMJ Publications.

Clifton S 1990. Prehospital assessment and management of head injury. *Top. Emerg. Med.* **11**: 7.

Commission on the Provision of Surgical Services 1986. Report of the working party on head injuries. Royal College of Surgeons of England.

Demetriades D, Charalambides D, Lakhoo M, *et al.* 1992. Role of prophylactic antibiotics in open and basilar fractures of the skull: a randomized study. *Injury* **23**: 377.

Driscoll P, Skinner D & Gwinnutt C (in press). The management of the multiply injured patient with a significant head injury in the emergency department. *Hospital Update.*

Eisenburg H, Foulkes M, Jane J, *et al.* 1991. Report on 'The Traumatic Coma data bank'. *J. Neurosurg.* **75** Suppl.

Gennarelli T 1983. Head injury in man and experimental animals: clinical aspects. *Acta Neurochir. Supp.* **32**: 1.

Gennarelli T, Spielman G, Langfitt T, *et al.* 1982. Influence of the type of intracranial lesion on outcome from severe head injury. *J. Neurosurg.* **56**: 26.

Gennarelli T & Thibault L 1982. Biomechanics of acute subdural haematoma. *J. Trauma* **22**: 680.

Gentleman D 1990. Preventing secondary brain damage after head injury: a multidisciplinary challenge. *Injury* **21**: 305.

Gentleman D & Jennett B 1981. Hazards of inter-hospital transfer of comatosed head-injured patients. *Lancet* **2**: 853.

Gentleman D & Teasdale G 1986. *Head and Spinal Trauma.* Surrey: Update-Seibert Publications.

Goldberg S 1988. *Clinical Neuroanatomy made Ridiculously Simple.* Miami: MedMaster.

Gloag D 1985a. Rehabilitation after head injury: (1) Cognitive problems. *Br. Med. J.* **290**: 834.

Gloag D 1985b. Rehabilitation after head injury: (2) Behaviour and emotional problems, long-term needs, and the requirements for services. *Br. Med. J.* **290**: 913.

Nicholson D, Hodgkinson D, Driscoll P, *et al.* (in press). The skull. In Nicholson D & Driscoll P (eds): *ABC of Assessing Emergency Radiographs.* London: BMJ Publications.

Suggestions from a Group of Neurosurgeons 1984. Guidelines for initial management after head injury in adults. *Br. Med. J.* **228**: 983.

Teasdale G, Galbraith S, Murray L, *et al.* 1982. Management of traumatic intracranial haematoma. *Br. Med. J.* **285**: 1695.

Teasdale G, Murray G, Anderson E, *et al.* 1990. Risks of acute traumatic intracranial haematoma in children and adults: implications for managing head injuries. *Br. Med. J.* **300**: 363.

Chapter 7

Facial, ophthalmic and otolaryngological trauma

Cindy LeDuc Jimmerson and Gabby Lomas

Objectives

The objectives of this chapter are that upon completion the reader will:

- realize the significance of facial injuries relative to injuries of the head and neck;

- appreciate that the vascular supply is bountiful in soft-tissue structures of the face and scalp but poor in structures of the outer ears, and that a different approach must be taken in evaluating and tending wounds in these areas;

- be able to list life-threatening complications that may occur with facial injuries;

- be able to describe principles of dressing application appropriate for facial, eye, nose and ear injuries.

■ Introduction

While injuries to facial structures are rarely life-threatening, the potential blood loss and the loss of the airway, due to secretions, bleeding and tissue oedema, must be considered for the potential risk that exists. Injuries to the eyes, ears and nose usually result from rapid deceleration accidents, such as motorcycle or car crashes, contact sports or violent altercations. One must be wary of the possibility of associated head and neck injuries and not be misled by the often disfiguring appearance of facial injuries. Many times the cosmetic value of the injury can lead the care-giver away from the more important issues of airway risk, blood loss and brain injury. Because the soft-tissue structures of the face are very vascular there is often a large amount of shed blood apparent with even a small wound, and maintaining haemostasis is important, although the priorities of the ABCs should never be second-rated.

■ Assessment

All patients who have suffered facial injuries should be observed for the following:

- adequate airway
- cervical spine injury
- bleeding
- level of consciousness
- scalp injuries
- asymmetry of facial structures
- difficulty in swallowing or talking
- missing or broken teeth
- malocclusion of the mandible
- cerebrospinal fluid leak from eyes, ears, nose and mouth
- visual acuity
- impaired hearing

Frequently the patient will have several of these signs in conjunction with a mechanism of injury that is quite clear. Obtaining adequate information from the pre-hospital personnel is strongly advised, to assist in making an early plan of care for the patient. Knowing whether the windscreen was fractured, whether or not the patient was wearing a seatbelt, or how far and onto what a patient fell can be very helpful in anticipating what severity of injury to expect. Penetrating injuries to the face and neck often result from violence and one should remember to examine the scalp and hair of the patient for entrance and exit wounds that may not be obvious.

It is generally a good idea to elevate the head of the bed between 15° and 30° to assist drainage of blood and secretions from the nasopharynx and to decrease the amount of oedema that is likely to develop. Until a cross-table cervical spine x-ray has been performed and satisfactorily interpreted to be normal, cervical spine precautions should be strictly enforced. The analogy of the head as a 'big melon on a skinny stalk' correlates nicely to the sus-ceptibility of the neck to injury when high velocity is applied to the head. When examining a patient wearing a cervical collar, it is important to use an additional pair of hands to stabilize the head and maintain cervical stability while the collar is removed and the underlying soft tissue and bony structures are observed and palpated.

☐ **Diagnosis**

Diagnosis of injuries of the face is made based on the physical examination and on x-rays of the patient. If the patient is awake and co-operative he may be helpful in locating lacerations, haematomas and abrasions that may be difficult to recognize under the 'gear' of resuscitation and the patient's clothing and hair.

☐ **General treatment**

General treatment for all facial injuries includes the stabilization and guaranteeing of the airway, haemostasis, the provision of supplemental oxygen and suction, nasogastric-tube evacuation of the stomach, the stabilization of fractures, and the protection of vital tissue. Most injuries benefit from ice and from elevation of the head of the bed when the patient's other injuries permit.

■ **Eye trauma**

Eye injuries should never take precedence over life-threatening injuries; a complete initial assessment of the patient should be done in the case of multiple trauma before initiating eye care.

Once the patient's condition has been established as stable, the eye should be cleaned, closely examined for lacerations, foreign bodies and haematomas. A visual acuity test should be performed and x-rays should be taken when the clinical examination suggests the possibility of bony injury, or injury to the adjacent sinuses (Figure 7.1). Contact lenses should be removed and, particularly with the unconscious patient, the corneas must be lubricated. When the patient is unconscious and the eye injury is minimal, taping the eyes closed to prevent dehydration may be adequate. Any fluid leaking from the eye should be checked for cerebrospinal fluid. If globe injury has occurred, suspicion of vitreous and aqueous humour leaking creates an ophthalmological emergency. An ophthalmologist should be consulted to evaluate the injury. Gentle pressure with a fluffy gauze pad should be maintained until the consultant arrives. Impaled objects should be removed *only* by a skilled ophthalmologist under surgical conditions.

☐ **Orbital rim injury**

If orbital rim injury is suspected, x-rays should be done and a visual acuity test performed. The patient should be observed closely for asymmetry of the

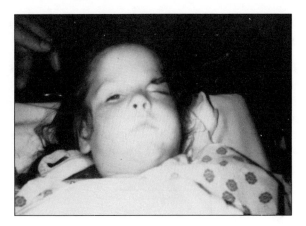

Figure 7.1 A penetrating eye injury

face and other deformities. 'Bulging' of one eye suggests an interruption of the support of the orbit. Any drainage should be examined for CSF, and periorbital ecchymosis (the classic 'black eye') suggests fracture and should be investigated. Emergency treatment requires ice and elevation if the patient's other injuries permit, and evaluation for surgical repair.

☐ **Eyelid laceration**

This condition is rare. Nevertheless, both eyelids must be examined and any trauma noted, particularly if it involves the lacrimal duct or margin. These injuries are associated with damage to the globe of the eye and to the face. Consequently these areas also must be thoroughly inspected.

Preparation for repair consists of irrigating with normal saline solution and cleaning the surrounding tissue. Surgical repair requires small sutures and good after-care instructions. Eyelids heal very quickly, and it is important that patients have sutures removed at the appropriate time to avoid excessive scarring. Usually the physician will recommend that sutures be removed from the eyelid repair 2–3 days post-injury. A reconstructive surgeon may need to be consulted if eyelid injury is extensive or involves tearing, as with animal bite injuries. Tetanus immunization is always recommended.

☐ **Injury to the globe**

Blunt injury to the eyeball may cause compression of the iris by aqueous humour, causing haematoma or pressure in the anterior chamber. The patient should have both eyes patched to decrease movement, be sedated and put on bed rest, and instructed concerning the importance of quiet and the severity of the injury. Diuretics and steroids may be given to decrease intra-ocular pressure. A combination of blunt injury to the globe and fracture of the orbital floor is known as a 'blow-out fracture'. On observation the examiner may notice periorbital haematoma, haemorrhage enophthalmos, diplopia, or limited eye movements. X-ray examination will confirm the diagnosis and dictate the patient's therapy.

This condition may be treatable by packing the maxillary sinus or surgical repair. The team leader should anticipate this, apply a cold pack to the eye, and begin preparing the patient for the appropriate procedure.

☐ Penetrating injury

Penetrating injury to the eye is an emergency. The patient should be reassured and instructed not to touch the impailing object or move his head. The offending object should be stabilized; then an x-ray to determine location made, both eyes patched, and the patient prepared for surgery.

■ Nose trauma

Nasal fractures occur frequently when the face sustains trauma, due to the nose's prominence and location. It may be the first and only structure injured, absorbing the energy of the injury. Conversely, it may be associated with major injuries to the face and head. Thorough examination must be made to avoid missing injuries to associated structures which may be more significant that the obvious nasal injury.

When deformity, oedema and/or epistaxis are noted, x-ray examination should be performed to identify fractures. Ice and elevation of the head of the bed can reduce swelling and bleeding. The patient should be considered for preparation for surgery, depending on the severity of the injury and the availability of the surgeon.

☐ Epistaxis

Epistaxis, or nosebleed, can present airway patency problems if the patient is unable to spit or swallow clots of blood in the oropharynx. The patient's ability to swallow and control secretions is an important observation in determining the significance of epistaxis. When estimating blood loss in a multiply injured patient, it is important to recall that a fair amount of blood from nosebleed can be swallowed and go unnoticed. Also, blood is very irritating to gastric mucosa, and patients with posterior nosebleeds who are swallowing even small amounts of blood frequently vomit. The team should keep this in mind and be prepared to log-roll the patient if his condition allows, or have suction on hand to remove the vomitus and protect the airway.

Anterior bleeding may be controlled by direct pressure for 6–7 minutes over the bleeding site, by packing the nose, or by cauterization with electrocautery or silver nitrate. The patient should be reassured and advised to rest quietly.

Posterior nosebleeds may be effectively treated with the insertion of a urinary catheter into the naris that is bleeding. The bulb is inflated with air (not water, due to the risk of aspiration if the bulb ruptures) and the catheter is gently snugged up to produce gentle direct pressure at the opening of the nasopharynx.

■ Ear trauma

Unlike the rest of the soft-tissue structures of the head and face, the ear does not have good vascularization. It is composed almost solely of cartilage and skin, with no muscle and little fat. Injuries of ears therefore tend not to heal well, and require special care in cleaning, suturing and dressing. Frequently injuries to the ears occur as a result of human or animal bites, and infection is a major concern. It is important to know the history of the event and to consider associated head injuries; any blood or fluid draining from the ears should be examined for cerebrospinal fluid and neurological checks should be made initially and repeatedly to rule out occult head injuries.

□ Laceration of the pinna

Generally these lacerations are repaired in the emergency department unless there is extensive tissue damage such as might cause poor cosmetic results. All lacerations should be repaired without the use of adrenaline in the local anaesthetic preparation to prevent increased vasoconstriction in this area of already poor circulation. The area to be repaired should be prepared very well to prevent infection, and the ear should be well padded with loose fluffy dressings that will avoid pressure on the injured ear and possible necrotic injury. Sometimes a complete amputation of a part of the ear occurs, and rapid surgical repair is the patient's only opportunity for saving the injured ear.

□ Haematoma of the pinna

Blunt injury to the ear may cause bleeding between the anterior and posterior layers of the pinna, causing haematoma or 'cauliflower ear'. Usually these injuries will appear hot, red and very painful, and will require aspiration.

☐ Tympanic membrane injury

A small sharp object or excessive pressure over the ear may cause the tympanic membrane to rupture. The conscious patient will usually describe a sudden onset of very sharp pain, tinnitus, vertigo, and possibly hearing changes in the affected ear. There may be bleeding from the ear, and again the medical team leader should confirm that the blood does not contain CSF. It is important not to put any objects into the ear to explore the injury; small lacerations usually heal on their own. If there is an unusual amount of bleeding, the patient may have a large injury that requires surgical repair.

■ Summary

Facial, eye, nose and ear injuries should first be considered as clues that the patient has been struck with sufficient force to have caused a brain or neck injury. Blood loss and potential airway compromise from oedema, blood clots and facial deformity due to fractures should be ruled out in the initial evaluation of the patient. Awareness and observation of ongoing blood loss and the potential for increasing soft-tissue oedema should always remain a concern until the patient is stable. Eye injuries must be considered an ophthalmic emergency until the vision-testing has been completed and all foreign bodies and penetrating objects have been removed by the appropriately skilled individual. Special dressing techniques for eye and ear injuries should be considered to maximize healing and prevent further damage during recovery.

■ References and further reading

Gardiner P 1979. *ABC of Ophthalmology*. London: BMJ Publications.
Hutchinson I, Lawler M & Skinner D 1991. Major maxillofacial injuries. In Skinner D, Driscoll P & Earlam R (eds): *ABC of Major Trauma*. London: BMJ Publications.
Hodgkinson D, Lloyd D, Nicholson D, *et al.* (in press) The face. In Nicholson D & Driscoll P (eds): *ABC of Assessing Emergency Radiographs*. London: BMJ Publications.
Ludman H 1981. *ABC of Ear, Nose and Throat*. London: BMJ Publications.
Ragge N & Easty D 1990. *Immediate Eye Care*. Aylesbury: Wolfe.

Sheehy S 1992a. Ear, nose, throat, facial and dental emergencies. In Sheehy S, Marvin J & Jimmerson C (eds): *Emergency Nursing, Principles and Practice,* 3rd edn. St. Louis: C V Mosby.

Sheehy S 1992b. Eye emergencies. In Sheehy S, Marvin J & Jimmerson C (eds): *Emergency Nursing, Principles and Practice*, 3rd edn. St. Louis: C V Mosby.

Sheehy S, Marvin J & Jimmerson C 1992. *Manual of Clinical Trauma Care: the first hour*. St. Louis: C V Mosby.

Chapter 8

Spinal trauma

Peter Driscoll, Olive Goodall
and Robert Harvey

Objectives

The objectives of this chapter are for members of the trauma team to understand:

- the types of forces responsible for spinal injury;
- the differences between primary, secondary and partial neurological damage;
- the differences between neurological and spinal shock;
- the assessment and management of the patient with a suspected spinal injury.

■ Introduction

Spinal cord injuries commonly affect the young, fit and active members of the society. Furthermore, in many cases the damage is only partial. Consequently some recovery is possible provided the patient is resuscitated appropriately. It follows that the trauma team must maximize this chance of recovery by maintaining adequate tissue oxygenation and stabilizing the spinal column correctly. A systematic guide to achieving these goals will be described in this chapter.

■ Applied anatomy

The vertebral column is made up of separate bones (vertebrae) which provide protection and support for the spinal cord whilst allowing mobility. Figure 8.1 demonstrates the features of a vertebra. These bones are held together by a series of ligaments, including the intervertebral discs (Figure 8.2). The vertebral column is also completely surrounded by paravertebral muscles.

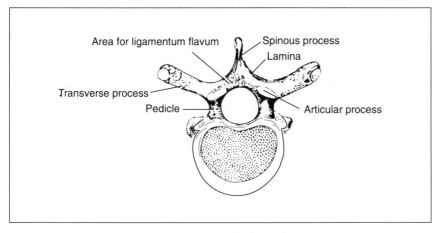

Figure 8.1a   Standard vertebra
Source: Adapted from © Last R 1985. *Anatomy: regionally applied*, 7th edn. Edinburgh: Churchill Livingstone. Reproduced by kind permission.

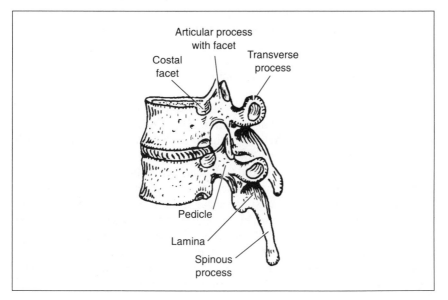

Figure 8.1b   Standard vertebrae
Source: © Last R 1985. *Anatomy: regionally applied*, 7th edn. Edinburgh: Churchill Livingstone. Reproduced by kind permission.

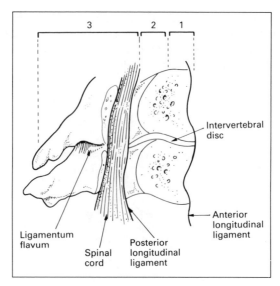

Figure 8.2   Cross-section of the vertebral column, including ligaments and discs

The stability of the vertebral column depends on the integrity of the ligaments mentioned. Schematically, they can be divided into three vertical complexes. The anterior complex consists of the anterior longitudinal ligaments and the anterior half of the intervertebral discs. The middle complex is made up from the posterior longitudinal ligaments and the posterior half of the intervertebral discs. The posterior complex is made up of the remaining intervertebral ligaments and joints (Figure 8.2), and is structurally the most important. If any two these complexes are torn the vertebral column will become unstable.

The spinal cord runs down the spinal canal to the level of the second (adult) or third (baby) lumbar vertebra. This region is called the cauda equina, and it is here that the spine splits into the nerve roots for the lower limbs. In a similar fashion to the brain, the spine is covered with three meningeal layers, blood vessels and CSF. The outer, dural, layer is separated from the bony canal by a space loosely filled with fat and blood vessels.

The size of this space varies, depending on the relative diameters of the spinal cord and the spinal canal. In the region of the thorax the space is very small because the spinal cord is relatively wide. In contrast, there is a large potential space at the level of C2. Consequently injuries in this area are not automatically fatal because there is a potential space behind the dens. This has been described in Steel's 'rule of three' (Box 8.1).

BOX 8.1   Steel's 'rule of three'

One-third of C1's spinal canal area is occupied by the odontoid, one-third by the intervening space and one-third by the spinal canal.

The space in the spinal canal may be reduced in some patients due to spinal stenosis (narrowing), or the presence of posterior osteophytes (bony outgrowths). An awareness of this space is therefore important because it controls the body's ability to adapt to injuries that further reduce the size of the spinal canal.

The spinal cord consists of bundles of nerve fibres transmitting impulses to and from the higher centres (Figure 8.3a). The posterior columns carry sensory fibres transmitting vibration, fine touch and proprioception. The cortico-spinal column carries motor fibres which do not cross over to the opposite side until they reach the medulla in the brain stem (see Chapter 6). In contrast, the spino-thalamic tracts, which carry pain, temperature and coarse-touch fibres, cross over within two vertebral bodies of entering the spinal cord (figure 8.3b). This feature, of certain fibres crossing the spinal cord, is important in interpreting the clinical signs after spinal injury.

■ Mechanisms of injury

Box 8.2 lists the incidents which commonly lead to spinal injury.

BOX 8.2   Common causes of spinal injury

- Road traffic accidents
- Sporting accidents
- Falls from a height
- Stab wounds to the back

Road traffic accidents (RTAs)

Road traffic accidents produce approximately 50 per cent of the spinal injuries in the UK. They can result from side, rear or front collision. Inspection of the windscreen may reveal a 'bulls-eye' pattern (see Figure 1.1) due to the patient's face or head hitting the glass. This is associated with neck and head injuries. Ejection from the car increases the chance of a spinal injury to approximately 1 in 13.

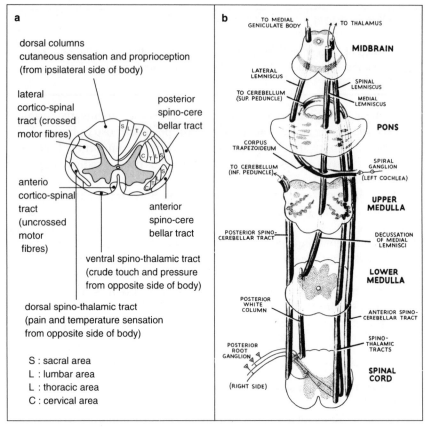

Figure 8.3a   Cross-section of the spinal column showing the long tracts

Figure 8.3b   Longitudinal diagram of the spine showing cross-over of spino-thalamic tract fibres

Source: © Last R 1985. *Anatomy: regionally applied*, 7th edn. Edinburgh: Churchill Livingstone. Reproduced by kind permission.

Rear-end collisions can produce hyperextension of the neck followed by hyperflexion (the 'whiplash phenomenon').

Unprotected victims such as pedestrians hit by cars or motorcyclists have a high chance of sustaining a spinal injury.

Sporting accidents

The sporting activities which are infamous for producing spinal trauma are rugby (especially after a collapse of the scrum), gymnastics, trampolining, horse-riding, skiing and hang-gliding. Diving is a common cause of neck injuries during the spring and summer months, particularly in young males who have recently drunk alcohol. The victim usually misjudges the depth of the water or dives from too steep an angle and hits his head on a solid surface.

☐ Forces that cause spinal injuries

The common feature of all the mechanisms leading to spinal injury is that the vertebral column is subjected to a series of forces. These can act either singularly or in combination to produce flexion, extension, rotation, lateral flexion, compression and distraction, with the commonest movements being those shown in Box 8.3.

BOX 8.3   Forces that may cause spinal injuries

- Hyperflexion
- Hyperflexion with rotation
- Hyperextension
- Rotation
- Compression

The vertebral column is usually injured at C5/C6/C7 and T12/L1. At these sites flexibility is reduced because the normal forward-facing (lordotic) curve changes to a backward facing (kyphotic) one.

Pure hyperflexion

Pure hyperflexion injuries in the adult frequently occur in the T12–L2 area and in the child at T4/T5. They are usually caused when the patient is wearing only a lap belt and is involved in a road traffic accident with a forward impact. Other common causes are the patient falling in a bent position, or a weight falling on top of his lower back. The forward movement leads to anterior crushing of the lumbar vertebral body and tearing of the posterior ligamental complex. If the vertebral column is distracted at the same time as being hyperflexed then the facet joints can slide forward on one another, but the articular surfaces will usually remain partly in contact with one another. This is known as *subluxation* and it occurs in addition to the injuries described above. However if there is support anteriorly, for example from a lap belt, then this does not occur. Instead there is considerable intervertebral pressure which can result in ligamental damage and the lumber vertebral bodies sustaining a horizontal fracture. The latter is known as a *chance fracture* and it usually occurs in the L1–L3 region.

Pure hyperflexion can occur in the cervical vertebrae but is less common because the forward movement is limited by the chin hitting the sternum. Extreme hyperflexion (e.g. diving accidents) can result in all the cervical ligaments being torn. In addition, the violent contact between two adjacent cervical vertebral bodies may be sufficient to fracture the anterior superior corner of the inferior vertebrae. This is known as a *tear-drop fracture* and it is commonly found in the C5/C6 region. In view of the associated ligamental damage, this condition leaves the patient's neck mechanically unstable.

Hyperflexion with rotation

Hyperflexion with rotation can cause significant disruption of the posterior stabilization elements of the vertebral column. This is responsible for 50–80 per cent of the cervical injuries. In mild situations the stabilizing elements are stretched, but in severe cases they can tear and the facet joints, lamina, transverse processes and vertebral bodies may fracture. In the cervical region the relatively flat facets may dislocate. At the same time the spinous processes of C6/C7 can be avulsed by the taut interspinous ligaments.

Hyperextension

Hyperextension tears the anterior stabilizing elements and can produce an avulsion fracture of the anterior inferior aspect of the vertebral body. Occasionally the posterior aspect of the vertebral body is crushed, with fragments of bone being pushed into the vertebral canal.

A special type of fracture occurs through the pars interarticularis of C2 following hyperextension with distraction or compression. This is known as the *hangman's fracture*, following judicial executions which produce hyperextension and distraction. In extreme cases the fracture gap widens and extends into the C2/C3 intervertebral disc. If there is a distraction component to the mechanism of injury, the vertebral body of C2 is displaced anteriorly and ultimately there is bilateral facet dislocation of C2 on C3.

Rotation

Rotational forces can tear the posterior longitudinal ligamental complex and so have a higher chance of producing instability. This may be associated with a unifacet dislocation. A common site for this type of injury is the T12/L1 junction.

Compression

Compression forces can only be applied to straight parts of the vertebral column, therefore only the cervical and lumbar parts are affected. They are occasionally severe enough to fracture the vertebral bodies and project bone fragments and soft tissue into the spinal canal. An example of this is seen commonly in C5 after diving accidents. In *Jefferson's fracture* the lamina and pedicles of C1 fracture when they are subjected to a compressive force between the occipital condyle and C2. In addition, the transverse atlantal ligament holding the dens in position can be torn. This will allow the skull and C1 to slide forward on C2. This lesion is not automatically fatal because of the potential space behind the dens (remember Steel's rule).

■ Pathophysiology

□ Primary neurological damage

This is a neurological injury resulting directly from the initial insult (Box 8.4). It is usually due to blunt trauma which produces abnormal movement in the vertebral column. In severe cases this leads to ligamental rupture and fractures of the vertebrae.

These movements reduce the space around the spinal canal and also allow bone and soft tissue to impinge directly on the cord (Box 8.4). The potential space around the spinal cord may already be small so the chance of neurological damage is increased.

BOX 8.4 Incidence of neurological injury following fractures or dislocations

Fractures or dislocations	Frequency (%) of neurological injury
Any	14
Cervical spine	40 (50–60 if unstable)
Thoracic spine	10
Thoraco-lumbar spine	35
Lumbar	3

Less commonly the primary spinal damage is caused by penetrating trauma. A localized area of injury is the usual result of stabbings. Much more extensive areas of destruction and oedema occur when the spinal cord is subjected to a large force such as a gunshot (see Chapter 10).

□ Secondary neurological damage

This is deterioration of the spinal cord after the initial insult. The three common causes are mechanical disturbance of the back, hypoxia, and poor spinal perfusion. These effects are additive.

Following an injury, the vertebral column may be mechanically unstable. In these cases the spinal cord could be further damaged by direct pressure or ischaemia if the vertebral column is moved inappropriately. However, secondary deterioration is not induced by careful and coordinated log-rolling of the patient.

Hypoxia can result from any of the causes mentioned in Chapter 3, but significant spinal injury on its own can also produce hypoxia. The reasons for this are listed in Box 8.5. The common underlying problem is usually a lack of respiratory muscle power following a high spinal lesion. Lesions above T12 will involve the intercostal muscles. Injuries above the level of C5 will also block the phrenic nerve and consequently paralyse the diaphragm.

BOX 8.5   Respiratory failure in spinal injury

Tetraplegic
- Intercostal paralysis
- Phrenic N. palsy
- Inability to expectorate
- V/Q mismatch (see Chapter 3)

Paraplegic
- Intercostal paralysis

Inadequate spinal perfusion results from either general hypovolaemia or a failure of the spinal cord to regulate its own blood supply. This failure in autoregulation can occur after cord injury. A fall in mean arterial pressure will therefore produce a reduction in spinal perfusion. Conversely, if the pressure is increased too much then a spinal haemorrhagic infarct could develop.

Secondary damage leads to interstitial and intracellular oedema which further aggravates the deficient spinal perfusion. As this oedema spreads, neurons are squeezed and an ascending level of clinical deterioration will be produced. With high spinal injuries, this process can lead to secondary respiratory deterioration.

☐ Partial spinal cord injury

These types of injuries are becoming more common.

Anterior

This is due to direct compression or obstruction of the anterior spinal

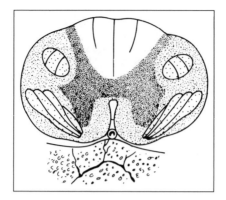

Figure 8.4 Cross-section of the spinal cord – anterior cord damage
Source: © Swain A, Dove J & Baker H 1991. Trauma of the spine and spinal cord. In
Skinner D, Driscoll P & Earlam R (eds): *ABC of Major Trauma*. London: BMJ
Publications. Reproduced by kind permission.

artery. It affects the spino-thalamic and cortico-spinal tracts (Figure 8.4),
resulting in a loss of coarse touch, pain and temperature sensation, and
flaccid weakness. This type of injury is associated with fractures or dislocations in the vertebral column.

Central

This is found usually in elderly patients with cervical spondylosis. Following
a vascular event the cortico-spinal tracts are damaged, with flaccid weakness resulting. In view of the anatomical arrangement in the centre of the
cord, the upper limbs are affected more than the legs and hands.

Sacral fibres in the spino-thalamic tract are positioned laterally to
corresponding fibres from other regions of the body (Figure 8.3). It follows
that anterior and central injuries, which are primarily affecting the midline
of the spinal cord, may not affect the sacral fibres. This leads to the
phenomenon of 'sacral sparing' in which sensation is lost below a certain
level on the trunk but pinprick appreciation is retained over the sacral and
perineal area (Figure 8.5).

Lateral (Brown-Séquard syndrome)

This condition results from penetrating trauma. On the side of the wound,
at the level of the lesion, all sensory and motor modalities are disrupted.
Below this level, however, there is a contralateral loss of pain and temperature sensation and an ipsilateral loss of muscle power and tone (Figure 8.6).

Posterior

This is a rare condition. It results in a loss of vibration sensation and
proprioception.

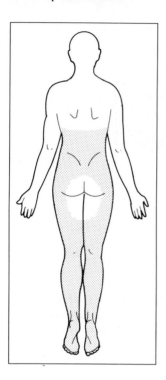

Figure 8.5   Sacral sparing
Source (Figures 8.5 & 8.6): © Harrison M 1990.
Neurological skills: a guide to examination and
management in neurology. London: Butterworths.
Reproduced by kind permission.

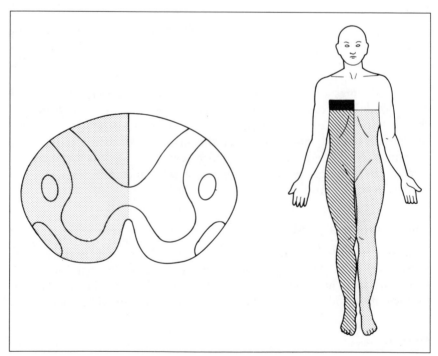

Figure 8.6   Cross-section of the spinal cord – Brown-Séquard syndrome

☐ Special types of shock

Neurogenic shock

Following significant injuries at or above T6 there may be impairment of the sympathetic nervous system. Consequently the vasomotor tone is lost; and if the lesion is high enough, sympathetic innervation of the heart ceases. The result is vasodilatation, hypotension, bradycardia and the loss of temperature control. This is called *neurogenic shock*. It is important to detect because the low blood pressure is not due to true hypovolaemia and should be treated with judicious fluid replacement (see later). The lack of awareness of this phenomenon caused a high percentage of Vietnam war spinal patients to be over-transfused, with significant pulmonary complications developing.

The lack of sympathetic tone also enhances the vagal effect produced by stimulation of the pharynx. This can lead to profound bradycardia.

With incomplete spinal injury some sympathetic control will remain, allowing a normal response to hypovolaemia.

Spinal shock

This refers to the totally functionless condition occasionally seen after spinal injury. The patient has generalized flaccid paralysis, diaphragmatic breathing, priapism, gastric dilatation, and the autonomic dysfunction associated with neurogenic shock. Beevor's sign – that is, movement of the umbilicus when the abdomen is stroked – may be present.

This state can last for days or weeks but areas of the cord are still capable of a full recovery. Parts which are permanently damaged give rise to spasticity once the flaccid state is resolved. Upper motor neuron reflexes will return, below the level of the lesion, if there has been a complete transection of the cord. This is seen as exaggerated responses to stimuli, but there will be no sensation.

■ Standby preparation

With the improvement in pre-hospital training, the ambulance personnel are becoming more aware of the importance of the mechanism of injury. This information is frequently being relayed to the receiving hospital. The team leader must analyse this message to ascertain the chances of spinal injury. For example, there is a 5–10 per cent chance of a cervical injury if the patient is unconscious and has been injured from a fall or road traffic accident.

The team needs to be made aware of the situation if there is a chance that the spine could be injured. Extra care should be taken by all team members to work in a coordinated fashion and not, inadvertently to move or twist any part of the vertebral column.

■ Assessment and management

□ Transfer of patient to trolley

A minimum of five people will be required to transfer the patient if he is not already on a backboard. One team member, usually one of the airway personnel, must stabilize the head and cervical spine with her hands and forearms. On this person's command, four of the team lift the patient vertically off the ambulance trolley, while keeping the spine perfectly level. The fifth member then removes this trolley, allowing the team to place the patient on the resuscitation trolley (see Figure 1.2). **At no time should the patient be subjected to a bending or twisting force.**

If a short spinal board is already in place, the patient still needs to be moved in the coordinated manner described without removing the board. The patient should not be moved by means of the board, if one of the short extraction devices has been used, as this can lead to uncontrolled spinal movement.

□ Primary survey and resuscitation

Patients with a spinal injury are often labelled early on as a specialist problem with the basic rules of trauma management forgotten. Deterioration is looked upon as an urgent need to transfer the patient to the specialist centre instead of managing the spinal hypoxia and hypoperfusion which are causing secondary spinal injuries. It is essential that the team leader does not allow this to happen. About 50 per cent of patients with damage to the spinal cord have other injuries as well.

The initial plan of action is the same as that described in the previous chapters. The individual team members must all work at the same time so that the ABCs are assessed and stabilized as quickly as possible.

(A) Airway and cervical spine

The skills described in Chapter 2 are used by the doctor and nurse to clear and secure the airway whilst simultaneously stabilizing the neck in the neutral position. This has to be carried out without the spine being subjected to any distracting or compression forces. The quickest way to perform this is for the nurse to hold the base of the patient's neck whilst supporting the head between her wrists and forearms (see Figure 2.2). Maintaining neutral alignment reduces the pressure on the spinal arteries and nervous tissue.

Motorcycle crash helmets must be gently removed by two members of the team so that the neck can be stabilized throughout the procedure (see Chapter 1).

Vigorous pharyngeal suction or airway manipulation can produce vagal stimulation if there is an associative cervical spine injury. This can be strong enough to precipitate asystole. In such cases pre-treatment with atropine is required. When the airway has been cleared, the retropharyngeal area is inspected. A haematoma here should increase one's suspicion of a cervical fracture.

The airway takes priority and so intubation is not contraindicated in the presence of cervical injury but inline stabilization must be maintained throughout the procedure. In skilled hands fibre-optic or blind nasal intubation may produce less cervical movement than oral intubation (see Chapter 2).

If a spinal injury is combined with unconsciousness there is an urgent need to secure the airway because aspiration pneumonitis markedly increases the morbidity and mortality of the patient. The chances of aspiration are enhanced in these patients because they usually have a paralytic ileus, the stomach is often full, and there is an increased risk of reflux from an incompetent gastro-oesophageal junction. Furthermore there is no premonitory sign of vomiting.

Once the airway has been cleared and secured, the neck is inspected for tracheal deviation, distended neck veins and wounds. The team leader should remember that injuries to the cervical spine are another cause of tracheal deviation (cf. tension pneumothorax, page 78). The cervical spine can be stabilized with a rigid collar, sandbags and tape or a commercially available apparatus (see Figures 1.4 and 1.5).

In the presence of a spinal injury the conscious patient can become extremely upset. The airway nurse must build up a relationship with the patient and be sensitive to his needs. Neck stabilization can also provoke feelings of claustrophobia in the trauma victim. Therefore, the same nurse must talk and explain the team's actions to the patient. This helps the patient to develop trust and confidence in the team.

The medical staff and nurses should not try to force down the head of the restless patient if he persists in trying to sit up. This type of action only serves to increase the forces acting on the cervical spine and so enhance the chance of injury. In such a situation a less satisfactory state is accepted whereby a rigid collar is put on the patient but the head is not anchored. At the same time, action is taken by the rest of the team to correct the cause of the restlessness.

(B) Breathing

Once the airway has been cleared and secured, the patient must be given 100% oxygen to breathe. It will be clear from the pathophysiology section above that the damaged spine is very sensitive to hypoxia. The types of methods used to administer a high inspired concentration of oxygen are described in Chapter 2.

For logistical reasons, it is usually the team leader who is responsible for examining the chest. Clothing is carefully removed and the thorax examined for the six immediately life-threatening conditions (see Chapter 3). Detection of a fractured sternum is important because it has a strong association with injuries to the thoracic spine in road traffic victims.

Arterial blood-gas measurements and assessment of the respiratory effort are needed. In those patients where intubation is inadequate, ventilatory support is commenced.

(C) Circulation

During the primary survey, the trauma team should not assume that signs or symptoms of shock are simple manifestations of the spinal injury. Even when a spinal injury exists, adequate perfusion needs to be maintained to limit secondary neurological damage.

The team should therefore carry out the normal tasks of the 'Circulation' part of the primary survey (see pages 21–22). Overt haemorrhage must be controlled by direct pressure and two large-bore IV cannulae inserted. After 20 ml of blood have been taken for laboratory tests, the cannulae are connected to two half-litre bottles of colloid. When these tasks have been completed the circulation nurse can measure and record the remaining vital signs (pulse, blood pressure, and core and peripheral temperature). Simultaneously, the circulation doctor must examine for evidence of shock (see Chapter 4).

Bradycardia with hypotension is not found in hypovolaemic shock but if present may be the first indication of a high spinal injury in an unconscious patient. Care must be taken not to over-hydrate these patients because pulmonary oedema can result. A central venous line should therefore be inserted early so that the effects of a fluid challenge on the central venous pressure can be monitored.

In the presence of an isolated cord injury a systolic blood pressure of 90 mmHg is acceptable but the optimum level is unknown. It is therefore important that the patient is observed to regain the normal signs of adequate perfusion.

(D) Dysfunction

This is assessed by the team leader when he or she has completed the examination of the chest. The pupils are tested and the gross neurological response (AVPU) recorded. During the testing asymmetrical weakness may become apparent. This should be noted by the team leader, but the definitive neurological examination must wait until the secondary survey.

(E) Exposure

Once A–D of the primary survey have been carried out, the remaining clothing can be removed, making sure the spine is not moved. It is important to remember to keep all trauma patients covered by a warm sheet when they are not being examined. This is both to prevent the patient's embarrassment and also to avoid the heat loss resulting from vasodilatation which occurs after high spinal injuries.

At the end of the primary survey the team leaders should check that all the allocated tasks have been completed, and that any immediately life-threatening condition has been corrected. If an arterial blood sample has not been taken or the patient has not already been connected to an ECG monitor, these tasks should now be done. Atropine should be given to the tetraplegic patient if the heart rate falls below 50/minute. The venous and arterial blood samples need to be sent to the appropriate laboratories and a radiographer requested to take the three basic x-rays (chest, pelvis and lateral cervical spine).

☐ Secondary survey

The patient must now be examined, in detail, from head to toe. This task, which is usually carried out by the medical team leader, has been described in detail in Chapter 1. He or she must remember that an abdominal injury may be masked in patients with spinal injuries because of the reduction in sensation. In these situations a diagnostic peritoneal lavage or abdominal CT scan can help in detecting intra-abdominal injury.

Throughout the secondary survey it is very important that the patient's vital signs continue to be monitored, so that any deterioration of his state can be detected and quickly brought to the team leader's attention.

The remainder of this section will concentrate on the spinal aspect of this examination. All neurological signs are to be taken seriously, and the team leader should never assume that they are a result of an old injury.

Most of the history-taking will be done at the end of the secondary survey, but if the patient is responsive the medical team leader should ask him how the injury occurred. This gives information about the mechanism of injury. It can also be compared with the witnesses' and ambulance personnel's accounts so that memory gaps can be detected. Most conscious patients with spinal injury will complain of pain in the region of the injury which radiates on movement. The team leader should also enquire if there is absent or abnormal sensation in the limbs and body. If there is no vertebral pain, the patient should be asked to cough and his heels tapped. This can occasionally reveal a painful area in the back. The patient is then requested to move each limb in turn, provided there is no pain or discomfort in the limb or spinal column.

A full neurological examination must be carried out including the cranial nerves and the higher functions. Each dermatome (Figure 8.7) is tested for sensitivity to pinprick (sharp or painful sensation) and cottonwool (fine touch). Ideally this should be carried out on both sides of the patient simultaneously so that the doctor can detect any asymmetry. The tone, power, coordination and reflexes should then be tested and any asymmetry noted. Muscular power can be classified (Box 8.6) to facilitate temporal comparison as well as variation between the right and left and upper and lower limbs.

BOX 8.6   The MRC scale for muscle power

0 – No flicker of movement
1 – A flicker of contraction but no movement
2 – Movement but not against gravity
3 – Movement against gravity
4 – Movement against resistance
5 – Normal power

Partial spinal injury

A complex situation can arise where there is partial spinal damage. As the presence of early spinal activity is very important in predicting recovery, care must be taken to detect these findings in the trauma patient (Box 8.7).

BOX 8.7   Recovery from partial spinal injury

Activity at 72 hrs	% walking after 1 yr
None	0
Partial sensory function	47
Motor activity present	87

In the unconscious patient, important signs can be detected which increase the chances that there is a spinal injury (Box 8.8).

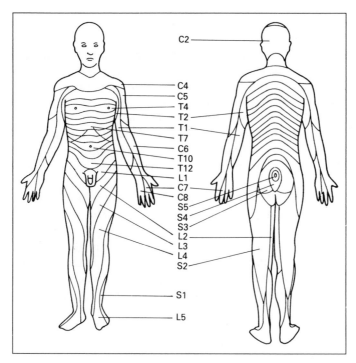

C2
C4
C5
T4
T2
T1
T7
C6
T10
T12
L1
C7
C8
S5
S4
S3
L2
L3
L4
S2
S1
L5

Figure 8.7 Dermatomes

BOX 8.8 Signs of spinal injury in the unconscious patient

- Diaphragmatic breathing
- Hypotension with bradycardia
- Flaccid areflexia (especially a flaccid rectal sphincter)
- Loss of reflexes below the level of the lesion
- Loss of response to pain below the level of the lesion
- Priapism (not necessarily a full erection)

If there is any spontaneous movement it must be noted and the following questions asked:

1   Is the movement truly spontaneous or is it secondary to painful stimuli?

2   Are all the limbs moving equally?

All trauma patients must have a rectal examination. This can be performed either with the patient supine or whilst he has been turned using the log-rolling technique (see below). During this the sphincter tone can be assessed and, in males, the bulbocavernosus reflex tested if spinal injury is suspected. This test involves squeezing the glans penis and detecting any increase in tone of the bulbocavernosus muscle at the base of the penis.

There is a negative response if there is no spinal injury, or if the state of spinal shock exists.

Following this peripheral examination, the vertebral column can be examined. Whilst the airway nurse maintains inline stabilization, the collar, tape and sandbags are removed. The team leaders will already have checked for any overt deformities during the primary survey. They should now reassess to make sure there has been no change and that haematomas, surgical emphysema, tracheal deviation and distended neck veins have not developed. The cervical spinous processes and paravertebral muscles are then palpated and any tenderness, malalignment, bogginess or spasm recorded.

The rigid collar is then reapplied and the team organized so that the patient can be log-rolled in a controlled manner. This requires a minimum of four people (see Figure 1.8). Upon the command of the person in charge of the neck (usually the airway nurse), the patient is rolled away from the team leader. **Care must be taken to ensure the vertebral column is not subjected to any twisting forces.** This requires all the personnel to move the patient simultaneously and by the same amount.

The medical team leader should then inspect the whole back and occiput. Wounds, deformities and marks are noted, and the chest and renal areas palpated for tenderness. The chest is auscultated and the spine and paravertebral muscles palpated for tenderness, malalignment, bogginess and spasm. Any debris and clothes are removed from the trolley and the pressure areas noted before the patient is rolled back in a coordinated fashion.

The Waterlow score should be recorded at this stage because care of the pressure areas starts in the A/E department (see Figure 1.9). This is especially important if the patient is potentially going to be in the same position for several hours as further tests are carried out.

The secondary survey finishes with completion of the patient's history (see Chapter 1). It is important that any previous medical problems affecting the spinal cord or vertebral column are accurately recorded. The doctor should also get as much information as possible about the mechanism of injury, the presence of neurological impairment post-incident, and the treatment provided. This will come from the ambulance personnel, the witnesses and the patient himself.

By the completion of the secondary survey, the trauma victim should have a naso- or orogastric tube and urinary catheter *in situ*. These tubes can help prevent bladder and gastrointestinal distension developing after spinal injury. Urinary catheterization must be performed under strictly aseptic conditions and the tube secured with tape to the abdominal wall or thigh. These actions will help reduce the incidence of infection.

□ **Radiological interpretation**

It is important that a discipline is followed when studying a radiograph so that multiple pathology is not missed. Therefore once the adequacy of the film has been determined, the authors advocate an ABCs approach to radiographic interpretation:

- *A* – Alignment
- *B* – Bones
- *C* – Cartilage and joints
- *s* – Soft tissue

This is usually carried out by the medical team leader. However, it is important that the nurse can read and describe a radiograph when she is working in areas of limited resources. The most important spinal x-ray is the lateral cervical view and this will now be used to demonstrate the ABCs principles of radiographic interpretation.

The lateral cervical spine radiograph

Adequacy of the film

Count the number of vertebrae visible and make sure T1 is visible

An adequate lateral cervical spine radiograph will detect approximately 80–90 per cent of cervical injuries. However, it is only 'adequate' when all the cervical vertebrae, as well as the C7–T1 joint, are visible. To get this type of view, the doctor must remove the sandbags and pull down on the upper limbs as the x-ray is being taken (see Figure 1.6). At the same time, a member of the trauma team is maintaining inline stabilization. In some cases the shoulders cannot be pulled down sufficiently to clear the C7–T1 junction – this is common when there is an injury to the upper limbs or where the patient is very muscular. In these cases a 'swimmer's view' can be taken. If this attempt fails to show the required area then either a CT scan or an oblique view of this area must be carried out.

Most of the diagnostic difficulties occur at the atlanto-axial and cervico-thoracic junctions. The latter is also the place where the majority of missed lesions occur.

(A) Alignment

Check the contours of the lateral view and the interspinous alignment (Figure 8.8)

The anterior and posterior longitudinal lines as well as the posterior facet margins should trace out a smooth contour from T1 to the base of the skull. The spinolaminar line should also be a smooth curve, except at C2 which can be posterior to the line by up to 3 mm. Normally, the spinous processes are nearly equidistant and converge to one point behind the neck of the patient. Divergence is an abnormal sign.

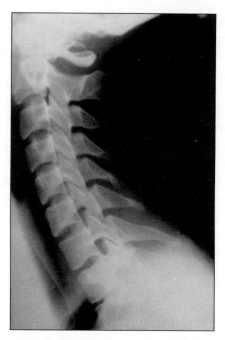

Figure 8.8 Lateral cervical radiograph
with the four longitudinal lines, the
spinal canal and the C1-dens gap
marked

A break in the contour of these lines may be due to displacement or
fracture of a vertebra. The commonest sites are C1/C2 and C6/C7. The
maximum displacement allowed is 3.5 mm. Slippage greater than this is
associated with cervical spine instability because it implies that the posterior
longitudinal ligament is torn.

If the vertebra has slipped less than a half of the width of a vertebral
body then a unifacet dislocation is usually responsible. If the displacement
is greater, then bilateral facet dislocation is present (Figure 8.9).

With hyperflexion injuries there can be an associated 'tear drop' fracture of the anterior superior corner of the vertebral body, a flexed posture,
widening of the interspinous gap, and narrowing of the intervertebral space
anteriorly and widening posteriorly.

Hyperextension of the neck can lead to avulsion of the anterior inferior
corner of the vertebral body, along with opening of the intervertebral space
anteriorly and narrowing posteriorly.

The simple loss of the normal cervical lordosis may be due to a variety
of conditions (Box 8.9) and therefore only indicates that the patient *may*
have sustained a cervical injury.

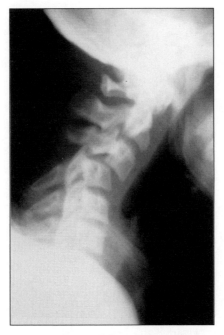

Figure 8.9 Bifacet dislocation

BOX 8.9 Causes of the loss of cervical lordosis

- Muscular spasm
- Age
- Previous injury
- Radiographic positioning
- Hard collar

(B) Bones

Check each vertebra for deformity

If C1 is examined carefully on the lateral view a fracture of the lamina and pedicles may be seen. This is produced by a compressive injury and is known as a Jefferson fracture. It is structurally unstable and a third of these injuries are associated with fractures of C2.

Fractures of the pars interarticularis of C2 (Hangman's fracture) can be quite subtle. Only in extreme cases is there anterior displacement of C2 on C3, opening of the posterior disc intervertebral space and bilateral facet dislocation (Figure 8.10). This condition produces cervical instability.

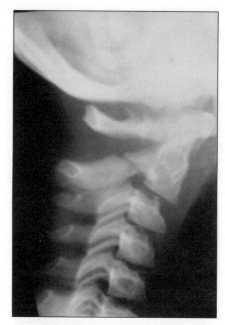

Figure 8.10   Fracture of the pars
interarticularis (Hangman's fracture)

With regard to C3–T1, the heights of the anterior and posterior aspects
of each vertebral body should be the same. A disparity of greater than 2 mm
is significant and implies that there is a compression fracture (Figure 8.11).
A disparity greater than 25 per cent can only occur if the middle and
posterior ligamental complexes have been torn. It is therefore a sign of
mechanical instability.

A 'tear drop' fracture must be distinguished from a simple avulsion
fracture. The former is associated with a significant rupture of the ligamental
complexes. The radiograph therefore shows interspinous widening and
marked soft-tissue swelling. In addition the height of the fragment of bone
is greater than its width. With avulsion fragments the width is usually
greater than its height.

Each spinous process must be checked for avulsion fractures. Then the
spinal canal can be assessed. This should be over 13 mm wide and is
measured from the posterior surface of the vertebral body to the spinolaminar
line (Figure 8.8). Narrowing of the canal occurs following dislocations and
compression fractures which displace segments of bone posteriorly (Figure
8.11). Pre-existing disease and degeneration may also lead to a narrowing of
the canal. In these situations there is a higher chance of the spinal cord being
damaged following any bone displacement.

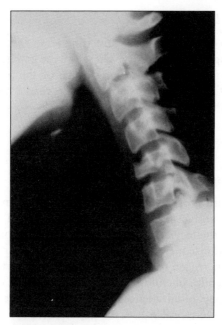

Figure 8.11   Crush fracture of C5

(C) *Cartilage and joints*

Check that the disc spaces are similar and even throughout

Narrowing of the anterior disc space with widening posteriorly indicates there has been a hyperflexion injury (Figure 8.9). Conversely hyperextension produces widening of the anterior disc space with narrowing posteriorly.

Check the facet joints for alignment and width

Normally the facet joint has parallel articular surfaces with a gap of less than 2 mm. Following a unifacet dislocation there is usually soft-tissue swelling and the vertebrae above the lesion are rotated so that both facet surfaces are seen on the lateral view. This feature is called the 'bow tie' sign. Below this level the vertebrae are normally aligned. A bifacet dislocation is associated with forward displacement of the vertebral body (over 50 per cent), widening of the interspinous processes, disc-space narrowing, and soft-tissue swelling. However, there is no rotation of the vertebrae (Figure 8.9).

Check the dens/C1 gap

It is important to remember that the transverse ligament may rupture without there being any bony injury. Therefore the gap between the anterior surface of the dens and the posterior surface of the anterior arch of C1 should be checked in all cases. It is normally less than 3 mm in the adult and less than 5 mm in the child.

(s) Soft tissue

Check the soft-tissue shadows

The 'rule of thumb' is that the gap between C1–C3 and the air shadow, caused by the oro- and nasopharynx, should be less than 7 mm (Figure 8.8). Below the level of the larynx the trachea is separated from the vertebrae by the oesophagus. Consequently the gap between the air shadow (trachea) and the bones is increased to 21 mm in the adult (1 vertebral body width) and 14 mm in the child. In children this gap can be wider due to crying, neck flexion and pre-sphenoidal adenoidal enlargement. The latter leads to an increase in the pre-vertebral soft-tissue gap at C1/C2.

In summary, the stability of the vertebral column is dependent on ligaments which cannot be seen on plain x-rays. Consequently the lateral cervical radiograph is checked for radiological clues of ligamentous injury. It is important to note that even with major spinal injury there could be little abnormal on the plane lateral radiograph.

Box 8.10 lists the features indicative of cervical instability.

BOX 8.10 Radiological findings associated with cervical spine instability

---

- Facet joint overriding
- Facet joint widening
- Interspinous fanning
- Greater than 25% compression of the vertebral body
- Over 10° angulation between vertebral bodies
- Over 3.5 mm vertebral body overriding with fracture

When a cervical spine injury is suspected two further radiographs can be taken (AP and open mouth views) but in most cases the patient will have to be taken to the x-ray department. This is only allowed, therefore, if the patient is haemodynamically stable and when the resuscitation has been completed.

These additional radiographs will detect a further 10–15 per cent of the cervical abnormalities. The 'recommended reading' list at the end of this chapter includes texts which will provide further advice on interpretation of these radiographic views.

Lateral thoracic and lumbar radiographs

The same system as previously described is used to interpret these two radiographs. Once the adequacy of the films has been determined, the 'ABCs' examination is carried out.

Adequacy

Check the adequacy and quality of the films. Count the vertebrae and make sure that all five lumbar vertebrae can be clearly seen along with the lumbosacral junction and also the thoracic vertebrae under investigation.

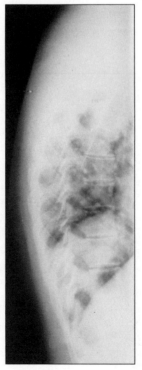

Figure 8.12 Normal lateral thoracic radiograph

(A) Alignment

The anterior and posterior longitudinal lines, as well as the spinolaminar line, should trace out smooth curves (Figures 8.12 and 8.13). These change from kyphotic to lordotic at the T1/L1 junction.

An anterior displacement greater than 25 per cent is usually due to a shearing injury. It is associated with fractures of the facets and tearing of all three ligamentous complexes. The spine is therefore mechanically unstable. Hyperflexion with rotation can also produce anterior displacement due to subluxation or dislocation of the facet joints once the ligaments have been torn. There are not necessarily any fractures to the vertebral bodies in contrast to the pure hyperflexion injury which leads to the fractures described previously.

(B) Bones

Each vertebra must be checked separately for deformity. An anterior/superior wedge fracture indicates that the spine has been subjected to either a hyperflexion or hyperextension injury. With hyperflexion there is associated

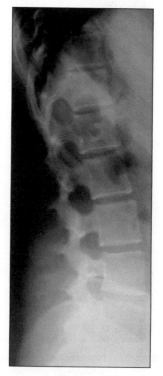

Figure 8.13 Normal lateral lumbar
radiograph

soft-tissue swelling, anterior disc-space narrowing, widening of the posterior disc space, loss of the anterior vertebral height, and, in extreme situations, subluxation of the facet joints.

Hyperextension injuries can lead to widening of the anterior disc space with fracture and posterior displacement of the posterior aspects of the vertebrae.

Chance fractures of the vertebral bodies are best seen on the lateral view and can extend into the laminae and pedicles.

There is usually a fracture of the vertebral body if the anterior vertebral body height is 2 mm less than the posterior height. A 50 per cent disparity is always associated with significant ligamentous damage. Gross disruption of the vertebral body usually indicates that there has been axial compression. This is associated with soft-tissue swelling, retropropulsion of bone fragments into the spinal canal, and anterior wedging.

Isolated fractures of the transverse and spinous processes can occur following direct trauma as well as being part of the pattern of injuries resulting from hyperflexion and hyperextension mechanisms.

(C) Cartilage and joints

The intervertebral disc spaces and facet joints must be checked in the manner described previously for the cervical spine.

(s) Soft tissue

This examination is carried out once the skeletal system has been assessed. Soft-tissue swelling can indicate the presence of an underlying bony or ligamentous injury.

Special radiology

Myelography can be done in conjunction with a CT scan to pick up spinal column or root compression. It is indicated when there is an unexplained deterioration since arrival, an anterior cord syndrome, or a partial cord syndrome which is not improving.

These tests should only be used when there are no contraindications for further investigations and when the patient is haemodynamically stable.

☐ Definitive care

Caution is needed before declaring a patient free from a spinal injury because palpation of the vertebral column is not a foolproof way of detecting vertebral damage. Furthermore, 17 per cent of cervical injuries show no radiological evidence of damage. Therefore, spinal stabilization must be maintained until specialist advice is obtained if a spinal injury is suspected from either the mechanism of the injury or the examination. It will depend on the hospital whether this advice comes from the neurosurgeons, the orthopaedic surgeons or a special centre. The local policy with regard to analgesia in the patient with a spinal injury can also be discussed and instituted.

Cervical injuries may require skeletal traction to reduce the degree of cord compression. Early surgery on the spine is controversial but it is considered if there is an unstable injury, neurological deterioration or a need to correct spinal deformity.

Recent work has shown the advantage of giving high doses of methylprednisolone in the first 24 hours, after spinal injury (Box 8.11).

BOX 8.11   The early use of methylprednisolone following spinal injury

---

- 30 mg/kg IV over 15 minutes immediately
- Then 5.4 mg/kg/hr for 23 hours

If other injuries are present then it is up to the team leader to decide on the management priorities for the patient. This may require abdominal or thoracic surgery. In all cases the spine must be stabilized and adequate oxygenation and perfusion maintained to prevent any secondary neurological damage. In the presence of a pure spinal injury, hypotension is usually corrected with no more than 0.5 to 1 litre of intravenous fluid. Those cases which do not respond may require vasopressors or inotropic support (see Chapter 4). These agents should only be administered if the systolic blood pressure remains less than 80 mmHg when the circulating blood volume has been restored (as indicated by appropriate invasive monitoring).

■ Summary

The management of a patient with a special injury should start at the scene of the incident and continue through to his rehabilitation. The basic principles of resuscitation still apply but it is crucial that the situation is not made worse by careless or uncoordinated handling of the trauma victim.

■ References and further reading

Baker J 1989a. The first-aid management of spinal cord injuries. *Seminars in Ortho*. 4: 2.

Baker J 1989b. The initial hospital management and resuscitation of patients with spinal cord injuries. *Seminars in Ortho.* 4: 15.

Bracken M, Shepard M, Collins W, *et al.* 1990. A randomized, controlled trial of methylprednisolone or naloxone in the treatment of acute spinal-cord injury: results of the second National Acute Spinal Injury Study. *N. Eng. J. Med.* 322(20): 1405.

Cohen A, Bosshard R & Yeo J 1990. A new device for the care of acute spinal injuries: the Russell extraction device (RED). *Paraplegia* 28: 151.

Driscoll P, Ross E & Nicholson D (in press). The cervical spine. In Nicholson D & Driscoll P (eds): *ABC of Assessing Emergency Radiographs.* London: BMJ Publications.

Driscoll P, Ross E & Nicholson D (in press). The thoraco and lumbar spine. In Nicholson D & Driscoll P (eds): *ABC of Assessing Emergency Radiographs.* London: BMJ Publications.

Folman Y & Masri W 1989. Spinal cord injury: prognostic indicators. *Injury* 20(2): 92.

Grundy D, Penny P & Graham L 1991. Diving into the unknown. *Br. Med. J.* 302: 670.

Hoffman J, Schriger D, Mower W, *et al.* Low-risk criteria for cervical-spine · radiography in blunt trauma: a prospective study. *Ann. Emerg. Med.* 21: 1454.

Majernich T, Bieniek R & Houston J 1986. Cervical spine movement during orotracheal intubation. *Ann. Emerg. Med.* 15(4): 417

Mirvis S, Diaconis J, Chirico P, *et al.* 1989. Protocol-driven radiologic evaluation of suspected cervical spine injury: efficacy study. *Radiology* 170: 831.

Mirvis S, Young J, Lim C, *et al.* 1987. Hangman's fracture: radiologic assessment in 27 cases. *Radiology* 163: 713.

Oller D 1990. The relationship between face or skull fractures and cervical spine and spinal cord injuries: a review of 13,834 patients. *34th Ann. Proc. AAAM.* 1: 315.

Ravichandran G & Silver J 1984. Recognition of spinal cord injury. *Hospital Update* 10: 77.

Shaffer M & Doris P 1981. Limitations of crosstable lateral view in detecting cervical spine injuries: a retrospective analysis. *Ann. Emerg. Med.* 10(10): 508.

Swain A, Dove J & Baker H 1991. Trauma of the spine and spinal cord. In Skinner D, Driscoll P & Earlam R (eds): *ABC of Major Trauma.* London: BMJ Publications.

Toscano J 1988. Prevention of neurological deterioration before admission to a spinal cord injury unit. *Paraplegia* 26(3): 143.

Wilberger S 1990a. Initial management of spine and spinal cord injury. *Top. Emerg. Med.* 11: 24.

Wilberger S 1990b. Radiologic evaluation of spinal trauma. *Top. Emerg. Med.* 11: 30.

Chapter 9

Extremity trauma

Peter Driscoll, Carl Gwinnutt
and Simon Brook

Objectives

The objectives of this chapter are for members of the trauma team to understand:

- the importance of different mechanisms of injury;

- the importance of pre-hospital information;

- the causes of life- and limb-threatening injury;

- the assessment of the patient with a skeletal injury;

- the management of the patient with a skeletal injury.

■ Introduction

Extremity trauma often has a marked visual impact and may distract the team away from other, life-threatening injuries. Injuries to the extremities are extremely common, with approximately 70 per cent of multiply injured patients having either fractures or dislocations.

To manage these patients appropriately, the trauma team has to be able to identify and treat life-threatening conditions before the limb-threatening ones. The latter should than be dealt with before the minor problems. However, minor injuries must not be ignored as they can give rise to prolonged morbidity and rehabilitation problems if not managed correctly in the resuscitation room. It follows that the same diligence and care spent on the serious injuries must be extended to the management of the minor problems at the appropriate time.

■ Applied anatomy

☐ Bone

The size, shape and consistency of bone varies with age. Old bones require less force to break them than young ones because they are more brittle and often osteoporotic. In children, fractures may involve the growth plate (epiphysis), which if not accurately reduced can subsequently lead to deformity (see Chapter 11).

Bone is a living tissue with a generous blood supply, and can bleed profusely after injury. Furthermore, blood loss from adjacent vessels and oedema in the surrounding tissues (Chapter 4) can be severe enough to cause hypovolaemic shock (Box 9.1). These volumes can be much higher if there is an open fracture (see later).

BOX 9.1   Approximate blood loss with some common closed fractures

- Pelvis: 1–4 litres
- Femur: 1–2.5 litres
- Tibia: 0.5–1.5 litres
- Humerus: 0.5–1.5 litres

Fractures are usually extremely painful because of the extensive sensory nerve supply to the periosteum. Analgesia will be required not only for humanitarian reasons but also because pain can reduce the tolerance of the patient to hypovolaemia (see Chapter 4).

☐ Nerves

In the limbs, nerves tend to lie close to the long bones in neurovascular fascial bundles (i.e. associated with blood vessels). This close proximity is particularly noticeable around joints. Consequently joints are prone to nerve damage following fractures and dislocations.

Nerves can be damaged in three basic ways (Box 9.2). All three will produce a disruption of impulse conduction, but the potential for recovery is highest if the nerve is being compressed: this is known as *neuropraxia.*

BOX 9.2   Causes of nerve injury

- Transection
  - penetrating trauma (see Chapter 10)
  - fracture
- Compression
  - soft-tissue swelling
  - fracture
  - splints
- Stretching
  - traction injury
  - high-energy transfer (see Chapter 10)

☐ **Arteries**

The arterial wall consists of three layers. Following trauma, the inner layer (intima) may be the only part of the artery damaged. This can be very difficult initially to detect clinically because distal pulses and capillary refill are maintained (see Chapter 4). More overt signs are seen only if a significant area of the lumen is occluded.

When all the layers of the artery are transected tranversely the vessel will go into spasm, due to constriction of the muscle fibres in the media, limiting the degree of blood loss. Conversely, if there is a partial or longitudinal laceration, the muscle spasm tends to keep the hole in the vessel open and blood loss continues.

☐ **Veins**

Veins have little muscle fibre in their walls and therefore cannot contract when they are damaged. Consequently, blood continues to leak from the lumen until direct pressure is applied.

☐ **Limb compartments**

The muscles in the limbs are grouped into compartments formed by fascial sheaths (Figure 9.1). Running within these compartments are the nerves and blood vessels which supply the limb. Following injury, muscle swelling is contained within these compartments and there is a rise in tissue pressure. Necrosis of nerves and muscles, resulting from tissue ischaemia, will ensue once the compartment pressure exceeds capillary pressure. This condition is known as the *compartment syndrome* and can result from a variety of causes (Box 9.3).

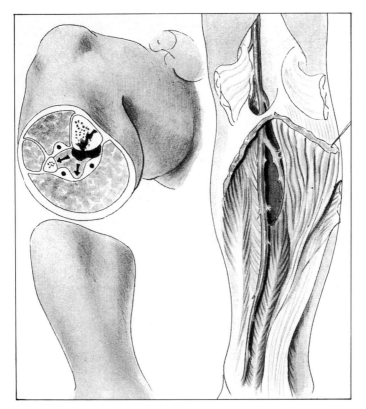

Figure 9.1 Cross-section of the lower leg, showing the compartments
Source: © Landon B, Driscoll P & Goodall J 1993. *The Atlas of Trauma Management*. Carnforth, Lancashire: Parthenon. Reproduced by kind permission.

BOX 9.3   Causes of compartment syndrome

- Crushing injury
- Open or closed fracture
- Prolonged compression of a limb in an unconscious patient
- Restoration of blood flow to a previously ischaemic limb

■ Pathophysiology

☐ Fracture

This is defined as a break or disruption in the normal physical continuity of a bone; it usually results from trauma. A fracture is termed 'pathological' if the bone has already been weakened by a disease process such as osteoporosis or tumour. Even minor forces may be sufficient to cause a break in these cases.

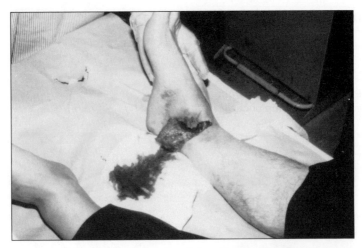

Figure 9.2   A compound fracture of the ankle

Open (compound) fractures

These have a surface wound which leads from the overlying skin to the fracture site (Figure 9.2). The skin damage can be produced by an external, blunt or penetrating source. Alternatively the wound may be caused by bone rupturing through the skin at the time of the injury.

Closed fractures

These have no overlying skin wound but there may still be extensive subcutaneous damage.

☐ Subluxation and dislocation

Trauma can lead to a partial (subluxation) or complete (dislocation) loss of congruity between the articulating surfaces of a joint. These may be associated with a fracture of one or more of the bones. As these combination injuries can rarely be diagnosed clinically, x-ray examination will be required in all cases.

☐ Crush injuries

These occur in a variety of ways (Box 9.4) and may result in muscle destruction secondary to ischaemia (rhabdomyolysis). In additional there is often associated bone damage (Figure 9.3).

BOX 9.4   Examples of crush injuries

- Trapped under fallen masonry
- Trapped in a car following a road traffic accident
- Prolonged use of the PASG (see Appendix 9.1)
- Prolonged compression of an extremity by the patient's own body (this is seen only in the unconscious patient)

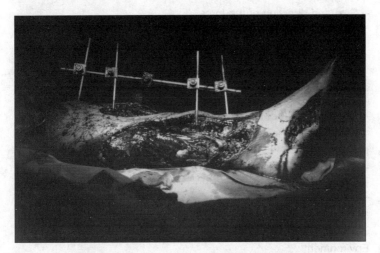

Figure 9.3   A crush injury of the lower leg
Source: © Mr R Harvey. Reproduced by kind permission.

The ischaemia results in loss of integrity of the muscle cells, and the intracellular constituents are released into the plasma, causing myoglobinaemia, and raised levels of potassium, phosphate and uric acid.

Until the limb is released, there is little systemic effect. However, once re-perfusion starts, plasma and blood leaks into the surrounding soft tissues. In severe cases this can cause hypovolaemia.

The combination of hypovolaemia and myoglobinaemia can lead to acute renal failure, and hyperkalaemia may precipitate a cardiac arrest. Ultimately the devitalized tissue has a high chance of becoming infected. This in turn results in the release of further toxins systemically.

■ Mechanisms of injury and pre-hospital information

In the trauma patient, a combination of forces may contribute to the pattern of injury. These can be direct, from blunt or penetrating trauma, or indirect, from rotational or shearing forces. Trying to put all these various forces together to determine how the patient was injured is complicated. However, a great deal of important information can be gained from a description of events and the ambulance personnel should be trained to obtain and pass on this information (Box 9.5).

BOX 9.5   Pre-hospital information required in extremity injury

- Time of the incident
- Mechanism
  - Size and direction of the force
  - For a road traffic accident:
    - Patterns of damage in the vehicle
    - Ejection from the vehicle
    - Position of the patient in the car
    - The use and type of any seatbelt
  - Pedestrian
  - Crushing injury
  - Fall from height

- Initial findings
  - Posture
  - Open fracture
  - Neurovascular supply
  - Soft-tissue damage (Figure 9.4)
  - Estimation of blood loss

- Environment
  - Temperature
  - Contamination
  - Duration
  - Flames; explosion; smoke

- Management
  - Nature
  - Effect

For example, in the case of Figure 1.1 the ambulance personnel might report: 'A frontal impact with a "bull's eye" pattern on the windscreen. The steering column was collapsed and there were indentations in the dashboard.'

The possible injuries sustained by the driver of a car in these circumstances are shown in Box 9.6. If the patient had been ejected from the car, there would be a greater chance of multiple injuries as well as a significant risk of neck and spinal damage.

A completely different pattern of injuries is produced in the patient who has fallen from a height and landed on his feet (Box 9.7).

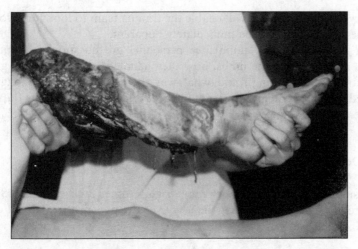

Figure 9.4   A degloving injury

BOX 9.6   Injuries to a car driver likely to result from frontal impact

- Facial fractures
- Obstructed airway
- Cervical injury
- Cardiac contusion
- Flail chest/fractured ribs
- Liver and/or splenic injury
- Fractured patella
- Fractured femur
- Posterior dislocation of the hip
- Acetabular fracture

BOX 9.7   Injuries likely to result from falling from a height

- Calcaneal compression fractures
- Ankle fracture
- Tibial plateau fractures
- Pelvic vertical shear fracture
- Vertebral wedge fracture
- Cervical injury
- Dissecting thoracic aorta
- Ruptured main bronchi

This type of information will enable the trauma team to look for secondary injuries which may not be immediately apparent.

It is essential that ambulance personnel are questioned about their initial assessment of the limbs, how they handled any problems (e.g. joint reduction and splinting), and what was the effect of these management procedures. This will give the team further indications concerning the extent of the tissue damage.

☐ Occult injuries

Occasionally an obvious injury may disguise other injuries (Box 9.8). It is therefore very important that the *whole* of the patient is examined during the secondary survey.

BOX 9.8 Examples of occult injuries

- A facial injury may overlie an unstable cervical spine
- A thoracic injury may be associated with a fractured shoulder girdle
- A muscular thigh can make difficult the detection of a femoral fracture
- An obvious injury on one side may draw attention away from an injury on the other side of the patient
- An obvious injury on the anterior aspect may draw attention away from an injury on the back of the patient

---

☐ Environment

Warm environments are conducive to infection and render the tissues more vulnerable to hypoxia. Cold environments increase the chances of hypothermia (see Chapter 13); and if the patient has been in water, wounds have a high chance of becoming infected.

■ Assessment and management

☐ Primary survey and resuscitation

This is carried out in the ABC manner described in Chapter 1. The team leaders must make sure that personnel do not become distracted from their tasks by a spectacular limb injury.

The aim of the primary survey is to identify and correct any immediately life-threatening conditions. With regard to extremity trauma, this means identifying and controlling massive haemorrhage (Box 9.9). Other extremity trauma is managed in the secondary survey.

BOX 9.9   Life-threatening orthopaedic injuries

- Traumatic amputation proximal to the knee or elbow
- Major vascular injury
- Pelvic disruption
- Haemorrhage from an open fracture
- Multiple long-bone fractures
- A severe crushing injury to the pelvis

Haemorrhage control

Any external bleeding point should have a pressure bandage placed over it by one of the circulation nurses, after the medical team leader has noted the degree of haemorrhage. Attempting to clamp vessels in the resuscitation room wastes time and may lead to further tissue damage.

Tourniquets increase tissue necrosis and are therefore reserved for cases where the limb is deemed unsalvageable. If the decision is taken to use them, one of the circulation nurses must note the time the tourniquet was inflated.

In cases of haemorrhage from major pelvic fractures, the medical team leader should consult the orthopaedic senior on call (if he or she is not a member of the trauma team) to determine whether the patient would benefit from stabilization of the pelvis by external fixation. The nursing team leader should know how to obtain the equipment for this procedure if it is not routinely stocked in the resuscitation room.

The PASG can be of some use in stemming the bleeding from a disrupted pelvis, while equipment and expertise are being assembled.

Intravenous fluid administration

Haemorrhage control should be accompanied by the insertion of two large-bore intravenous lines. When choosing the site for these cannulae, care must be taken to ensure that they are not placed distal to vascular or bony damage as this would allow the infused fluid to leak. Initially 1 litre of colloid should be given, followed by blood if the state of the patient or his response indicates a need (see Chapter 4).

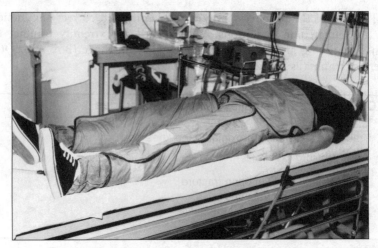

Figure 9.5   PASG around a patient's legs and abdomen

Exposure

Rings and all other constricting jewellery must be removed during the exposure phase of the primary survey. Care must be taken removing clothing, because movement of a fractured limb may not only cause severe pain, but also exacerbate bone and soft-tissue injuries. In certain units, patients will arrive with a PASG suit already on and inflated (Figure 9.5). **It is extremely important that this suit is not suddenly deflated because circulatory collapse could be precipitated.** A fuller description of this garment is given in Appendix 9.1 at the end of the chapter.

☐ Secondary survey

With regard to the extremities, the objectives of the secondary survey are to identify and manage any limb-threatening conditions. Minor injuries can be dealt with once this has been achieved. *Limb-threatening injuries* are defined as injuries that will result in the loss of function of part or all of a limb (Box 9.10).

The limbs are examined using a 'look, feel and move' technique.

BOX 9.10   Limb-threatening injuries

- Vascular injury proximal to the elbow or knee
- Major joint dislocation
- A crush injury
- An open fracture
- A compartment syndrome
- A fracture with a major nerve injury

Look

All the extremities must be inspected for swellings, deformities, bruising, wounds, marks and skin colour. The affected limbs should then be compared with the corresponding areas on the opposite side. Shortening or rotation usually indicates that there is a proximal fracture or dislocation.

Feel

The assessor should gently feel the limbs, noting any tenderness, crepitus, or vascular impairment (Box 9.11). Patients may also complain of altered sensation. Abnormalities relating to any of these parameters can be caused by local or systemic problems and must be reported to the medical team leader.

BOX 9.11   The 'P' signs of vascular impairment

- *P*allor or *P*urple discoloration of the skin
- *P*erishing-cold skin
- *P*rolonged capillary refill
- *P*ain
  - sudden onset (e.g. emboli or trauma)
  - increased with passive movement (e.g. compartment syndrome)
- *P*araesthesia
- *P*aralysis
- *P*ulse absent or diminished distally

Limb ischaemia quickly affects the peripheral nerves and decreases all types of sensation. Consequently, a finding of general sensory loss in a limb or hand/foot should initially be considered to be due to an ischaemic cause.

It is important to remember that the presence of distal pulses does not rule out vascular compromise or injury. In contrast, a diminished pulse should always be assumed to be due to a vascular injury until it has been excluded.

The assessing clinician must never assume a poor pulse to be due simply to 'vascular spasm'.

Certain factors increase the chances of there being a vascular injury (Box 9.12).

BOX 9.12 Factors increasing the chances of a vascular injury

■ Major joint dislocation
■ Penetrating trauma (especially if a high-level energy transfer was involved)
■ Local contusions
■ Fractures
  – especially humeral-supracondylar region
  – distal femur
  – proximal tibia
  – comminuted open tibia

Portable dopplers can be useful in monitoring peripheral blood flow to an extremity in the resuscitation area. However, if a vascular injury is suspected, arteriography remains the definitive investigation of choice.

Move

Although fractures of long bones are usually obvious (Box 9.13), a systematic survey of all the limbs must be carried out to detect any occult damage, particularly if the patient is unconscious. Adjacent joints must also be checked for associated injuries. Initially, if the patient is conscious, the medical team leader must ask him to move his limbs one at a time, and any weakness and limitation in movement accurately assessed. Careful passive movement is then carried out. This is contraindicated in the situation where the patient refuses to move a limb or where there is an obvious fracture.

BOX 9.13 Clinical signs and symptoms of a fracture

■ Deformity
■ Abnormal movement
■ Crepitus
■ Palpable edges of fractured bones
■ Pain (increased on movement)

As fractures are discovered, the affected limb is splinted, and the distal pulses are checked to ensure that there is no distal vascular impairment.

The nursing team leader must ensure that all the clinical findings have been recorded. This documentation is helped greatly by using pre-drawn body charts on the trauma sheet to record the injuries (see Figure 1.10).

Initial management during the secondary survey

Skin lacerations

Wounds must be inspected for site, size, depth and damage of associated structures (see Chapter 10). Gross contamination can then be removed and the skin defect covered with a sterile dressing. To avoid the pain and contamination of repeated inspections of the wound, a Polaroid™-type photograph is useful. The need for tetanus prophylaxis should be considered at this stage (see Chapter 10).

Fractures and dislocations

Fractures of long bones are usually obvious, but nevertheless a systematic survey of all the limbs must be carried out to detect any occult skeletal damage (Box 9.10). The adjacent joints must also be checked for associated injuries.

Fractures or dislocations which are compromising the distal circulation or surrounding soft tissues must be reduced before the area is x-rayed (Figure 9.6), particularly when the hip, knee, ankle, shoulder and elbow are involved. In these areas marked vascular compromise can occur. However, reducing any bony deformity is very painful and analgesia will be required in the conscious patient (see later). It is essential to record both the pre- and post-reduction neurovascular status from both the medical and the legal points of view.

Following reduction, a lack of improvement in the distal circulation indicates that there may be a vascular injury requiring either further investigations or surgical intervention. It is essential that the advice of a vascular surgeon be obtained urgently.

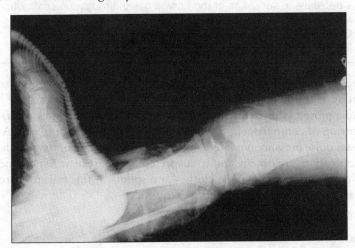

Figure 9.6 X-ray of the crushed lower leg. This radiograph should never have been taken – the limb should have been straightened out before it was x-rayed

If the circulation has improved, a splint should be applied to immobilize the joint above and below the fracture site, and one of the circulation nurses must continue to monitor the perfusion of the limb. Any alterations in the parameters listed in Box 9.8 must be reported to the medical team leader.

It is not advisable simply to rest a fractured limb on pillows. Even though this makes observation easier, it does not help immobilize the injury whilst the patient is being moved. There is therefore potential for further injury, bleeding and pain.

Dislocations have a higher chance than fractures of producing nerve damage and the distal tissues must be tested for sensation, sweating and motor power. However, it must be remembered that muscles can be innervated proximally, so the motor power can be present when sensation has been disrupted.

Compartment syndrome

If an abnormally high compartment pressure is not relieved, ischaemia of muscles and nerves occurs causing a Volkmann's contracture and paralysis. Any limb that has been significantly injured, with or without an underlying fracture, may be affected in this way.

The changes indicating that the compartment pressures are high are listed in Box 9.14; they are best monitored by the circulation nurse.

BOX 9.14   Signs of a compartment syndrome

- Increasing pain in the limb
- An increase in pain on passive movement of the distal limb
- The compartment may feel tense
- A decrease in sensation of the nerves going through the compartment
- Weakness in the affected muscles
- A decrease in pulse pressure in the distal limb (*late* sign)

The trauma team should try to detect this syndrome when pain is the main symptom. It follows that the unconscious patient is more at risk of having an undiagnosed compartment syndrome, and where facilities exist, direct monitoring of compartment pressures should be used (Figure 9.7). A fall in the distal pulse pressure is a late sign and indicates imminent tissue ischaemia. The immediate treatment for a suspected compartment syndrome is to remove all constricting bands, clothes and splints. If this fails to restore the circulation, an urgent fasciotomy is required.

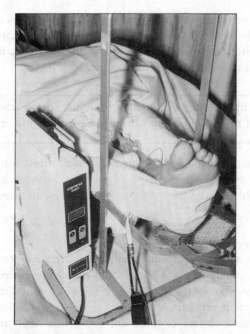

Figure 9.7 Measurement of compartment pressures
Source: © Mr S Royal. Reproduced by kind permission.

hypovolaemia which must be managed in the primary survey. During the secondary survey, the stumps of the amputated extremity should be carefully handled to avoid dislodging blood clots and thereby precipitating further blood loss.

Any amputated limb or digit should be considered for reimplantation. These tissues are only viable for 4–6 hours if they are kept at room temperature, but can last up to 18 hours if cooled. The limb or digit should therefore be wrapped in gauze, moistened with saline, and placed in a waterproof bag and then put into *melting* ice. Care must be taken to ensure that the appendage is not in direct contact with blocks of ice as this can lead to 'frostbite' of the soft tissue. Advice from the local reimplantation specialist can then be sought. The amputated limb or digit and the patient must travel together if transportation to a specialized centre is required.

Crush syndrome

In this group of patients, resuscitation should be carried out bearing in mind the possibility that acute renal failure may develop. In all such cases, the patient's urine should be checked for myoglobin. This is seen clinically as a dark-red or smoky-brown discoloration of the urine. Initially treatment consists of intravenous fluids to restore the circulatory volume. Prevention of acute renal failure depends on maintaining a urine output of 60–150 ml/hr with a pH of 6.5. Occasionally diuretics may be needed to achieve this. Ultimately, the facilities of an intensive care unit are required to monitor and maintain this alkaline diuresis.

One of the circulation nurses must continue to monitor the nature, quality and quantity of the urine output during the primary and secondary survey.

The management of a hyperkalaemic cardiac arrest is beyond the scope of this book: the interested reader is advised to consult the 'further reading' list at the end of this chapter.

Analgesia

As limb injuries are often extremely painful, analgesia is required to manage these patients appropriately. However, in extremity injuries care must be taken to ensure that systemic analgesia does not mask the symptoms of rising compartment pressure.

Good communication, explanation and gentle handling are important preliminaries to pain relief. Correct immobilization of the limb can also be very effective. For example, traction splints (see below) are particularly good at reducing the pain associated with a fractured femoral shaft.

Entonox

This gaseous mixture of 50% oxygen and 50% nitrous oxide can be effective as a short-term analgesic agent, for example during splinting. It is contraindicated when there is a pneumothorax or a fracture to the base of the skull.

Systemic analgesia

Morphine sulphate is an extremely effective analgesic agent. It is best administered intravenously, having been diluted with normal saline to produce a solution of 1 mg/ml. This is then given in small increments until the patient's pain is relieved. The circulation nurse who is monitoring the peripheral vascularity of the affected limb should also monitor the analgesic and respiratory depressant effect of the administered medication, particularly if it is suspected that any other drugs or alcohol have already been taken.

There is no place for oral or intramuscular analgesia in the trauma patient because both sites have poor perfusion. This leads to limited absorption of the drug initially and bolus absorption following resuscitation. As opiates may cause nausea and vomiting, the circulation nurse should administer an antiemetic (e.g. metoclopramide) intravenously with the opiate.

Regional analgesia

This can be extremely effective if skilfully administered to the patient suffering limb trauma. However, it can totally desensitize a limb and so mask the signs of rising compartment pressures. When there is a possibility of a compartment syndrome developing, therefore, this type of analgesia should be administered only at the discretion of a specialist. The nurse monitoring the limb after the regional anaesthesia has been administered must also be very sensitive to any circulatory changes.

Splints

Upper-limb fractures can be immobilized in simple short splints in the position of function. In all cases, the splints should protect the infusion site but leave it exposed so that cannula displacement or 'tissuing' of the IV fluid can be noticed quickly. Hands should be splinted in a position of function by having the patient grip a bandage roll and then bandaging around it.

Fractures of the femoral shaft are effectively immobilized in traction splints which counter the spasm of the quadriceps muscles (Figure 9.8). These devices are simple to apply and are effective at reducing pain, bleeding and deformity.

Vacuum splints or box splints (Figure 9.9) are used for fractures below the knee. The former are extremely useful since the pressure of the vacuum can be controlled and the splints are not circumferential, they are radiolucent and they will conform to the limb deformity.

Once the splint has been applied, one of the circulation nurses must serially reassess the neurovascular condition of the limb and document her findings.

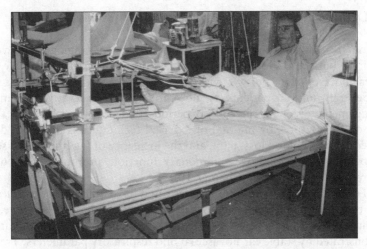

Figure 9.8 A traction splint used for a fractured femur
Source: © Mr R Harvey. Reproduced by kind permission.

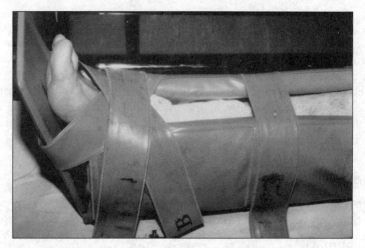

Figure 9.9   A box splint on a fractured ankle

Antibiotics

These should be given intravenously and according to the departmental protocol. Prior to administration, the nursing team leader should find out about allergies and medications taken by the patient before the injury.

By the end of the secondary survey all the information required to complete AMPLE (see Chapter 1) should have been collected. The extent and priority of the injuries can then be determined so that a definitive care plan for the patient can be carried out.

☐ Definitive care

During this phase, specialist investigations such as angiography will be required, but these should only be carried out if the patient is stable from the cardiorespiratory point of view.

Severely injured patients do not thrive on 'conservative' regimes of management, involving prolonged periods of traction or bed rest. Early fixation of fractures by internal or external techniques is preferred due to the reduction in blood loss, pain, and the incidence of fat emboli and sepsis. Early mobilization improves pulmonary function, promotes faster union, and reduces infection (see Chapter 10).

Trauma patients with limb injuries often have other major injuries and need transport to specialist facilities in the same hospital or elsewhere. This should only be done when the patient has been adequately resuscitated as demonstrated by stable cardiovascular and respiratory parameters. Traction splints may not fit ambulances or helicopters and the logistics of urgently transporting these patients need to be thought about in advance. When transportation is prolonged, due consideration must also be given to the patient's pressure areas, with appropriate turning and adjuncts.

Psychological support

Patients are only too well aware of the implications of losing a limb in terms of their ability to live at home, their independence, their work, their social activity and their body image. Appropriate support for the patient and relatives, from the time of their arrival, facilitates their long-term psychological rehabilitation.

■ Summary

A continuity of care of the trauma patient with an extremity injury extends from the scene of the incident right through to rehabilitation. The initial management is aimed at optimal resuscitation. Therefore the life-threatening problems must be treated before limb-threatening and minor conditions are assessed. This facilitates the patient's definitive care and increases his chances of early rehabilitation.

■ Appendix 9.1: The pneumatic anti-shock garment (PASG)

This trouser-shaped compression garment is commonly used in North America and South Africa, but rarely in the UK.

□ Indications

- Blunt abdominal trauma leading to an exsanguinating intraperitoneal or retroperitoneal haemorrhage.
- Pelvic fractures.

□ Procedure

Putting it on

The patient's immediately life-threatening problems are managed appropriately and the vital signs recorded. The suit is then laid flat onto the stretcher, backboard or trolley.

Using the log roll-technique (page 30), the patient is placed on the PASG, and the leg and abdomen sections closed (Figure 9.5). The air tubes can then be connected. Before the trouser legs are inflated, the vital signs should be measured again. The legs are inflated one at a time, followed by the abdominal section if the patient's haemodynamic condition has not improved. **The team must remember to measure the patient's blood pressure, *not* the pressure reading in the trousers.**

If the PASG has been inflated to maximum – that is, if the pop-off valves have been activated – then no further air should be pumped into the suit. The maximum time the PASG can be left on, at this level, is 30 minutes.

It is very important that the patient is continuously monitored while the suit is in place so that any complications can be noted early on.

Taking it off

Deflation should not take place until:

- two intravenous lines are in place and fluid is being infused;
- the patient's vital signs are being accurately and continuously monitored;
- the patient is haemodynamically stable or in the operating room with the fully prepared surgical team;
- the team leader instructs the team to commence deflation.

Deflation is carried out slowly. Should the blood pressure fall by 5 mmHg, the procedure is halted and the infusion accelerated until the blood pressure is restored. Initially the abdominal part is deflated, next one leg and then the other. If there is sudden fall in the blood pressure, the PASG must be reinflated and the hypovolaemia corrected.

☐ Contraindications

Left ventricular failure and pulmonary oedema are *absolute* contraindications. Relative ones are a ruptured diaphragm, a CNS injury or an intrathoracic injury.

☐ Complications

- Compartment syndrome (this can occur with or without fractures being present).
- Increasing dyspnoea.
- Limited access to the abdomen.

■ References and further reading

American College of Surgeons Committee on Trauma 1993. Extremity trauma. In *Advanced Trauma Life Support Course for Physicians*. Chicago: American College of Surgeons.

Fulde G & Harrison P 1991. Fat embolism – a review. *Arch. Emerg. Med.* 8(4): 233.

Herron D 1990. Emergency department nursing management of patients with orthopaedic fractures resulting from motor vehicle accidents. *Nurs. Clin. N. Am.* **25**: 71.

Hoppenfield S 1976. *Physical Examination of the Spine and Extremities*. Norwalk: Appleton & Lange.

Mansfield A & Wolfe J 1993. Trauma. In Wolfe J (ed.): *ABC of Vascular Diseases*. London: BMJ Publications.

McRae R 1991. *Practical Fracture Treatment*. London: Churchill Livingstone.

Nicholson D & Driscoll P (eds) (in press). *ABC of Assessing Emergency Radiographs*. London: BMJ Publications.

Paris R & Trautman D 1992. Pain management. In Sheehy S, Marvin J & Jimmerson C (eds): *Emergency Nursing, Principles and Practice*, 3rd edn. St. Louis: C V Mosby.

Wald D 1989. Upper extremity injuries. *Emergency* **21**: 25.

Willett K M, Dorrell H & Kelly P 1991. Management of limb injuries. In Skinner D, Driscoll P & Earlam R (eds): *ABC of Major Trauma*. London: BMJ Publications.

Chapter 10

Soft-tissue trauma

*Corinne Siddall, Peter Driscoll
and Tim Hodgetts*

Objectives

The objectives of this chapter are for the members of the trauma team to understand:

- the importance of the mechanism of the soft-tissue injury;

- the factors affecting wound healing;

- the assessment of a soft-tissue injury;

- the management of a soft-tissue injury;

- tetanus prophylaxis.

■ Introduction

The assessment of soft-tissue trauma and its subsequent care is an important part of the nurse's role in the trauma team. It is vital that wound care is supported by sound clinical knowledge, based on researched principles, and guided by standardized, realistic and flexible protocols.

Most of the wounds encountered are minor and uncomplicated, and require little attention in the resuscitation room. However, extensive, neglected or infected wounds, and those that involve deeper structures, may require intensive treatment within the emergency department.

■ Applied anatomy and pathophysiology

The principal soft tissue in the body is the skin. This is composed of two main layers, the epidermis and the dermis (Figure 10.1). The outer layer, the *epidermis*, is the first line of defence for the body, and is made up of dead, keratinized cells which are continually shed in a process called *desquamation*. A basement layer of living cells divides continually to form the cells of the epidermis, which are pushed slowly to the surface.

Beneath the epidermis lies a tough and highly elastic layer, the *dermis*. It consists of fibrous and elastic tissue, and encloses many specialized skin structures (Figure 10.1).

Further soft tissue is found under the skin, with varying amounts of fibrous elastic, muscle and adipose tissue. Running through this are blood vessels, nerves, tendons and ligaments.

With increasing age, there is a decrease in the amount of collagen in the skin and subcutaneous tissues as well as a weakening of the elastic fibres. These changes reduce the tensile strength of skin and so allow extensive lacerations to develop with minor trauma. Similar effects are seen following long-term steroid use.

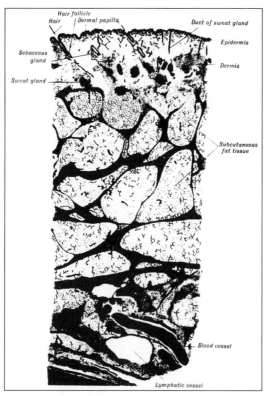

Figure 10.1 Cross-section of skin and subcutaneous tissue: blood vessels, sensory nerve endings, sweat glands, hair follicles, sebaceous glands and lymphatics can be seen

Source: © Bloom W & Fawcett D 1970. *A Textbook of Histology*. London: W B Saunders/ Baillière Tindall. Reproduced by kind permission.

The skin has many vital functions (Box 10.1). It is therefore clear that any disruption to the integrity of the skin may interfere with some, or all, of these actions.

BOX 10.1 Skin functions

- Protects the underlying tissues from infection, radiation, dehydration, direct trauma and corrosive chemicals
- Helps in temperature regulation
- Acts as a sense organ
- Produces vitamin D
- Determines the individual's appearance

■ Mechanisms of injury

Soft-tissue injuries can be divided into 'blunt' or 'penetrating', depending on their cause. Often a combination of both types occurs, a particular example of which is blast injuries, which will discussed later.

The degree of damage that results is directly dependent on how much energy is transferred to the tissues from the agent causing the injury.

☐ Blunt trauma

In blunt trauma, the force is spread over a wide area. This minimizes the energy transfer at any one spot and so reduces tissue damage. Nevertheless, when high energies are involved (see 'Blast injuries' below), considerable tissue disruption can be produced. In low-energy impacts, the clinical consequences are dependent on the organs involved (cf. 'Diffuse axonal injury' in Chapter 6).

Blunt trauma gives rise to three types of forces: shearing, tension, and compression.

Shearing

This results in lacerations and abrasions, and occurs when there are two forces acting in opposite directions.

Skin lacerations following blunt trauma tend to produce irregular wounds which have a higher chance of infection. They are also associated with more damage to the surrounding tissue and excessive scarring compared with low-energy penetrating trauma (see below).

Abrasions involve the removal of the outer layer of skin and have all the problems associated with blunt-trauma lacerations. This type of wound can be of any size and frequently it is contaminated. Significant abrasions can be managed in the same way as burns (see Chapter 12).

Tension

This occurs when a force hits the skin at an angle of less than 90°. It gives rise to avulsions and flap formation because skin is torn away from its subcutaneous base. This type of injury is associated with more tissue damage and necrosis than that found after a shearing mechanism.

Compression

In these cases, the force hits the skin surface at 90°, crushing the underlying tissue. This usually results in significant damage and necrosis of the skin.

The site of impact can often be identified by the presence of a contusion, a haematoma (if a significant number of blood vessels have been damaged), and possibly a breach in the skin. In themselves these injuries are not life-threatening, but they can indicate the site of possible underlying visceral injury.

☐ Penetrating trauma

The clinical consequences of penetrating trauma are dependent on both energy transfer and local damage.

The amount of energy transferred to surrounding tissues

Several factors affect the degree of energy transfer to tissues surrounding the track of the missile (Box 10.2).

BOX 10.2   Factors that affect energy transfer from a missile

- The kinetic energy of the missile
- The mean presenting area of the missile
- The missile's tendency to deform and fragment
- The density of the tissues
- Mechanical characteristics of the tissues

The amount of kinetic energy of the missile (KE) is proportional to its velocity (v) and its mass (m):

$$KE = m \times v^2/2$$

It follows that if the missile has a high velocity (e.g. a rifle bullet), then it will carry a considerable amount of kinetic energy, even though its mass may be small. It is important to realize that the crucial speed is the *impact velocity* (i.e. the speed of the missile when it hits the patient), not its initial velocity (i.e. the speed of the projectile when it leaves the barrel of the gun). Unlike the bullet, a knife has a much lower KE because, even though it has a larger mass, it is travelling at a much lower speed.

The neighbouring tissues will be injured when the missile's KE is transferred. If the missile impacts in the tissue and fails to exit, *all* the KE will be transferred, and the maximum amount of damage will have been achieved for that particular missile. Military bullets tend to tumble (and sometimes fragment) once they enter tissues: this enables them to slow down rapidly and so maximize their energy transfer. Many of the fragments resulting from civilian explosions are irregular in shape; this not only means that they travel more slowly than aerodynamic fragments in the air, but also that they will quickly give up their KE if they hit a person.

With high-energy transfer, neighbouring tissues are pushed away from the missile track (Figure 10.2). Two cavities therefore develop. The permanent cavity is formed by the immediate destruction of tissue in the direct path of the missile. The temporary cavity lasts only a few milliseconds and is due to the continuing movement of surrounding tissues. Its size can reach thirty to forty times the diameter of the missile, depending on the amount of energy transferred to these tissues and their elastic properties. As the energy wave dissipates, the tissues rapidly return to their normal position.

'Cavitation', as it is known, has three consequences. Firstly, there is functional and mechanical disruption of the neighbouring tissues. The extent is related to energy transfer and to the tissue characteristics (Figure

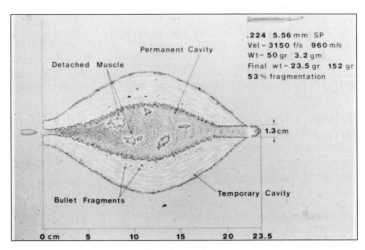

Figure 10.2   Cavitation from a high-energy transfer impact
Source: © Professor J Ryan. Reproduced by kind permission.

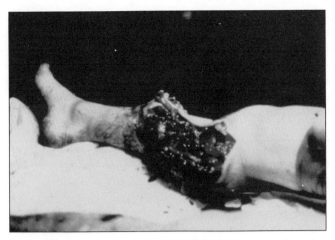

Figure 10.3   A leg injury following a high-energy transfer impact
Source: © Professor J Ryan. Reproduced by kind permission.

10.3). Solid organs, such as the liver and spleen, sustain more damage than the lungs and other low-density organs such as muscle, skin and blood vessels. These tissues have greater elastic properties and so can 'ride the punch' created by the energy transfer. In so doing, they minimize the amount of damage they sustain. It is important to remember that tissues may be severely damaged beyond the visible, permanent cavity.

Secondly, a core of any clothing that was originally over the skin surface is carried in front of the missile deep into the wound. The higher the velocity of the projectile, the finer the shearing of material and the more widely it is spread. Further contamination can be caused by other debris being sucked into the wound from the negative pressure at the missile's exit site. These grossly contaminated wounds have a high chance of becoming infected.

Thirdly, as a general rule, if a missile traverses a narrow part of the body, then the exit wound is usually larger than the entry one. This is due to the temporary cavitation effect extending along the wound track. Conversely, the temporary cavitation effect would have finished if the missile had given up enough KE to behave as a low-energy missile before it left the body. There are no absolute certainties, however, and variations in the relative sizes of exit and entry wounds are well recognized.

Local damage

A skin incision, produced by low-energy penetrating trauma (e.g. a stab wound), results in a wound with little oedema and inflammation, which heals quickly and with minimum scarring. However, one should not dismiss low-energy transfer injuries as being unimportant – some can be fatal, as for example a stab wound to the heart. Therefore the significance of the penetrating wound is dependent on the individual organ involved, and the extent of the injury.

The depth of penetration of the missile is dependent on many of the factors already discussed (Box 10.3). It follows that slow-moving small projectiles (e.g. shotgun pellets fired from over 10 metres) may only penetrate superficial tissues.

BOX 10.3   Factors that affect the penetration of a missile

- The impact velocity of the missile
- The mass of the missile
- The mean presenting area of the missile
- The density of the tissues
- Mechanical characteristics of the tissues

☐ **Blast injuries**

Following the detonation of a bomb, there is a sudden release of considerable energy. Initially, this leads to an almost instantaneous rise in pressure in the surrounding air. This band of very high pressure is known as the *shock front* (or blast wave) and it moves *through* the surrounding air. Travelling faster than the speed of sound, it rapidly spreads out in all directions, but gets weaker as the distance from the edge of the band to the epicentre of the explosion increases:

Energy of the shock front = $1/d^3$

where d = the distance from the epicentre of the explosion to the edge of the shock front.

As with all waves, the shock front can 'bounce off' solid surfaces, such as walls (or even internal viscera). These reflected waves can augment incoming waves and so increase the amount of pressure around these structures. This is one of the reasons why explosions in confined areas can be so devastating.

The duration of the pressure wave is dependent on the *type* and *amount* of explosives involved in the incident, but it is usually in the order of several milliseconds or less.

Behind the shock front comes the *blast wind*. This is movement of the air itself. As the blast wind rapidly spreads out from the epicentre, it carries fragments, either from the bomb or from surrounding debris. In view of the velocity at which they are travelling, many of these fragments can produce 'high-energy transfer' wounds.

Bomb blasts therefore can injury people in a variety of ways, as described below.

Primary effect

This is a result of the shock front. It mainly affects air-containing organs such as the lung, the bowel and the ears. Once the band of pressure hits the surface of the body it causes distortion. The magnitude as well as the rate of onset of this distortion has a direct effect on the extent of the tissue damage. It is now thought that the most important parameter is how quickly the distortion develops. The higher the rate, the bigger the pressure wave traversing the body. It is these waves which produce most of the damage associated with 'blast' lung, gut (see Figure 5.4) and tympanic membrane (Box 10.4), with most of the pathology occurring at the air/tissue boundary.

BOX 10.4   Pathological features of 'blast' lung, gut and tympanic membrane

- Haemorrhage into alveolar spaces
- Damage to alveolar septae
- Stripping of bronchial epithelium
- Emphysematous blebs produced on the pleural surface
- Contusion of the gut wall
- Leakage of blood into the gut lumen
- Perforation
- Rupture or congestion of the tympanic membrane

If these pulmonary changes are extensive, a ventilation-perfusion (V/Q) mismatch will develop and hypoxia will result (see Chapter 3). High blast pressures can also lead to air emboli, and if these obstruct the coronary or cerebral arteries sudden death can occur.

Secondary effect

In civilian explosions, most of the injuries are caused by the bomb's secondary effects. These secondary injuries are a result of the direct impact of the fragments carried in the blast wind. As most of the fragments are irregularly shaped, their velocity rapidly declines with distance from the epicentre. Therefore, high-energy transfer wounds are more likely in those who were originally close to the detonation. In view of their location, these victims will also have sustained the full force of the shock front.

Nevertheless, in most explosions the lethal area for fragments is much greater than that for the shock front. At distances outside this area, considerable damage can still be produced by these fragments. The patient usually presents with multiple, extensive wounds, of varying depth, these wounds being grossly contaminated. As the distance increases, the wounds become more superficial.

Tertiary effects

This is a result of the dynamic force of the wind itself. It can be so great as to carry all or part of the patient along with it. This results in impact (deceleration) injuries and, in extreme cases, avulsive amputations. In civilian explosions, the latter is usually seen only in those victims close to the detonation. It therefore occurs mainly in those who die at the scene from the associated primary and secondary effects of the explosion.

In addition to these effects, the patient may also sustain injuries from falling masonry as well as fires, toxic chemicals and flash burns (see Chapter 12). Acute and chronic psychological disturbances resulting from explosions are also well recognized.

■ The healing process

□ The four phases of wound healing

Phase 1: The traumatic inflammatory response (0–3 days)

Several minutes after injury there is activation of the platelets and the clotting system. Histamine and other enzymes are also released from the damaged tissue and mast cells. These cause local capillary vasodilatation. At the same time leucocytes are drawn into the wound and an exudate of serum is formed. Later on macrophages and polymorphonucleocytes appear in the wound and start the process of repair.

This increased cellular activity and blood supply is the reason why the wound initially has a red, hot and swollen appearance.

Phase 2: The destructive phase (2–5 days)

Macrophages are large cells with the ability to remove and digest dead tissue and bacteria from the wound. They attract more macrophages to the wound and encourage the collection of fibroblasts. The latter cells produce collagen, which is the principal structural protein of the body. Eventually new blood vessels begin to grow from the wound edges, heralding the onset of the next phase.

Phase 3: The proliferative phase (3–24 days)

Granulation tissue (i.e. fresh collagen and new blood vessels) develops in the wound. As this phase continues, the wound becomes stronger as the collagen is organized.

Phase 4: The maturation phase (24 days – 1 year)

The scar changes in appearance in this stage, from red to pale pink, because of the continuing organization of the collagen as well as the decrease in vascular supply. Though the strength of the wound has increased, the maximum level is not attained for 6 to 12 months.

Contraction of the wound and epithelialization are of particular importance when there has been tissue loss or destruction. However, these features come into play after the end of the secondary phase, and so do not concern the trauma team. They will not be discussed further here, but the interested reader should consult the articles listed in the 'Further reading' section at the end of this chapter.

☐ **Problems with wound healing**

Under optimum conditions, the body's inherent compensatory mechanisms will deal effectively and efficiently with most wounds. Nevertheless, several factors can interfere with these ideal conditions (Box 10.5). This can lead to delays in, or even prevention of, the wound healing.

BOX 10.5   Factors that affect wound healing

- Poor vascular supply
- Chronic disease (e.g. cancer, liver disease, renal failure, anaemia and inflammatory bowel disease)
- Chronic use of steroids, cytotoxics, anticoagulants, anti-inflammatories (e.g. aspirin)
- Inadequate nutritional status
- Infection

The chance of wound infection is increased under certain conditions (Box 10.6). The trauma team must try where possible to minimize or eliminate these so that the wound can heal quickly, with minimal scar formation.

BOX 10.6   Features that increase the chance of wound infection

---

- Wound over 6 hours old at presentation
- Poor vascularity
- Crushing or maceration of the surrounding tissue
- Necrotic surrounding tissue
- Wound contamination with foreign material
- A high-impact force
- Inadequate cleansing and irrigation of the wound
- Incorrect wound cleansing agent
- The use of local anaesthetic with adrenaline
- Inadequate haemostasis
- Excessively tight sutures
- Inappropriate wound dressings

■ Assessment and management

☐ Primary survey and resuscitation

The initial assessment must take the form of a primary survey and resuscitation period specifically aimed at the diagnosis and treatment of the immediately life-threatening injuries (see Chapter 1).

(A) Airway and cervical spine control

The airway must be cleared and secured whilst inline cervical stabilization is maintained (see Chapter 2). Particular care should be taken in those patients with bony or soft-tissue injuries to the facial area and neck, as these can lead to airway compromise.

The acute psychological effects of an explosion on the patient may be marked. Symptoms include apathy, withdrawal, hallucinations, irritability and agitation, and they may be associated with autonomic disorders. It is important that the treatment for this condition begins as soon as possible, with the pre-hospital personnel, and then the airway nurse, providing constant support and reassurance.

(B) Breathing

One of the circulation nurses, along with the medical team leader, must specifically look for the six immediately life-threatening thoracic conditions (see Chapter 3).

It is extremely important that patients who present with wounds to the chest or back have their chests completely exposed so that a full inspection and assessment can be carried out. The commonly seen 3 cm stab wound may be more sinister than at first appears.

(C) Circulation

This evaluation is described in Chapters 1 (pages 21–22) and 4 (pages 126–128).

With regard to patients with soft-tissue trauma, one of the circulation nurses must control any significant external haemorrhage. Rapid blood loss is primarily stemmed by direct pressure on the wound. This can be followed by pressure bandaging and elevation of the extremity if appropriate. The clamping of the ends of bleeding vessels should be avoided because it causes trauma which may render microsurgery impossible. The use of tourniquets is also widely discouraged as these can lead to anaerobic metabolism in distal tissues.

At this stage, the team should estimate blood loss from clinical observation of the patient, information on blood loss at the site of the incident, and inspection of the patient's clothing and dressings. It must be remembered that these estimates are prone to errors (see Chapter 4).

(D) and (E) Dysfunction and Exposure

These evaluations are carried out in the manner described in Chapter 1.

☐ Secondary survey

This combines a detailed head-to-toe assessment with the collection of information on factors which will affect the patient's management.

With regard to soft-tissue injuries, the important aspects of the history and examination are as follows:

History (AMPLE)

(A) Allergies

(M) Medicines

In particular:
- steroids;
- anticoagulants;
- cytotoxics.

(P) Past medical history

In particular:
- diabetes mellitus;
- arteriosclerosis;
- other chronic diseases;
- AIDS;
- hepatitis status;
- alcohol consumption;
- tetanus immunization status.

(L) Last meal

(E) Event

In particular:
- mechanism of injury;
- time of injury;
- pre-hospital assessment:
  - environment
  - contamination
  - deformity
  - wound site and size
  - blood loss
  - neurovascular status
  - associated injuries;
- pre-hospital care and result.

Examination

Adequate wound examination relies on an understanding of the normal anatomy in the area of the wound. The team can then anticipate which structures may be damaged, and plan appropriate management.

The vascular and neuromuscular systems distal to the wound should be examined first. This is particularly important in areas where these structures run close together and are superficial – for example, the wrist, elbows, hands, feet and ankles. Wounds in these sites have a high chance of damaging underlying tendons, nerves and vessels. The team should be aware that small nerves can be completely transected but still retain their ability to conduct sensation for several hours. This makes assessment difficult and increases the importance of direct inspection of the wound later on.

Wounds in the neck, thorax, abdomen or back may be associated with underlying visceral injury. This must be excluded by assessing the patient's clinical state as well as by conducting further diagnostic tests. In some cases surgery may be required to fully exclude visceral damage. Appropriate x-rays should be carried out, along with a full fracture assessment, if an underlying bony injury is suspected (see Chapter 9).

The wound itself can then be gently examined under adequate lighting. A sterile technique is needed, with full protection for the staff involved (see Chapter 19). As the wound is painful, examination usually requires the administration of a local anaesthetic (LA), unless nerve damage is suspected. In this case a specialist should examine the patient prior to the LA being administered.

The wound's parameters (site, size, depth, width) must be determined. The depth is best assessed under direct vision. **Blind probing of wounds with a metal instrument must not be carried out as haemorrhage and tissue damage can result.**

A note should be made of the degree and nature of any contamination because foreign bodies in wounds can:

- impair healing;
- increase the risk of infection;
- produce a painful scar;
- lead to a poor cosmetic result.

Wounds sustained by falling onto glass and gravel, and penetrating injuries and wounds caused by explosive forces or high pressure, may all hide foreign materials. Many will be superficial, and foreign bodies can be adequately removed with thorough wound cleansing under local anaesthetic. However, material which is more deeply embedded or extensive in nature will usually require a general anaesthetic. X-rays can be helpful when the foreign bodies are radio-opaque (e.g. 90 per cent of glass is visible on x-rays), but less dense materials (e.g. wood) are rarely seen.

Finally, the degree of maceration of the wound edges and the presence of any necrosis in the surrounding tissues must be assessed.

By the end of the secondary survey, the medical and nursing team leaders should know if the patient requires a general anaesthetic for his soft-tissue injuries (Box 10.7).

BOX 10.7   Reasons for a general anaesthetic

- In order adequately to examine and cleanse the wound (e.g. following gross contamination)
- For adequate and effective closure of the wound (e.g. in children and in cases of multiple lacerations)
- To remove complex foreign bodies
- To remove foreign bodies from areas where there are vital structures in close proximity (e.g. the neck, the joints, the hands and the feet)

The team should also be aware if specialist help is required (Box 10.8).

BOX 10.8   Reasons for specialist help

- There are complex wounds in cosmetically crucial areas (e.g. the face and the eyelids)
- It is necessary to exclude or repair underlying visceral damage
- It is necessary to manipulate or fix underlying fractures
- To repair tendon, nerve or vascular damage
- Skin grafting is required
- There is gross contamination, or repair would be too time-consuming to be undertaken in the resuscitation room

---

☐   Definitive care

The definitive management of the patient's wounds presents many challenges to the trauma team. They cannot have the same approach as surgical personnel because they are not dealing, in the main, with people who have been prepared physically and psychologically for the appearance of a wound.

The ultimate aim is optimal healing and restoration of function, with minimal scarring and maximal recovery of tensile strength. These targets should be reached with the minimum discomfort to the patient. Therefore, before starting their wound management, the trauma team leaders need to decide whether they have the knowledge, the skill, the resources, the facilities and the time to deal adequately with the patient's soft-tissue injuries. If they do not, then specialist help must be summoned. As this may require transfer of the patient to another hospital, all immediately or potentially life-threatening conditions must be corrected initially.

The management of wounds of the trauma victim is carried out in several stages (Box 10.9).

BOX 10.9   Stages in wound management

- The use and administration of local anaesthetic
- Wound preparation
- Methods and principles of wound closure
- Wound dressings

The use and administration of local anaesthetic

Adequate wound preparation cannot be effectively achieved without the use of some form of anaesthesia. Few patients can tolerate the necessary scrubbing and débridement required to clean heavily contaminated wounds.

Anaesthesia is most frequently given by local infiltration into or around wound edges. Regional nerve blocks (see later) may be considered in two situations: firstly, when a large area is involved, as this will reduce the amount of anaesthetic agent required; and secondly, when there is a local area of sepsis – direct injection of the local anaesthetic in this circumstance is painful and ineffective, and disseminates the infection.

The most commonly used local anaesthetic agent in the UK is lignocaine hydrochloride. It is provided in various concentrations, but a 1% solution (10 mg/ml) is adequate for most wounds. It is also effectively absorbed by mucous membranes, and it is available in solutions of 2–4% concentrations for use as a surface anaesthetic.

The maximum dose is 3 mg/kg, consequently one should not exceed 180 mg (18 ml of 1% lignocaine) for a 60 kg patient. Usually 10 ml of a 1% solution is all that is required. If the maximum dose is exceeded, toxic side-effects can result (Box 10.10), with the central nervous system signs usually preceding those of the cardiovascular system.

BOX 10.10   Side-effects of lignocaine

CNS: nausea, vomiting, tremor and convulsions
CVS: bradycardia, hypotension and cardiac arrest

Large amounts of lignocaine should not be injected into inflamed or infected tissue, because it may be rapidly absorbed by the increased blood supply to the area. This can result in systemic side-effects.

In patients with multiple lacerations, excess amounts of lignocaine may be used inadvertently if each wound is injected separately. To avoid this, the maximum allowable dose must be determined before any injections are started. To avoid a toxic dose being given, it may be necessary to use a 0.5% solution, a regional block (see later) or even a general anaesthetic.

In certain situations adrenaline is added to the local anaesthetic. This produces powerful vasoconstriction, which goes some way towards providing temporary haemostasis and prolonging the duration of action of lignocaine. However, this combination should only be used in well-vascularized areas. It is prohibited in areas where there is no collateral blood supply distal to the injection site as there is a danger of precipitating tissue necrosis (Box 10.11).

BOX 10.11   Sites where adrenaline is contraindicated

- Fingers
- Toes
- Nose
- Ears
- Penis
- Flap lacerations

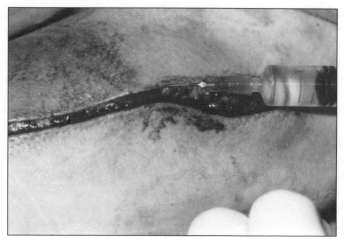

Figure 10.4   A local anaesthetic injection into a wound

Adrenaline is also thought to lower resistance to infection and therefore should not be used in heavily contaminated wounds.

Local anaesthesia is obtained by direct infiltration of the subcutaneous tissues through the open wound edges (Figure 10.4). This limits further surface trauma and prevents the injection of foreign materials which may be contaminating the skin surface. It is important to remember to aspirate for blood before injecting any local anaesthetic agent – this prevents the accidental administration of an intravascular bolus.

Once it has been determined that the needle is in a safe position, **the anaesthetic agent is injected in a continuous flow** *as the needle is withdrawn.* Never inject as the needle is being inserted because, again, an intravascular bolus may be administered.

The local anaesthetic is infiltrated parallel to the wound edges, enough to slightly raise the dermal tissues. A slow rate of infiltration is recommended as this is less painful.

Anaesthesia is usually achieved within 5 minutes if the tissue is healthy. Regional anaesthesia for infected tissue takes longer, requires more anaesthetic agent, and may be incomplete.

In certain cases, the distortion of the skin edges causes a problem in closing the wound. To avoid this a regional block can be used (Box 10.12). The most common type is the digital nerve block ('ring' block), which is used in the management of many types of finger injuries. There are many other regional nerve blocks (see the 'Further reading' section at the end of the chapter): each requires training, skill and a working knowledge of the peripheral nervous system if it is to be applied safely and effectively.

BOX 10.12   Advantages of a regional anaesthetic block

- Less anaesthetic agent is required
- It is less painful than local infiltration
- It does not produce distortion of the wound edges

Before any further procedures are carried out, the adequacy of the anaesthesia should be determined by touching the area with a needle. The patient will be aware of tissues being moved but there should be no pain.

Wound preparation

Adequate preparation provides the best possible environment for optimum wound closure and healing. It consists of several stages, with some or all being required for most wounds (Box 10.13).

BOX 10.13   Stages in wound preparation

- Skin preparation
- Wound
  - inspection
  - irrigation
  - scrubbing
  - débridement
- Removal of surrounding hair
- Securing haemostasis

In skilled hands, the majority of traumatic wounds can be managed adequately in the resuscitation room. However, heavily contaminated wounds, which need extensive cleaning or débridement, will require a general anaesthetic. This includes wounds sustained as a result of blast injuries, or those with deep foreign bodies *in situ*.

Removal of surrounding hair

The belief that shaving hair from around the edges of a wound reduces infection is no longer valid. Indeed the opposite appears to be the case. Razor blades damage the hair follicles and even the epidermis, providing access and substrate for bacterial growth. If hair has to be removed, it is recommended that it is clipped with a pair of sharp scissors. Eyebrows should never be cut as there is usually significant alteration in appearance with new growth.

Skin preparation

Grease, oil and other contaminants must first be removed with tap water or the appropriate solvents, prior to the administration of local anaesthetic. The skin surrounding the wound is then cleaned with an antibacterial solution.

Wound inspection

The wound's parameters should now be thoroughly rechecked and the involvement of any vital structures confirmed. In limb trauma, this can be facilitated by producing an avascular field by inflating a sphygmomanometer cuff. A pressure higher than systolic should be used to prevent venous ooze. Prolonged tourniquet application is not recommended, particularly in the shocked patient, because tissue necrosis can result: a note must therefore be made of the time when the compression was first applied.

Irrigation

Once the skin surface has been 'cleaned', foreign materials, bacteria and detached tissues should be removed from the wound.

The ideal irrigation agent should be economical and non-toxic, have a broad antibacterial activity and promote wound healing. Although there are many wound irrigation solutions available, recent comparison studies have failed to show that any one agent is more effective than the others. Normal saline is therefore widely used.

Studies also indicate that the effectiveness of removing foreign material depends on the volume and pressure of the irrigating fluid. High-pressure irrigation is defined as a force of 8 psi: this can be achieved by delivering the fluid directly into the wound, through a 16–14 g cannula and 50 ml syringe. In experimentally infected wounds, this type of irrigation has been shown to produce a significant reduction in the infection rate when compared with low-pressure irrigation.

Despite these advantages several objections have been raised (Box 10.14).

BOX 10.14 Potential disadvantages of high-pressure irrigation

- Foreign bodies and surface bacteria may be driven more deeply into the wound
- Tissue defences may be damaged
- The team personnel may be contaminated in the rebounding spray of the irrigating fluid

---

Although the benefits of high-pressure irrigation are thought to out-weigh its disadvantages, it should nevertheless be used with caution, and with all the personnel involved taking universal precautions (see Chapter 19).

Scrubbing

This may be required to clean the wound adequately. Gently scrubbing a wound with a fine, porous sponge soaked in the cleansing agent minimizes tissue damage and is undoubtedly useful in dealing with grossly contaminated areas. This can also reduce subsequent 'tattooing' of soft tissue by removal of impregnated foreign material. However, it must be noted that excessive scrubbing can cause further tissue damage, leaving the wound more prone to infection.

Débridement

This term has led to much confusion because in Europe it means leaving the wound open, but in North America and Sweden it is used to indicate the removal of devitalized tissues.

The excision of definitely, or potentially, necrotic tissue is widely considered to be the single most important factor in managing the contaminated wound because this reduces the chances of wound infection (Box 10.15).

BOX 10.15   Why devitalized tissue potentiates wound infection

- It acts as a culture medium
- It promotes bacterial growth
- It inhibits leucocyte functions including phagocytosis
- It provides anaerobic conditions

Tissue excision is carried out using a scalpel blade or a pair of sharp scissors. Occasionally, viable tissue also has to be removed to achieve an optimum closure and a cosmetic appearance to the wound.

For obvious reasons, a general anaesthetic should be used if an extensive operation is expected. An example of this is the high-energy transfer wound: this must be assumed to be grossly contaminated with foreign debris as well as containing devitalized tissue. All debris and dead or non-viable tissues should be removed and the wound left open. In these particular injuries, skill and clinical experience is required because it can be difficult to determine what is 'viable' tissue. Minimal excision is appropriate only if the bone and neurovascular structures are intact and the patient is being managed in a fully equipped hospital. A more radical wound-excision policy is recommended if the trauma team is working on war wounds under field conditions.

Securing haemostasis

The process of local anaesthetic administration, wound irrigation and tissue excision always causes fresh bleeding. This is usually controllable by direct pressure on the wound and elevation of the extremity, if appropriate. If this fails, the selective placement of vascular sutures can be used. Attempting to clamp off bleeding vessels is not advised as it can cause further tissue damage and may prevent microsurgical repair if this is subsequently deemed necessary.

Methods and principles of wound closure

Once the wound preparation has been completed, a decision can then be taken with regard to the method of its closure (Box 10.16).

BOX 10.16   Methods of wound closure

- Primary closure by suture
- Secondary closure by suture
- Skin tape/staples/adhesives

It is widely accepted that the infection rate increases in proportion to delay in treatment, and the degree of wound contamination. However, each wound should be considered on an individual basis as to its suitability for either primary or delayed closure.

Suture

This is the most common technique used for wound closure. The suture material is classified on its physical properties, the main one being whether it can be naturally absorbed by the body. Several characteristics of the suture can influence the tissue reaction and consequently affect the rate of wound healing (Box 10.17).

BOX 10.17   **Properties of the suture that affect the level of tissue reaction**

- The amount of material implanted
- The use of organic thread
- The capillarity of the thread

'Capillarity' is the capacity of the material to soak up fluid. This increases the chances of bacterial infection. Consequently, a non-absorbable suture with a high capillarity (e.g. silk) can give rise to chronic wound infections.

The non-absorbable types (e.g. nylon and silk) are used commonly in skin closure, but they can also be used in certain types of visceral and subcutaneous repair. Synthetic materials usually produce considerably less tissue reaction than organic sutures (e.g. silk).

Non-absorbable sutures are manufactured either as multifilament or monofilament fibres. The former consists of several filaments of thread twisted or braided together. A monofilament is a single, homogeneous strand of material: this makes knots harder to tie, but tissue reactions are minimal because, in comparison with the multifilament type, the monofilament has a lower capillarity and less of the suture is left in the wound.

Absorbable suture material – such as catgut, Dexon® (polyglycolic acid) and Vicryl® (polyglactin) – are used for certain types of subcutaneous or mucous membrane repair. Once implanted, the suture material is gradually destroyed by the body's enzyme system. The time taken to absorb catgut is dependent on:

- the amount of material;
- local infection;
- individual variation;
- the presence of proteolytic enzymes.

Synthetic absorbable materials (Dexon® and Vicryl®) are degraded by hydrolysis, and produce less of a tissue reaction than catgut. In contrast to the latter, their absorption time is not influenced by local infection and proteolytic enzymes.

It is important to note that the strength of the absorbable suture is reduced long before the material is completely removed. For example, catgut will lose its tensile strength within days, but it will remain in the wound for up to 40 days. The inflammatory reaction to catgut may cause lysis of the collagen, which further reduces the strength of the tissues supporting the suture. In contrast, the tensile strength of Dexon® and Vicryl® decreases only slightly during the first week after implantation.

Following this week there is a gradual and progressive fall, such that at 21 days the absorbable suture has approximately 20 per cent of its original strength.

BOX 10.18   Potential risks associated with suturing

- An early inflammatory reaction in the tissue due to the trauma of suturing
- Impaired blood supply and tissue necrosis if the sutures are too tight
- Inversion of the skin edges leading to wound dehiscence
- High infection rate associated with braided, multifilament sutures (e.g. silk)

Suture materials are available in a range of strengths, with corresponding needle sizes. The choice is left largely to departmental preferences, although a fine nylon suture (e.g. 6/0) is usually desired for facial repairs. Thicker nylon sutures (e.g. 4/0 and 3/0) are commonly reserved for wounds over joints or where tissues are thicker, such as on the scalp.

Suture technique

1   The needle is clamped by the needle holders approximately one-third of the way along from the suture.

2   Blunt forceps, or preferably skin hooks, are used to stabilize the skin edges.

3   The first suture is placed in the middle of the wound, so producing two lacerations of equal length (Figure 10.5). Subsequent sutures are placed

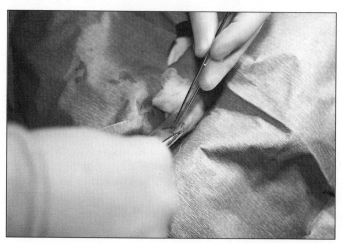

Figure 10.5   The first suture into the middle of the wound

in the middle of these lacerations. This technique helps prevent excess stitches being used.

4 The point of the needle is inserted at 90° to the skin, and close enough to the wound edge to 'bite' into healthy tissue. If they are placed too close to the wound edges, sutures can tear through skin when they are tightened.

5 The needle is advanced, with a twisting motion of the wrist, through the tissues and the bottom of the wound.

6 The needle point should emerge at a point equidistant from the wound edge to its insertion. This enables the wound edge to be everted when the suture is tied. The thread is then pulled through the wound until a short, free end is left.

7 The suture can now be tied using a 'double throw'. This is performed by coiling the thread around the needle holder twice, then grasping the free end of the suture and pulling it through the two loops. As the 'throw' is tightened, it is kept flat and brought to one side of the wound edge. Since the first throw determines the degree of edge approximation and wound tension, particular care must be taken in its placement.

8 The second part of the knot is a 'single throw'. This is carried out in a similar fashion to the double throw, but with only one coil, and in the opposite direction. This single throw secures the first throw and completes the knot.

9 Additional single throws, in alternating directions, may be added for extra security. This is commonly required when using a monofilament suture.

10 When the knot has been completed, the thread is cut leaving approximately 5 mm spare to enable the suture to be removed.

11 The size and location of the wound will dictate the number of sutures required. The wound must have adequate edge approximation and tension. If necessary, stitches should be removed and replaced. For cosmetic reasons, several small sutures, placed close together, are preferable to big sutures, widely spaced.

12 The correct time for removal of stitches is a balance between two opposing factors – cosmetics, and the tensile strength of the wound. A detailed discussion on this problem is beyond the remit of this book, but the interested reader should refer to the articles listed in the 'Further reading' section at the end of this chapter.

Secondary closure by suture

This should be considered when the wound:

- is heavily contaminated;
- contains devitalized tissue;
- requires extensive débridement;
- is more than 8 hours old.

It follows from this list that wounds resulting from high-energy transfer should be managed by secondary closure. Such injuries require all the wound preparation techniques described previously. They are then loosely dressed with saline-soaked gauze and covered with a sterile, occlusive dressing. (In the military situation well-fluffed dry gauze is used, as this is less likely to impede drainage). **Heavy or extensive packing should never be used because it leads to further tissue necrosis, tearing of fragile blood vessels, and impairment of drainage.** The patient should then be prescribed antibiotic cover and instructed to return in 3–4 days. The wound can then be reassessed to ensure that all the non-viable tissue has been removed. Delayed closure can then be carried out. This type of wound closure does not affect healing or scarring.

Skin taping

This should be reserved for superficial wounds, whose edges are dry and do not gape, and deeper lacerations in areas of low skin tension, when the edges will reapproximate easily (Box 10.19, Figure 10.6).

BOX 10.19   Advantages and disadvantages of skin tapes

Advantages
- Anaesthesia is not required
- The cosmetic effect is excellent
- Skin sensitivity is rare
- The procedure is less traumatic for young children
- The procedure is quick to carry out
- The tape can be removed by the patient himself

Disadvantages
- Haemostasis is required
- Wound edges can invert
- Tapes are commonly removed inadvertently by children
- Tapes cannot be used in areas of high skin tension, or on palms, soles, joints or hairy skin

---

Staples

These are used mainly for linear lacerations and wounds in areas of low skin tension, where they can provide a rapid and strong reapproximation of the

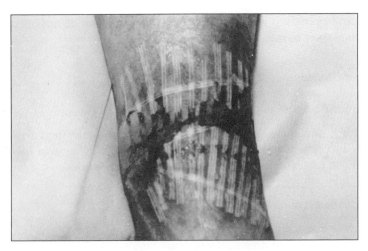

Figure 10.6 Skin tapes in position

skin edges. In view of their expense and lack of versatility, they are rarely used in resuscitation rooms in the UK.

Skin adhesive

This is a methyl-2-cyanoacrylate monomer (Histoacryl®) and it is applied, as a series of small drops, to the opposing surfaces of the wound. The latter are then held together for a few seconds until the glue dries. The disadvantages of this technique are that absolute haemostasis is essential, and the glue may delay healing because it can act as a barrier between the wound edges.

Wound dressings

In view of the large amount of research into this subject, it is now possible to choose an optimal dressing for any particular wound. The decision depends upon an adequate assessment of the type and location of the wound, as well as a thorough knowledge of wound healing and types of dressings available. Simply following departmental traditions and personal preferences should be resisted. It is important that each unit reads the relevant research and conducts their own clinical trials in order that the most appropriate dressing can be chosen for each particular wound.

The ideal dressing has the following properties:

- it removes excess exudate;
- it stems haemorrhage;
- it provides protection and insulation;
- it is non-toxic and free of contamination;
- it allows gaseous exchange;

- it can be removed without causing trauma, pain and disturbance of new granulation tissue.

Types of dressings

Haemostatic agents

Kaltostat™ and Surgicel™ are valuable as primary dressings to manage actively bleeding wounds, especially lacerations involving skin loss to the digits. Each can be left *in situ* until a dry scab has formed.

Non-adherent wound contact dressings

These were originally designed to overcome the problems of the traditional gauze and cottonwool dressings which are highly absorbent, but which tend to stick to the wound.

Jelonet™ and Paratulle™ are non-medicated and non-adherent dressings made from cotton or cotton/viscose weaves impregnated with soft white paraffin. Silicon N-A™ is a knitted viscose dressing coated with silicon; its manufacturer claims that it has superior qualities of non-adherence.

There is much research and discussion surrounding the relative merits of medicated *tulle gras* dressings, mainly concerning the relative non-adherent properties of each and the degree of release of antimicrobial agents onto the wound surface. The following examples are by no means exhaustive. Bactigras™ and Inadine™ are impregnated with antimicrobial agents and are used for infected grazes, burns, bites and lacerations, and as a prophylactic treatment for wounds subject to a high risk of infection. Bactigras™ is a cotton-weave fabric impregnated with soft paraffin containing 0.5% chlorhexidine. Inadine™ is a knitted viscose fabric impregnated with polyethylene glycol containing 10% povidone-iodine. There are other medicated dressings containing different anti-microbial agents and antibiotics.

In all cases an absorbent backing, such as Regal™ or Melolin™, should be applied to stop the exudate accumulating in the non-adherent dressing.

Tetanus prophylaxis

The tetanus immunization status of all trauma victims, along with any allergic reactions, should be elicited at the end of the secondary survey. It is important to determine whether the patient has had a full tetanus course in the past and when the last tetanus booster was given.

Tetanus prophylaxis can then be provided for particular patients with tetanus-prone wounds (Box 10.20).

BOX 10.20   Tetanus-prone wounds

- Wounds that are more than 6 hours old
- Wounds with irregular edges
- Wounds that are large and deep
- Wounds caused by burns, crush and blast injuries
- Wounds contaminated with soil, faeces or saliva
- Wounds in which signs of early infection are present
- Wounds with large areas of devitalized tissue
- Wounds resulting from animal or human bites

Patients who require tetanus prophylaxis in the resuscitation room (Box 10.21) should be provided with a card documenting their status in order that they can complete the immunization programme. Tetanus toxoid and human tetanus immunoglobulin are both given intramuscularly, but *different sites must be used.*

BOX 10.21   Tetanus prophylaxis

	Tetanus-prone wound?	
	Yes	No
Immune status	Further action	Further action
1	None	None
2	1 dose toxoid	None
3	1 dose toxoid *and* human antitetanus immunoglobulin 250 IU IM	1 dose toxoid
4	Complete course toxoid *and* human antitetanus immunoglobulin 250 IU IM	Complete course toxoid

---

Categories of immune status
1 – Previous complete course of toxoid or booster < 5 years ago
2 – Previous complete course of toxoid or booster 5–10 years ago
3 – Previous complete course of toxoid or booster > 10 years ago
4 – No complete course or immune status unknown

■ Summary

To facilitate optimal wound healing, the trauma nurse must utilize information gained from the mechanism of injury, the clinical state of the patient, and a detailed assessment of the wound. Only then can the skills and procedures required to manage the soft-tissue injury be put into effect.

■ References and further reading

Cooper D 1990. Optimizing wound healing. A practice within nursing's domain. *Nurs. Clin. N. Am.* **25**(1): 165.

David J 1986. *Wound Management – a comprehensive guide to dressing and healing.* London: Martin Dunitz.

Dimick A 1988. Delayed wound closure: indications and techniques. *Ann. Emerg. Med.* **17**(12): 1303.

Edlich R 1984. Current concept of emergency wound management. *Em. Med. Repts* **5**: 22.

Edlich R, Custer J, Madden J, *et al.* 1969. Assessment of the effectiveness of irrigation with antiseptic agent. *Am. J. Surg.* **118**: 21.

Edlich R, Rodeneaver G, Morgan R, *et al.* 1984. Principles of emergency wound management. *Ann. Emerg. Med.* **17**(12): 1284.

Eriksson E 1979. *Illustrated Handbook in Local Anaesthesia.* London: Lloyd-Luke.

Fackler M 1988. Wound ballistics: a review of common misconceptions. *JAMA* **259**(18): 2730.

Hall J & Cooper G 1992. The pathophysiology of blast injury. *Clin. Int. Care* **3**: 4.

Holmlund D, Tera H, Widerg Y, *et al.* 1978. *Sutures and techniques for wound closure.* New York: Naimark & Barba Medical and Surgical Publications.

Maynard R, Cooper G & Scott R 1989. Mechanisms of injury in bomb blasts and explosions. In Westerby S (ed.): *Trauma: pathogenesis and treatment.* Oxford: Heinemann Medical Books.

Nightingale K 1990. Making sense of . . . wound closure. *Nursing Times* **86**(14): 35.

Rigault D & Deligny M 1989. The 1986 terrorist bombing experience in Paris. *Ann. Surg.* **209**(3): 368.

Ryan J, Cooper G, Haywood I, *et al.* 1991. Field surgery on a future conventional battlefield: strategy and wound management. *Ann. R. Coll. Surg.* **73**: 13.

Simon R & Brenner B 1982. *Procedures and Techniques in Emergency Medicine.* Baltimore: Williams & Wilkins.

Spalding T, Stewart M, Tulloch D, *et al.* 1991. Penetrating missile injuries in the Gulf War 1991. *Br. J. Surg.* **78**(9): 1102.

Stevenson T, Thacker J, Rodenheaver G, *et al.* 1976. Cleansing the traumatic wound by high-pressure syringe irrigation. *JACEP* **5**(1): 17.

Thomas S 1990. *Wound Management and Dressings.* London: Pharmaceutical Press.

Trott A 1988. Mechanism of Surface Soft Tissue Trauma. *Ann. Emerg. Med.* **17**(12): 1279.

Westerby S (ed.) 1985. *Wound Care.* London: Heinemann.

Chapter 11

Trauma in the elderly, in pregnancy and in paediatrics

Cindy LeDuc Jimmerson, Peter Driscoll,
Carl Gwinnutt and Terry Brown

Objectives

This chapter concentrates on the special aspects of trauma management required to offer optimal care to the elderly, pregnant or paediatric patient. The objectives are that upon completion of this chapter, the trauma team will be able to describe the characteristics of each of these groups with respect to:

- anatomy and pathophysiology;

- response to injury;

- assessment and management.

Trauma in the elderly

■ Introduction

The general improvement in lifestyle which has occurred this century has resulted in people living longer and remaining physically active. However, the environment we have created (e.g. our housing) is geared towards younger people who are more agile, with relatively little consideration towards the elderly, particularly in terms of safety. It is not surprising, therefore, that this group of the population, whilst trying to maintain an independent lifestyle, have increased chances of sustaining injuries as a result of declining performance in their vision, hearing, reflexes and

283

musculoskeletal system. Furthermore, deterioration in sensation increases their susceptibility to burns whilst occasionally masking their perception of minor trauma completely.

■ Anatomy and pathophysiology

The decline with age in the body's ability to respond to injury is one of the reasons why the mortality rate for trauma is highest in the over-60s, even though they have fewer injuries. However, response is dependent upon a number of factors, including the patient's medical history, nutritional status, physical, emotional and social activities. The team must take these into account when they carry out the initial assessment and resuscitation of the elderly trauma victim.

□ Respiratory system

There is a generalized decrease in lung volume and compliance with age, which may be aggravated by the coexistence of chronic pulmonary disease. These changes, along with a reduced ability to cough, limit the patient's ventilatory reserves and increase the risk of pneumonia after injury. Arterial blood gases show a moderately decreasing oxygen tension (PaO_2) with advancing age, with other parameters remaining as for the younger patient.

□ Cardiovascular system

There is a decrease in cardiac function, which may be worsened by the presence of ischaemic heart disease. The vascular system is less elastic and the autonomic response to shock is impaired. These changes significantly reduce the elderly patient's ability to mount a compensatory response to trauma. The increased use of medications in this age group may further impair the response to shock. Blood pressure may therefore be a poor indicator of the degree of fluid loss. Although dysrhythmias are more common in the elderly, the team leader must always rule out hypoxia or cardiac trauma as the cause.

□ Renal system

Renal function declines with age and the kidneys become less effective at retaining water in the presence of hypovolaemia. This is secondary to reduced ADH secretion and diminished renin-angiotensin activity, both of which normally limit urine formation. Consequently, while the kidneys are perfused urine is produced, which can exacerbate fluid and electrolyte loss and potentially interfere with the assessment of fluid resuscitation.

Unfortunately, if acute renal failure develops as a result of prolonged hypoperfusion, the outcome is worse than in younger patients.

☐ Nervous system

There is a generalized deterioration in the sensory system with age, and the elderly are particularly dependent upon devices such as glasses and hearing aids. Degeneration within the CNS may cause memory problems, dementia, and deterioration in cognitive function. Intracranial haemorrhage must always be considered as a possible cause of unconsciousness in the elderly patient.

☐ Musculoskeletal system

Degenerative changes in bones and joints and ligamentous ossification lead to reduced flexibility of the skeleton, which may contribute to or worsen the injury. The vertebral column is particularly at risk and narrowing of the spinal canal may jeopardize the spinal cord. Osteoporosis is more common in women and results in bones fracturing after minimal trauma. Care must be taken in these circumstances with routine splinting and securing techniques.

■ Assessment and management

☐ Primary survey and resuscitation

(A) Airway and cervical-spine control

Elderly patients are often edentulous, but may occasionally have loose, inconveniently placed or very carious teeth. Along with resorption of the mandible and lax cheek muscles this may make maintenance of the airway more difficult. If intubation is required, arthritis of the temporo-mandibular joint may limit mouth opening. Soft tissues are more prone to injury, particularly the turbinates, which may bleed profusely. Care must be taken with the cervical spine, even when clinically and radiologically intact, so that iatrogenic injury is avoided.

(B) Breathing

It is often difficult to support ventilation using a facemask in the elderly for the reasons already stated. Furthermore, their reduced respiratory reserves mean that hypoxia ensues rapidly and therefore mechanical ventilation with 100% oxygen should be started early. However, the chances of causing a pneumothorax are significantly higher in this group of patients and the team leader should be constantly aware of this. Repeated assessment of breath sounds and observation of the patient's chest for equality of movement and the development of surgical emphysema are important to ensure early recognition of this complication should it occur. As soon as possible serial arterial blood gases should be performed to ensure adequate oxygenation and ventilation. Because of the potential problems the assistance of an anaesthetist should be sought early in the management of these patients.

(C) Circulation

Warmed fluids should be infused, but the patient's response must be continuously and accurately monitored by the circulation personnel because of the reduced tolerance to both hypovolaemia and overload. In addition to the vital signs and urinary output, invasive monitoring should be established early, using expert help if necessary, in order to optimize cardiovascular function. The insertion of a urinary catheter must be carried out in a strictly aseptic manner as these patients have an increased risk of developing infection.

(D) Dysfunction

Anxiety, disorientation and confusion in the elderly trauma patient should be treated initially by ensuring adequate cerebral perfusion with oxygenated blood rather than assuming this is the patient's normal mental state. Impaired sensory function, particularly deafness, may produce inappropriate responses and make assessment difficult.

(E) Exposure

The susceptibility of the elderly to greater injuries from a given force means that they must always be completely undressed to ensure that injuries are not missed. However, they are also very prone to hypothermia, so appropriate measures must be taken to prevent this being worsened or added to the patient's list of problems.

☐ Secondary survey

A full head-to-toe examination is warranted as a result of the inability of the elderly to withstand trauma. In view of the patient's intrinsic immobility due to degenerative diseases and the possible frailty of the skeleton from osteoporosis, care should be taken to maintain the anatomical position that is normal for each patient. Extra care must be taken during log-rolling.

Padding of bony prominences during transportation is essential to prevent skin breakdown. It is the responsibility of the nursing team leader to anticipate such complications and avoid them: patients will often not notice contact pressure because of decreased pain perception.

AMPLE

The patient's history is particularly important in the elderly. Polypharmacy is common and it is important that the medical team leader learns what medications are being taken as these may have a direct bearing on either the patient's response to injury or resuscitation. As patients get older they are more likely to have other diseases and information must be sought from the family, ambulance personnel or previous hospital records. Occasionally it may be possible to obtain information directly from the patient. However, because hearing may be less acute, members of the team must remember to speak clearly to the patient, preferably looking directly at him as they speak, allowing the patient to lip-read. They should watch the reaction during the conversation to ensure that the patient comprehends what is being said; the response to such communication will also provide further information on the patient's sensory and cognitive abilities.

■ Summary

Sensory overload, short-term memory impairment and senile dementia are common in the elderly. These patients must be allowed an appropriate amount of time to process information and formulate answers to questions. Sensitivity to these concerns can greatly assist the patient in accepting many of the intrusive procedures associated with resuscitation and subsequent hospitalization, thereby helping to maintain self-esteem.

The patient's dignity must always be respected throughout the resuscitation period (whether he is conscious or not) and during admission procedures. This contributes significantly to the trauma victim's emotional outcome, as fear of becoming dependent is a serious problem for the elderly patient.

Trauma in pregnancy

■ Introduction

Trauma in pregnancy is special because there are always at least *two* patients. However, because the foetus is totally dependent upon the maternal cardiovascular system for the supply of oxygen, the best method of ensuring its well-being is by treatment of the mother. Although the same principles are used, there are notable differences in the response of a pregnant woman to injury and resuscitation. These are due to anatomical and physiological changes which begin with the onset of pregnancy and increase in number and significance with time.

■ Anatomy and pathophysiology

□ Respiratory system

The capillaries of the upper airway are engorged, leading to an increase in the soft-tissue bulk in the larynx, narrowing of the airways and an increased fragility of the mucous membranes. These are worsened by the presence of eclampsia. There is also enlargement of the breasts and the soft tissues of the face, due to fat deposition.

During pregnancy tidal volume may increase by as much as 20 per cent, but the respiratory rate is generally unchanged. This 'hyperventilation' of pregnancy results in $PaCO_2$ of approximately 30 mmHg. Residual volume falls during pregnancy as the uterus and its contents enlarge, thereby diminishing oxygen reserves (see Chapter 3).

□ Cardiovascular

Blood volume increases between 40 to 50 per cent by the 34th week of pregnancy. This is due predominantly to an increase in plasma volume, with a smaller increase in red cell mass. This disparity results in a physiological anaemia during pregnancy. Heart rate increases during pregnancy, eventually reaching a rate about 20 beats per minute more than normal. Both systolic and diastolic blood pressures fall by 5–15 mmHg during the second trimester, returning to near pre-pregnant levels at term. Cardiac output increases early, reaching 20–30 per cent above normal shortly after the end of the first trimester. The ECG may show flattening or inversion of T waves in III, aVF and the chest leads, along with left-axis deviation during a normal pregnancy.

Aortocaval compression

During late pregnancy a supine or semi-recumbent posture allows the weight of the foetus to compress the maternal aorta and vena cava. The latter causes reduced venous return and can reduce cardiac output by up to 40 per cent. In some women the aortocaval compression is concealed and the blood pressure maintained by a compensatory increase in the peripheral vascular resistance (see Chapter 4).

A further complication of inferior vena cava compression is an increase in uterine venous pressure. This will enlarge any placental separation which has occurred.

☐ Renal system

The increased cardiac output causes an increased renal blood flow leading to lower plasma levels of urea and creatinine than normal. Glycosuria is a common finding in normal pregnancy.

☐ Nervous system

Pregnancy can cause dizziness and fainting. During the third trimester, changes in balance and movement can also occur, but the special senses are not usually affected.

Pre-eclampsia is a complication of pregnancy characterized by the presence of oedema, hypertension and proteinuria. It is more common in the primigravid patient and is rare before the 28th week of pregnancy. If untreated it may progress to eclampsia with worsening of the above signs along with headaches, drowsiness, hyper-reflexia and seizures.

☐ Gastrointestinal tract

Gastric emptying is delayed and the gastro-oesophageal sphincter is less competent. There is an increased incidence of hiatus hernia and the intestines are displaced to the upper abdomen.

☐ Uterus and placenta

It is not until the beginning of the second trimester (12th week) that the gravid uterus ascends from the protection of the bony pelvis. It reaches the umbilicus by the 20th week and its maximum height, the costal margin, by the 36th week. The thick uterine wall initially offers the foetus some protection from trauma but this is lost by the third trimester when the uterus becomes stretched and thin.

Blood flow to the uterus increases during pregnancy and can reach 700 ml/min. It follows that a significant haemorrhage can result from an injury that tears the uterine vessels. In view of the anatomical position of the uterus, this haemorrhage may also be concealed.

The placenta is less elastic than the uterine muscle and may shear off the uterus during trauma. This is known as a *placental abruption*, and if severe will cause the death of the foetus and may lead to loss of amniotic fluid into the maternal circulation (*amniotic fluid embolism*). This is characterized by dyspnoea, cyanosis, hypotension, chest pain and excessive bleeding from minor wounds. The last may be the initial presenting sign.

☐ Musculoskeletal system

Ligaments are softened during pregnancy due to the effect of oestrogens. This is particularly noticeable in the pelvis, with widening of the symphysis pubis and relaxation of the sacroiliac joints.

■ Assessment and management

☐ Primary survey and resuscitation

Resuscitating the mother is the best way of resuscitating the foetus. The management of the trauma victim is the same whether the patient is pregnant or not, however the trauma team should be expanded to include an obstetrician, an obstetric nurse and, if there is any likelihood of emergency delivery, a paediatrician.

(A) Airway and cervical-spine control

The delay in gastric emptying and the relaxation of the gastro-oesophageal junction both lead to an increased risk of regurgitation and aspiration. Early consideration should therefore be given to protecting the airway with a cuffed endotracheal tube. However, intubation may be more difficult in the pregnant patient, particularly secondary to breast enlargement, as may be application of a semi-rigid collar. Cricoid pressure should be used in an attempt to minimize the risk of regurgitation (see Chapter 2).

(B) Breathing

High concentrations of oxygen are particularly important in order to ensure foetal oxygenation. If ventilation is required, it is important to remember that mild 'hyperventilation' should be employed ($PaCO_2$ 30 mmHg).

(C) Circulation

The increased blood volume and ability to redirect blood from the placental to systemic circulation allow the mother to lose up to one-third of her circulating volume before developing the classic signs of shock. The amount of blood lost may be underestimated by relying on normal parameters. Furthermore, the vasodilatation that occurs with pregnancy causes the patient's skin to be warm and pink and dry, even with such a large blood loss. It follows that larger volumes than normal of warmed intravenous fluid and blood will usually be required.

Meticulous monitoring of the mother's vital signs and her response to intravenous fluids, and the early use of CVP monitoring, will assist with resuscitation.

Aortocaval compression may cause or worsen hypotension. To prevent this, patients in the second and third trimesters must be log-rolled onto their left side providing there is no spinal injury. Alternatively, the right hip can be elevated using a sandbag, pillows or a Cardiff wedge, and the uterus manually displaced to the left. The best method is to have the patient secured to a long spinal board so that these manoeuvres can be achieved without twisting the vertebral column.

As well as normal laboratory tests, blood should be taken for a Kleihauer test to determine whether there has been any leak of foetal blood into the maternal circulation. If this has occurred in the Rhesus-negative patient then prophylactic anti-D should be given to prevent Rhesus sensitization. Any foetal anaemia resulting from the leak is rarely severe enough to threaten the foetus.

The PASG can be used, though only the leg compartments should be inflated if the patient is in the second or third trimester.

(D) Dysfunction

Eclampsia can occur in late pregnancy, producing a variety of signs and symptoms, particularly a reduction in the level of consciousness. The medical team leader must ensure that this is not misinterpreted as resulting from a head injury. Blood pressure may or may not be elevated in these cases.

(E) Exposure

This examination should be carried out so that a full assessment of the abdomen and genital tract can be made.

☐ Radiology

Urgent radiology is not contraindicated in pregnancy but uterine radiation should be minimized by using lead shields.

☐ Secondary survey

Abdomen

The fundal height, uterine shape, presence of foetal movement, uterine contractions and any tenderness must be noted. An irritable uterus may be due to inadequate uterine oxygenation and if untreated may lead to pre-term labour.

Abdominal pain, tenderness or palpation of two abdominal masses suggests uterine injury and is an obstetric and trauma emergency, as maternal shock and foetal death can develop very rapidly. The dilated uterine veins may also be torn when the pelvis fractures. The presence of this injury should therefore alert the team leaders to the risk of massive retroperitoneal haemorrhage.

A vaginal examination is essential because it will enable the uterus, the cervical os and the presentation of the foetus to be assessed. It may also detect leaked amniotic fluid and local trauma. In view of its importance, the vaginal examination should be carried out by the obstetric member of the team.

Placental abruption occurs in 1–5 per cent of minor maternal injuries and 20–50 per cent of major ones. Bleeding is due to damage to the maternal venous sinuses. The severity of the signs (Box 11.1) is related to the degree of separation, but foetal distress may occasionally be the only sign. Close foetal monitoring is therefore required (see below). This should be continued for at least 48 hours because the onset of an abruption may be delayed.

BOX 11.1   Signs of placental abruption

- Maternal hypovolaemic shock
- Abdominal tenderness
- Increasing fundal height
- Uterine irritability
- Vaginal bleeding
- Foetal distress

Abdominal trauma in late pregnancy may damage the bladder because of crowding of pelvic structures. More commonly, spontaneous voiding occurs because of the increased pressure on the bladder. It is important that the urine is collected so that it can be differentiated from amniotic fluid that may have leaked from a premature rupture of the membranes.

Diagnostic peritoneal lavage can be carried out in pregnancy provided that the site of the incision is changed slightly. This is described in detail in Chapter 5.

Foetus

Foetal assessment must be carried out by skilled personnel during the secondary survey, when the mother has been resuscitated. The objectives are to detect signs of distress which include:

- a heart rate under 110 bt/min;
- loss of beat-to-beat variation;
- inadequate acceleration in heart rate following uterine contractions;
- late deceleration once the uterine contraction has finished.

Pelvic ultrasonography can be used to detect the presence of a foetal heart beat after seven weeks of pregnancy. Later on in the gestation the placental position, the liquor volume and the presence of intra-amniotic haemorrhage can also be assessed by ultrasonography. A cardiotocograph compares uterine contraction and foetal heart rate and is used to detect foetal distress during late pregnancy.

AMPLE

As with all trauma victims, a detailed history should have been obtained by the end of the secondary survey. Information with respect to allergies, medications, past medical history, last meal, events and environment must be known by the team leaders. Past medical history in this group of patients should also include details of the last menstrual period to allow gestational age to be estimated and compared with fundal height.

The mechanism of injury (i.e. the event) is important. As the gravid uterus develops, it becomes an easier target for penetrating trauma. Although the foetus may die following this type of injury, the mother may survive because by the third trimester the uterus acts as a shield for the rest of the abdominal contents. Blunt trauma at this late stage of pregnancy can result in uterine rupture with significant haemorrhage. Maternal mortality is high, but it usually results from associated injuries.

The risk of pre-term labour is increased with burn injuries, and the fluid requirements may increase beyond those cited in the standard fluid resuscitation tables (Chapter 12).

■ Caesarean section

An emergency Caesarean section should be considered in the situations listed in Box 11.2, where the release of aortocaval compression will have a beneficial effect on the maternal circulation and the foetal prognosis will not improve by waiting.

BOX 11.2   Reasons for an emergency Caesarean section

- A viable foetus in distress
- Foetal signs suggesting viability, but the mother:
  - is moribund
  - has died within the last few minutes

■ Summary

The best treatment for the foetus is by treatment of the mother. However, the conscious pregnant patient will be worried about the state of her unborn child. This anxiety may be compounded by the team's preoccupation with her rather than the foetus. It is important that the airway nurse quickly establishes a rapport with the patient so that these worries can be alleviated.

Trauma in paediatrics

■ Introduction

Over half of all deaths occurring between the ages of 1 and 15 are due to trauma. Motor vehicle accidents remain the primary cause, but fatalities from falls and sport are also important in the 0–4 and 5–14 age groups respectively. Multisystem injuries are more common in children because the energy transferred at impact is absorbed over a smaller area and internal organs are closer together. Children also vary enormously in their size and therefore a wide variety of equipment is essential to manage them appropriately.

■ Anatomy and pathophysiology

Clearly there is a gradual change from paediatric to adult anatomy and physiology with the major differences being in the very young. This section will concentrate on these young victims.

□ Respiratory system

The important anatomical differences between infants and adults which affect the management of the airway are shown in Box 11.3.

BOX 11.3   Comparison of paediatric and adult airways

- Infants under 6 months are obligate nose-breathers
- The head, compared to the body size, is relatively larger
- The occipital prominence is larger
- The tongue is relatively larger and the oral cavity relatively smaller
- The soft tissues of the oral cavity and pharynx are more delicate
- The larynx is at the level of C3 (adult C5/C6) and has an opening that is orientated more anteriorly
- The trachea is short and both main bronchi have the same vertical alignment

---

The chest wall is very compliant and significant internal damage can occur with minimal signs of external injury. For example, pulmonary contusions can occur without fractures of the overlying ribs.

Infants have a small functional residual capacity, a high closing volume and a high level of oxygen consumption (see Chapter 3). Respiratory rates vary considerably with age (see Table 11.1).

Table 11.1   Vital signs in a normal child who is not crying

Age (years)	Respiratory Rate (breaths/min)	Pulse (bt/min)	Systolic BP (mmHg)	Blood volume (ml/kg)
< 1	30–40	120–140	70–90	90
2–5	20–30	100–120	80–90	80
5–12	15–20	80–100	90–110	80

□ Cardiovascular system

Table 11.1 demonstrates the variation in blood volume and cardiovascular vital signs with age in normal children.

As the volume of blood in young children and babies is small, the importance of any bleeding source must not be underestimated. Haematomas and lacerations, especially in the scalp, can result in the loss of a significant percentage of the child's blood volume.

The normal systolic blood pressure can also be estimated using this formula:

$$\text{systolic blood pressure} = 80 + (2 \times \text{age}) \text{ mmHg}$$

After significant blood loss, children can maintain their blood pressure for a longer period of time than adults. The primary response is the development of a tachycardia accompanied by vasoconstriction. Consequently, by the time the child's blood pressure falls, he may have lost as much as 40 per cent of his circulating blood volume.

BOX 11.4   Signs of hypovolaemia in children

- Tachycardia – *an early sign*
- Anxiety – *an early sign*
- Poor skin colour and sweating
- Poor capillary refill
- Increased, shallow respiratory rate
- Hypotension – **a late sign of shock in children**

The lack of concurrent disease in children limits the chances of damage to the aorta following deceleration injuries. However, the mediastinum is more mobile than in adults, and children are less tolerant of a tension pneumothorax because of the enhanced effect on venous return and subsequent cardiovascular compromise.

☐ **Renal system**

The kidney is relatively insensitive to aldosterone and ADH. Consequently, low levels of urine output will be maintained even in the presence of hypovolaemia. A relatively greater urine output of 2 ml/kg/hr therefore indicates adequacy of resuscitation.

☐ **Nervous system**

Raised intracranial pressure resulting from diffuse brain oedema is the commonest cause of death in children with head injuries. In the very young, open fontanelles and mobile sutures enable the brain to adapt to any expanding intracranial mass. Consequently a bulging fontanelle or sutural diastasis is an important clinical sign. Once these compensation mechanisms have been exhausted there is a rapid clinical deterioration. As these cranial openings close with age, this compensatory ability gradually diminishes.

Extradural haematomas are not common in children under 2 years of age and are not usually associated with seizures. In contrast, subdural haematomas are usually seen in babies under 1 year of age and commonly cause seizures.

☐ Musculoskeletal system

Compared with the adult cervical spine, the child's neck is weaker, the facet joints more horizontal, and the ligaments more flexible. Consequently significant movement of the relatively large head on the cervical spine can lead to facet dislocation or subluxation (see Chapter 8).

Bones in childhood are more pliable than those in adults. They therefore have a tendency to bend rather than fracture when subjected to a force. If the cortical margins remain intact this is known as a *torus injury*. A *greenstick fracture* occurs when one of the bone's surfaces fractures whilst the opposite surface bends.

Longitudinal growth of bone occurs mainly at the junction between the metaphysis and epiphysis. If this 'growth plate' is damaged following trauma, therefore, developmental abnormalities can result. A commonly used classification for injuries to the growth plate is shown in Figure 11.1. As a general principle, the risk of developmental deformity increases as the classification number increases.

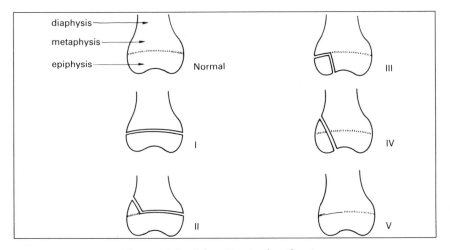

Figure 11.1 Salter-Harris classification

☐ **Abdominal organs**

The diaphragm is more horizontal, which has the effect of displacing the liver and spleen below the costal margin, reducing protection by the ribs. There is also less overlying muscle and fat offering protection. The bladder rises further out of the pelvis and is more exposed to injury.

☐ **Thermoregulatory changes**

The combination of a relatively large body surface area, thin skin and a lack of subcutaneous fat enables children to lose heat very rapidly, especially when wet. This leads to an increase in tissue metabolic activity as the body tries to prevent the core temperature falling (see Chapter 13). The resulting increase in oxygen consumption puts further stress on the compromised circulation of the trauma victim (see Chapter 4).

☐ **Psychological**

Regressive psychological behaviour is common in the young trauma victim who is unable to understand the stress and pain and the unfamiliar environment. This can lead to long-term abnormal psychological development. The team must therefore quickly develop a supportive relationship with the patient so that psychological trauma can be minimized.

■ **Assessment and management**

In the initial assessment of the paediatric patient it is important to consider the growth and development that is appropriate for the child's age. Observations of his language, activity level and interaction with his parents, as well as vital signs, are important to note.

(A) Airway and cervical spine

The principles of paediatric airway management with cervical spine control are the same as in adults (see Chapter 2). However, the equipment and techniques used have to take account of the unique anatomical features (Figure 11.2).

The large occiput pushes the cervical spine into a degree of flexion when the patient is supine; combined with a small, flexible airway, this leads to buckling of the trachea. Maintaining the child's head in the 'sniffing' position reduces this risk.

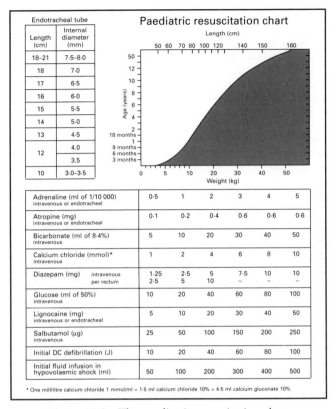

Endotracheal tube		
Length (cm)	Internal diameter (mm)	
18–21	7·5–8·0	
18	7·0	
17	6·5	
16	6·0	
15	5·5	
14	5·0	
13	4·5	
12	4·0	
	3.5	
10	3·0–3·5	

Paediatric resuscitation chart

Adrenaline (ml of 1/10 000) intravenous or endotracheal	0·5	1	2	3	4	5
Atropine (mg) intravenous or endotracheal	0·1	0·2	0·4	0·6	0·6	0·6
Bicarbonate (ml of 8·4%) intravenous	5	10	20	30	40	50
Calcium chloride (mmol)* intravenous	1	2	4	6	8	10
Diazepam (mg) intravenous per rectum	1·25 2·5	2·5 5	5 10	7·5 –	10 –	10 –
Glucose (ml of 50%) intravenous	10	20	40	60	80	100
Lignocaine (mg) intravenous or endotracheal	5	10	20	30	40	50
Salbutamol (µg) intravenous	25	50	100	150	200	250
Initial DC defibrillation (J)	10	20	40	60	80	100
Initial fluid infusion in hypovolaemic shock (ml)	50	100	200	300	400	500

* One millilitre calcium chloride 1 mmol/ml = 1·5 ml calcium chloride 10% = 4·5 ml calcium gluconate 10%

Figure 11.2 The paediatric resuscitation chart
Source: © Oakley P 1988. Inaccuracy and delay in decision making in paediatric resuscitation and a proposed reference chart to reduce error. *Br. Med. J.* **297**: 817.
Reproduced by kind permission.

Whilst holding the jaw the airway personnel must take care not to press on the soft tissues beneath the chin as this leads to obstruction of the airway. The fingertips must remain on the mandible.

The finger-sweep technique is contraindicated in children because trauma to soft tissues in the oral cavity may cause bleeding and airway obstruction. Foreign bodies may be impacted within the cone-shaped larynx, causing complete respiratory obstruction. Subsequent removal is both urgent and difficult. The airway personnel should therefore remove all foreign matter, under direct vision, using suction or Magill forceps.

For the same reasons, a Guedel airway should be inserted into a child's mouth the correct way up under direct vision into the pharynx, using a suitable tongue depressor.

A circular facemask is the optimum shape for a baby as this allows a good seal to be created. In the unconscious child, however, and in one whose airway is compromised, early intubation should be considered to maintain and protect the airway and facilitate adequate ventilation of the lungs.

Intubation

A detailed description on paediatric intubation is beyond the scope of this book, but this interested reader should consult the 'Further reading' section at the end of this chapter. In summary:

1   Preparation for intubation is the same in adult and paediatric cases (see Chapter 2).

2   If the infant is under 1 year, a straight-bladed laryngoscope may be used, placing the tip **behind** the epiglottis, lifting both this structure and the tongue forward to reveal the larynx.

3   An uncuffed endotracheal tube is used in children below 10 years of age; a small leak detected on ventilation indicates the correct size. The size of the tube is calculated either from the patient's age or better still by reference to a nomogram (see Figure 11.2).

4   Verification of correct placement is very important and should be carried out repeatedly, in the same way as that described for adults (see Chapter 2), as small tubes are easily dislodged, particularly when the patient is moved. In children, however, the endotracheal tube has an equal chance of going down either bronchus because of their similar alignment.

5   Throughout these procedures the cervical spine must be immobilized using the techniques described in Chapter 1. Manual immobilization must be maintained if, as commonly happens, an appropriately-sized collar cannot be found.

Cricothyroidotomy

Needle cricothyroidotomy is the technique of choice in children under 12 years of age as damage to the cricoid cartilage would remove the only complete supporting ring of cartilage in the trachea, causing it to collapse. Furthermore, healing is associated with tracheal stenosis.

(B) Breathing

Air swallowing is common in stressed and crying children. This leads to gastric dilatation and increases the risk of vomiting and aspiration. It also compromises ventilation by splinting the diaphragm and reduces venous return by compressing the vena cava. Early placement of a gastric tube is therefore essential in all injured children.

The team leaders must be aware of the normal respiratory rate in children and how this varies with age (Table 11.1).

Appropriately-sized equipment must be used. Facemasks and self-inflating bags of 240 ml and 500 ml are used for infants and children respectively; the latter can also be used to ventilate via an endotracheal tube. The non-rebreathing valve should be pressure-limited to prevent pulmonary barotrauma. The aim should be to deliver 100% oxygen, hence reservoir bags should always be used. Mechanical ventilators can be used, but if in doubt they are best left to the experts. The final guide to adequacy of ventilation is analysis of arterial blood gases.

A member of the airway team should regularly assess ventilation by looking for chest movement and listening for breath sounds bilaterally. Regular examination also alerts the team to any developing lung pathology.

(C) Circulation

In addition to the usual tasks, one of the circulation nurses must measure the child from head to toe so that an estimation of the patient's age and weight can be made (Figure 11.2).

Seriously injured children require aggressive fluid administration. Unfortunately the error of inadequate fluid resuscitation in children is commonly made and can have fatal consequences. One member of the team must therefore control any external haemorrhage by direct pressure at the same time as the circulation doctor gains intravenous access. If percutaneous cannulation is not possible, an intraosseous needle should be inserted (see Chapter 4). In older children a venous cutdown can also be carried out (see Chapter 4).

All fluids used in paediatric resuscitation must be warmed. They are given in boluses based on the patient's body weight, and must be warmed prior to use to prevent iatrogenic hypothermia. In the UK, 20 ml/kg of plasma should be infused over 10 minutes and the patient then reassessed. (In North America 20 ml/kg of Ringer's lactate is used instead.) If there is no improvement the fluid bolus needs to be repeated. If the child remains shocked after the second bolus, 20 ml/kg of whole blood (or 10 ml/kg packed cells) should be administered and the source of the bleeding urgently sought.

The pneumatic anti-shock garment (PASG) can be used on children, but only one paediatric size is available. It is designed to fit a child of about 8 years of age and weighing 25 kg. Care needs to be taken when applying this suit that ventilation is not inhibited by placing the abdominal compartment too high on the child. It must remain below the level of the diaphragm.

The techniques used to monitor the urine output vary with the age of the child and with local policies: these must be known by the team leaders. Infants up to the age of 2 have an average output of 2 ml/kg/hr; children generally make 1 ml/kg/hr. Restoration of adequate organ perfusion is indicated by the urine output, vital signs and capillary refill all returning to normal. At this stage the intravenous fluids can be continued at a rate of 5 ml/kg/hr.

(D) Dysfunction

The brief neurological examination has to be interpreted in the light of the child's age. Vomiting and fits tend to be more common in children but are usually self-limiting. If they persist or worsen, a significant intracranial injury must be suspected.

(E) Exposure

Care must be taken to minimize heat loss as this can occur rapidly in children. Core temperature must be recorded regularly, using either a low-reading rectal thermometer or an infra-red tympanic temperature probe. The hypothermic child can be rewarmed during resuscitation by putting warm blankets around and under him to help reduce heat loss. The use of overhead infra-red lights and water-filled or electrical heating blankets are other helpful non-invasive techniques (see Chapter 13). Using warmed IV fluid, peritoneal lavage fluid and humidified oxygen will also reduce the risk of cooling the child during the resuscitation.

☐ Secondary survey

Mini-neurological examination

When the team is dealing with a paediatric patient, the verbal component of the Glasgow Coma Scale has to be modified. Several special coma scales have been devised to accommodate the differences in age and development in children. One example is the Phoenix Children's Hospital scale, shown in Box 11.5. It is important that the scale used by the team is documented for later reference.

Assessment of the peripheral nervous system can be difficult in infants because primitive responses have to be distinguished from spinal pathology. Experience is also required in interpreting the spinal radiographs so that developmental features are differentiated from fractures and ligamentous damage (see Chapter 8). It is also important to remember that 50 per cent of children with a significant spinal injury have normal radiographs.

Abdominal

Most injuries to the abdomens of children are blunt, therefore a good history and physical examination are essential.

Because of the potential for causing both physical and psychological damage, **rectal and vaginal examinations should be limited to those cases where essential, and only performed by a member of the medical team who is going to act on the result.**

BOX 11.5   Phoenix Children's Hospital's paediatric coma scale

---

Eye opening
Spontaneous	4
To speech	3
To pain	2
No response	1

Best motor response
Spontaneous	6
Localizes to pain	5
Withdraws to pain	4
Flexion to pain (decorticate)	3
Extension to pain (decerebrate)	2
No response	1

Best response to auditory/visual stimulus (age < 2 years)
Social smile, orientated to sound, follows objects	5
Cries, consolable	4
Inappropriate, persistent cry	3
Agitated, restless	2
No response	1

Best verbal response (age > 2 years)
Orientated	5
Confused	4
Inappropriate	3
Incomprehensible word	2
No response	1

In the haemodynamically stable child with abdominal injuries, the CT scan is used instead of a diagnostic peritoneal lavage (see Chapter 5). The reason for this is the increased rate of complications and false negatives in lavages carried out on children.

If a CT is not available, a diagnostic peritoneal technique as described in Chapter 5 should be used. With children it is important that the lavage fluid is warm and only 10 ml/kg used.

Musculoskeletal

Limb injuries in children are not uncommon but because of the immaturity of the bones may require comparison x-rays to diagnose.

Injuries in and around joints may result in vascular compromise. In particular, the brachial artery has a high risk of damage following a supracondylar fracture in a child. Detailed examination of the neurovascular status of all injured limbs is therefore essential (see Chapter 9).

AMPLE

Blunt trauma is the commonest mechanism of injury in children and in view of their smaller size, it leads to a high incidence of multisystem injury.

The principles of assessing a child with a penetrating injury are the same as those described for adults (see Chapters 1 and 10). However, penetrating injury is not common in childhood.

When assessing an injured child the team leaders must always consider the possibility of child abuse. Common signs which may indicate this are listed in Box 11.6. In such cases the appropriate authorities must be informed. The policy determining this will vary from unit to unit, and must be known by the team leaders.

BOX 11.6   Signs of non-accidental injury

- Inappropriate delay in attending hospital
- The history of the incident does not correspond with the injuries
- The history of the incident varies
- Lack of concern by the child's guardian
- Abnormal interaction between the child and his guardian
- Unusual injuries (e.g. bite marks and cigarette burns)
- Signs of sexual abuse
- Retinal haemorrhages
- Torn frenulum
- Long-bone fracture in children under 3 years
- Previous injuries which cannot be appropriately explained

☐ **Emotional support**

Managing a critically injured child is emotionally demanding. The team leaders must be sensitive to the needs of the patient, the relatives and their own personnel.

The airway personnel are often best placed to provide continuous comfort to the conscious patient as well as an explanation of what is happening. Parents need to be considered as well, and be given truthful, regular information about the resuscitation by the relatives' nurse (see Chapter 16).

☐ **Pain relief**

Adequate analgesia is important for both humanitarian and physiological reasons (see Chapter 4). After the primary survey and resuscitation, intravenous morphine can be used, usually 50–100 µg/kg, titrated against the patient's pain (providing there are no contraindications).

■ References and further reading

Advanced Life Support Group (in press). *Advanced Paediatric Life Support (UK): student manual*. London: BMJ Publications.

American College of Surgeons Committee on Trauma 1993. *Advanced Trauma Life Support Course for Physicians: instructor manual*. Chicago: American College of Surgeons.

Bobb S 1988. Trauma in the elderly. In Cardona V, *et al.* (eds): *Trauma Nursing*. Philadelphia: W B Saunders.

Henao F, Daes J & Dennis R 1991. Risk factors for multiorgan failure: a case-control study. *J. Trauma* **31**(1): 74.

Kinsella S, Whitwam J & Spencer J 1992. Reducing aortocaval compression; how much tilt is enough? *Br. Med. J.* **305**: 539.

Kiwerski J 1992. Injuries to the spinal cord in elderly patients. *Injury* **23**(6): 397.

Kolberg S & Harmon S 1988. Pediatric trauma. In Cardona V, *et al.* (eds): *Trauma Nursing*. Philadelphia: W B Saunders.

Kravitz M, Elliott S, Wessman M, *et al.* 1985. Thermal injury in the elderly: incidence and cause. *J. Burn Care Rehabil.* **6**: 487.

Lloyd-Thomas A & Anderson I 1991. Paediatric trauma: secondary survey. In Skinner D, Driscoll P & Earlam R (eds): *ABC of Major Trauma*. London: BMJ Publications.

McKenna P, Welsh D & Martin L 1991. Paediatric bicycle trauma. *J. Trauma* **31**(3): 392.

Morton R & Phillips B 1992. *Accidents and Emergencies in Children*. Oxford: Oxford University Press.

Nash P & Driscoll P 1991. Trauma in pregnancy. In Skinner D, Driscoll P & Earlam R (eds): *ABC of Major Trauma*. London: BMJ Publications.

Ninan G & Puri P 1993. Late presentation of traumatic rupture of the diaphragm in a child. *Br. Med. J.* **306**: 643.

Scalea T, Simon H, Duncan A, *et al.* 1990. Geriatric blunt multiple trauma: improved survival with early invasive monitoring. *J. Trauma* **30**: 129.

Schlag G, Krosl P & Redl H 1988. Cardiopulmonary response of the elderly to traumatic and septic shock. *Perspec. Shock Res.* Alan Liss, Inc.

Schwartz G 1986. Trauma during pregnancy. In Schwartz G, Safer P & Stone S (eds): *Principles and Practice of Emergency Medicine*. Philadelphia: W B Saunders.

Sheehy S, Marvin J & Jimmerson C 1989a. Pediatric trauma. In Sheehy S, Marvin J & Jimmerson C (eds): *Clinical Trauma Nursing: the first hour*. St. Louis: C V Mosby.

Sheehy S, Marvin J & Jimmerson C 1989b. Trauma in pregnancy. In Sheehy S, Marvin J & Jimmerson C (eds): *Clinical Trauma Nursing: the first hour*. St. Louis: C V Mosby.

Shock N 1983. Aging of regulatory mechanisms. In Cape R (ed.): *Fundamentals of Geriatric Medicine*. New York: Raven Press.

Smith S 1988. The pregnancy trauma patient. In Cardona V, *et al.* (eds): *Trauma Nursing*. Philadelphia: W B Saunders.

Waller J 1974. Injury in the aged. *NY State J. Med.* **74**: 2200.

Chapter 12

Burns

Cindy LeDuc Jimmerson, Peter Driscoll and Carl Gwinnutt

Objectives

The objectives of this chapter are for members of the trauma team to be able:

- to define burn shock;

- to list the most common mechanisms of burn injuries;

- to discuss the three types of respiratory problems associated with smoke inhalation;

- to describe the recommended order of resuscitation efforts;

- to determine fluid resuscitation volumes based on burn size and depth, using standard formulae;

- to determine fluid resuscitation volumes for a patient with an electrical burn;

- to discuss wound care for surface burns.

■ Introduction

The complexity of the body's response to a burn injury challenges the nursing and medical staff both in the resuscitation and definitive care phases, due to the complexity of the physiology and the relationship to other injuries.

The presence of pain and possible disfigurement represent an emotional challenge both to the team members and to the patient. Mechanically it can be difficult to position the patient comfortably, especially when precautions are taken for associated injuries. It may even be arduous performing usually uncomplicated nursing procedures such as securing an intravenous line to burned skin.

■ Pathophysiology

Perhaps the most important factors in the initial responses to a burn are the cellular changes. It is only at a later stage that the respiratory, cardiovascular and immune systems are affected (see Chapters 3 and 4). Therefore the team should begin treatment early and not delay until alterations in the respiratory and cardiovascular functions have been recorded.

☐ Cellular response to burn injury

The normal host defence response to skin injury is a release of histamine and other vasoactive substances which increase cell-wall permeability and attract white blood cells and plasma protein so that infection can be fought (see Chapter 10).

Fluid shifts occur immediately after a burn injury with leakage of intravascular water, salt and protein into the interstitial space. Loss of circulating plasma volume leads to haemoconcentration (increased haematocrit) and hypovolaemia, the severity of which increases with the severity of the burn. In a significant burn (over 15 per cent of the total body surface area), the capillary leak may be systemic, causing generalized oedema and a significant fall in blood volume.

☐ Shock associated with burn injuries

The effect on the circulation is directly related to the size and severity of the burn wound. The body compensates for this loss of plasma with an increase in peripheral vascular resistance, and the patient will appear cool, pale and clammy, and urine output will fall. However, this compensation will only be effective in maintaining circulation for a period of time depending on the severity of the burn and the presence of other injuries. Ultimately the patient will demonstrate signs of hypovolaemic shock as the cardiac output falls (see Chapter 4).

A burn of greater than 25 per cent of the total body surface area (TBSA) almost always requires intravenous fluid administration to expand the depleted vascular volume. It has been accepted since the 1930s, however, that burn shock can occur with a burn involving a little as 15 per cent TBSA, as a result of complicating factors such as age, pre-existing disease and other major injuries. In these circumstances, a burn of 25–40 per cent becomes a potentially lethal injury.

☐ Carbon monoxide (CO) intoxication

Carbon monoxide intoxication is the biggest cause of death in people caught in house fires, or other types of closed-space fires.

Carbon monoxide affects the body in two ways. Firstly it inhibits the cellular cytochrome oxidase system, causing inhibition of cellular metabolism. Secondly, it has 200 times the affinity for binding to haemoglobin compared with oxygen, and therefore blocks the ability to transport oxygen to active tissues, thereby causing cellular hypoxia. This is usually demonstrated firstly in alterations in the patient's mental state, ranging from mild anxiety or nervous behaviour to drowsiness and eventual unconsciousness. The inhibition of the cytochrome oxidase system in the brain, resulting in a rise in ICP, is another cause for extended periods of unconsciousness. Carbon monoxide also combines with myoglobin in the patient's muscle cells, causing weakness.

Patients who have been in a closed-space fire, or who have a history of having inhaled smoke during the rescue phase, should be observed closely for signs of hypoxia. Carboxyhaemoglobin (COHb) should be measured on admission to assess the severity of exposure and help predict potential complications. However, as the carboxyhaemoglobin level declines as soon as the patient begins to breathe air or oxygen, the medical team leader must take into account the time delay between carbon monoxide exposure and the blood sample being taken. A nomogram is available to enable the carbon monoxide level at the time of exposure to be estimated. (The interested reader should consult the references at the end of this chapter for details on this subject.)

Treatment of any patient who has been involved in a fire should include high-flow oxygen therapy until carbon monoxide intoxication is ruled out. The duration of the patient's exposure to carbon monoxide is significant, as short exposures to a high concentration may cause high carboxyhaemoglobin levels without causing significant metabolic effects (usually acidosis with bicarbonate deficit). These are usually more severe in patients with low-level exposures of a longer duration. Carboxyhaemoglobin levels greater than 10 per cent are significant, and levels greater than 50 per cent are generally lethal.

Hyperbaric oxygen is the treatment of choice for symptomatic carbon monoxide exposure. This not only forces the oxygen molecules onto the haemoglobin, it also shortens the half-life of carbon monoxide and decreases intracranial pressure and cerebral oedema. As prolonged untreated carbon monoxide poisoning can cause residual neurological sequelae, rapid identification and hyperbaric treatment are essential.

The carboxyhaemoglobin level must be measured if there is a history of unconsciousness for an unknown reason, particularly when the event raises suspicion of carbon monoxide being present at the scene, for example when there has been machinery exhaust in a closed space.

☐ Response of the respiratory system to inhalation injury

The lungs themselves are rarely injured from 'burning' (even with blast injuries that cause air to be inspired under pressure). Usually laryngeal spasm occurs from the heat of the inspired gases, thereby protecting the lower airway and lungs from exposure.

The upper airway may receive thermal burns, and tissue swelling can develop very rapidly in these vascular tissues, particularly the mouth and oropharynx, and cause acute respiratory obstruction. Oedema from these injuries can also involve the vocal cords. Dramatic changes in the patient's ability to maintain his airway have been observed over a short period of time following this type of injury. Documentation from the pre-hospital care providers concerning the mechanism of injury and the changes in respiratory status en route to hospital allows the team to anticipate airway problems.

The lung parenchyma is frequently damaged by inhaled gases or chemicals that are released by the fire or explosive event in which the patient has been involved. Common sources of these are building and home decorating materials, particularly polyvinyl chloride (PVC), polyurethane and urea-formaldehyde, as well as acrylic fibres and nylon. Symptoms may be absent initially, but develop with time and rehydration during the resuscitation period. The lung responds initially with irritation (bronchospasm), inflammation and progressive oedema. The reaction frequently includes a decrease in surfactant levels and a decrease in pulmonary macrophages, and may result in haemorrhagic tracheobronchitis. This leads to a decrease in lung compliance, seen as an increase in the work of breathing and an impairment of diffusion through the alveolar membrane (see Chapter 3).

Intense observation of the burn patient's respiratory status is required to identify early symptoms such as rapid respiration, coughing, haemoptysis, and signs of poor perfusion. Adult respiratory distress syndrome (ARDS; see Chapter 3) may develop over a period of 24–48 hours.

In view of the very large surface area of the lung, fluid requirements for resuscitation may increase by as much as 50 per cent of the calculated values if a severe inhalation injury has been sustained. The severity of the injury will not be related to the TBSA burn size, but rather to the length of time and the intensity of exposure to the inhalation. Again, accurate information from the pre-hospital care providers about these conditions is vital in planning the patient's care and anticipating respiratory complications.

☐ Cyanide poisoning

When the polyurethane foam in modern furniture burns, a thick black smoke is produced. This contains not only a mixture of corrosive substances, but also cyanide gas. Like carbon monoxide, cyanide blocks cellular metabolism by inhibiting the cytochrome system. This leads to tissue hypoxia.

At very low concentrations the patient will complain of headaches and dizziness. Usually the inhaled concentration of cyanide is such that the victim becomes dyspnoeic and rapidly loses consciousness.

Plasma for cyanide levels should be taken. This measurement takes time, however, and an arterial blood sample must be taken and the saturation of haemoglobin with oxygen *measured* (not calculated) using a co-oximeter. Plasma lactate can also give the team an indication of the degree of tissue hypoxia, but again this is not immediately available.

The management of these patients is the same as that described for carbon monoxide poisoning. This includes hyperbaric oxygen in appropriate cases. In addition, specific antidotes for cyanide poisoning must be administered: these include amyl nitrate, dicobalt edetate and sodium thiosulphate. Local policies vary with regard to these antidotes and these policies must be known by the team leaders.

☐ Special types of burns

Thermal burns

These are the most common types of burns and are caused by heat from flames, scalds, contact with hot surfaces, or flashes. Burn-prevention programmes have been very effective in reducing the number of burn injuries seen in the past forty years, but hot-fluid scalding remains the most frequent mechanism of burns. Children who are unfamiliar with the danger of hot liquids and the elderly population are the most frequent victims. Scalding injuries also remain the most prevalent industrial burns.

Chemical burns

Acids and alkalis release energy in the form of heat when they come into contact with biological tissue. Alkalis produce the most damage because they penetrate into deeper tissues. Acids react with the tissue surface to produce a barrier which inhibits further penetration.

Electrical burns

There are several factors that affect the severity of the injury:

- the type of current (AC or DC);
- the voltage of the shock;
- the duration of the contact;
- the resistance of the tissues;
- the pathway along which the current travels.

Although the entrance and exit wounds are treated as thermal wounds, they do not give an accurate indication of the extent of the burn as the electrical current will have travelled through the tissues along the path of least resistance. As skin is highly resistant, the current travels preferentially along arteries, veins, nerves, bones and tendons. This causes progressive tissue loss as the circulation to some undamaged tissues will have been destroyed, leading to cellular hypoxia and necrosis. Thus the true extent of the tissue damage cannot be measured initially.

■ Assessment and management

□ Pre-hospital care

The patient's resuscitation begins with the first intervention after injury. A good relationship with the pre-hospital personnel ensures that the transition from the incident site to the hospital setting is smooth, unified and a true 'team approach'. This can be helped by planning with pre-hospital services to achieve a standardized approach to the major-burn patient.

Information that should be relayed by the pre-hospital personnel includes the following:

1 Name, age, weight.

2 Mechanism of injury:
  - How did it happen?
  - Is there suspicion of an inhalational injury?
  - Were any other injuries sustained?
  - Were there other victims involved?

3 History:
  - When did it happen?
  - Can witnesses, friends or family members give more information about the event?

4 First vital signs and any changes that have occurred.

5 Condition of airway.

6   Level of consciousness.

7   Treatment administered by pre-hospital service and the patient's response.

8   Past medical history.

9   Estimated time of arrival.

When safe to do so, the patient should be moved from the scene of the incident to an area of safety. Here burning, hot or smouldering clothing can be drenched with water and removed, provided it is not adhering to the victim's skin. In addition, high-flow oxygen must be administered as soon as possible if there is evidence of inhalation or if the patient was found in an enclosed environment.

Normally elaborate dressings are not required in the pre-hospital phase. If the journey time is expected to be greater than an hour, however, sterile foam dressings should be wrapped around the burns (Roehampton dressings).

☐ Primary survey and resuscitation

The most important rule in assessing a patient who has been badly burned is to remember to **treat the patient's life-threatening problems first.** Usually these are not the burn wound. Even when the patient presents with a significant burn and a great deal of pain, the team must recall the basic priorities of trauma care: airway, breathing, and circulation. In most cases this means that the team will treat the burn wound last. An exception is when there are chemical burns. In these cases there are simultaneous priorities to stop the burning process as the airway is being secured. The patient's clothing or other contaminated coverings should then be removed. Dilution of the chemical by irrigation needs to begin immediately, with precautions being taken so that other members of the team are not contaminated by splashes or by the water rinsing away from the patient's body (see Chapters 15 and 19).

The principles of the initial assessment are discussed in detail in Chapter 1. However, consideration of the special problems associated with that initial examination of the burn victim will now be covered.

(A) Airway

The assessment and management of the patient's airway is the first priority because ensuring good ventilation from the beginning of resuscitation, through the critical care phase, is vital to the patient's outcome.

The airway personnel must anticipate the development of oedema from the response to the thermal injury, the complication of smoke inhalation, and the possibility of facial, oral and upper airway burns. Meticulous observation of the respiratory status of the critically burned patient is therefore essential so that subtle signs can be detected early.

The signs listed in Box 12.1 should raise suspicions of potential airway obstruction.

BOX 12.1   Signs of impending airway problems

- Difficulty in controlling secretions
- Carbonaceous particles in the sputum
- Hoarseness
- Difficulty in breathing and swallowing
- Burns of the tongue
- Singed facial hairs
- Blisters around the nose and mouth

Early airway management with endotracheal intubation should be considered in those patients with any of the features listed in Box 12.1 (Figure 12.1). Although the oral route is preferred, to allow visualization of the vocal cords and correct placement of the tube, nasotracheal intubation may also be considered if the oral route is impossible.

Intubation in these cases is often done as an emergency and is frequently difficult because of the complications mentioned before. The airway nurse and doctor must therefore have anaesthetic training. For further details the interested reader should consult Chapter 2.

Surgical airways are usually avoided because of the complications with oedema and infection.

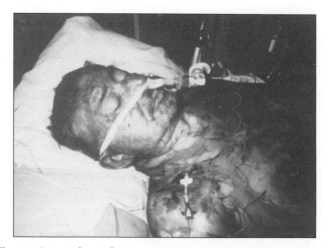

Figure 12.1   A burned patient requiring endotracheal intubation to protect the airway

(B) Breathing

The patient's ability to ventilate adequately is an observation which should be repeatedly assessed during resuscitation of the burn patient so that problems can be anticipated and avoided, particularly those arising from the inhalation of smoke and toxic gases. It is insufficient simply to determine that the patient is breathing on his own.

Patients who are breathing adequately must receive high-flow oxygen by a suitable facemask. Tracheal intubation is indicated if the patient is unable to ventilate adequately as a result of inhalational injuries, a reduced level of consciousness due to carbon monoxide poisoning, or other injuries. Intubation allows the airway personnel to ventilate the patient with 100 per cent oxygen using a bag-valve apparatus or a mechanical ventilator. As always following this manoeuvre, appropriate checks of tube placement and ventilation must be made (Chapter 2).

Measurement of arterial blood gases to ensure success in ventilation should be repeated at least every 30 minutes throughout the resuscitation, and frequently during the intensive care phase.

Escharotomy

One group of patients in whom ventilation must be carefully monitored is those with circumferential chest burns. These burns extend around the thorax, and as tissue oedema develops, a constricting girdle forms. If patients with this type of injury develop increasing difficulty in breathing – such as decreased chest expansion and rapid, shallow ventilation, along with increasing oedema of the chest wall and tight leathery skin – then escharatomy must be considered. This involves making relieving incisions through insensitive skin in areas of full-thickness burns to allow chest expansion.

Escharotomy: procedure

Preparation for this procedure includes providing vascular clamps, diathermy and whatever other forms of haemostasis the physician requires, as blood loss can contribute to hypovolaemia. The circulation nurse must be prepared to assist with this procedure in the resuscitation room, or at the patient's bedside after admission if problems arise.

Longitudinal incisions are made in the mid-axillary line through the burnt skin until the wound gapes open. If this fails to release the tension, transverse incisions should be carried out over the anterior chest wall. Once haemostasis has been obtained, absorbent dressings can be applied to the wound.

(C) Circulation

The primary task of the circulation personnel is to insert two large-bore intravenous cannulae to ensure rapid access to the circulation. If possible, the long saphenous vein should be avoided because of the risk of thrombosis and the poor flow through it due to vascular spasm. The placement of cannulae through burned skin is acceptable if this enables a large vein to be cannulated. A cannula that has been placed through burned skin may need to be sutured in place or secured using gauze bandaging, as adhesive tape is usually ineffective.

Once the cannulae are in place 20 ml of blood should be removed for haematocrit, full blood count, urea and electrolytes, cyanide and carboxy-haemoglobin (if relevant), and group- and crossmatching.

Estimation of hypovolaemia

One of the circulation nurses must record the patient's vital signs whilst intravenous access is being obtained. An increase in irritability and signs of cerebral hypoxia may be the first subtle clues of inadequate oxygen delivery. Tachycardia, tachypnoea, delayed capillary refill (greater than 2 seconds) and a decrease in blood pressure are important signs of hypovolaemia (see Chapter 4). Nausea, vomiting, paralytic ileus and a haematocrit of above 50 per cent are other indications of a low-flow state. These parameters must be monitored frequently so that the response to treatment can be assessed.

One of the best methods of monitoring the adequacy of tissue perfusion is urinary output. In the burn patient who has large and fluctuating fluid demands, close observation of the amount of urine that is being produced can provide a clear indication of how well the kidneys are being perfused. From this information the team leaders can estimate the degree of perfusion of other organs, such as the heart, lungs, and liver.

'Adequate' urinary output in a burn patient who is being volume-resuscitated is generally accepted to be 50 ml/hour in the adult patient. However, the patient with a major electrical burn can be expected to have significant amounts of myoglobin in the urine as a by-product of muscle tissue destruction (see later). In these circumstances urinary output should be maintained at 2–3 times normal, that is 100–150 ml/hr. Urinary output in children with burns should be 20–30 ml/hour (or about 1 ml/kg/hour), and for infants 2 ml/kg body weight/hour.

Whenever possible, invasive monitoring devices should be kept to a minimum because of the risk of septicaemia developing in the immuno-compromised burn patient.

Estimation of burn size

Whilst team members are obtaining access to the circulation, the team leader must make an assessment of the magnitude of the burn. Both the size

and depth of the burn are very important in determining the fluid requirements of the patient as well as in predicting his future progress. It is
therefore essential that the medical team leader evaluates these requirements
as accurately as possible. He or she should also determine whether there are
any unusual burn patterns that may suggest abuse or foul play, and whether
there are circumferential burns in other areas, particularly the limbs, that
may require escharotomy.

Careful recording of the findings of the assessment of the burn patient
must be carried out *throughout* the resuscitation and definitive care phase.
Burn wounds often extend, as oedema and poor circulation cause additional
cell destruction. Meticulous recording will help detect this phenomenon as
it occurs and thus allow the team to address the problem as early as
possible.

It is recommended that both the burned surface area and the unburned
area are measured. This allows a check of comparable percentages, thereby
improving the accuracy of the estimate. Simple erythema is considered as
unburnt tissue.

As there are three standard methods of estimating the burn area, with
varying levels of accuracy, it is important that the one used is recorded. The
Lund and Browder chart (Figure 12.2) can be coloured at the bedside and
computed in a quieter setting. The less accurate Rule of Nines (Figure 12.3)
is helpful for making quick, gross estimates of burn size, and is the method
usually used by the pre-hospital services. The team leaders should remember
that for children the Rule of Nines must be modified for age. In the infant,
the head and neck represent 19 per cent of the total body surface area and
each lower extremity is assigned only 14 per cent. When correcting this
formula for age, reduce the head size by 1 per cent per year of age and add
0.5 per cent per leg for each year of age.

If burns are inconsistent over a body area, it is helpful to recall that the
palmar area of the patient's hand is approximately 1 per cent of his body
surface area. This general guideline may also help in estimating the overall
burn area.

Electrical burns pose a special problem because the area of skin burned
is not an accurate reflection of the true size of the burn. As the injury is not
initially measurable, different criteria are used for fluid resuscitation of
patients with electrical burns (see later). Entrance and exit wounds need to
be identified and treated as the thermal injuries.

Fluid requirements following a thermal burn

Several standard fluid resuscitation formulas for burn shock have been
developed. Provided the fluid contains 130–150 mmol Na^+/l, the actual
fluid is less important than its commencement. It is therefore important that
the nursing and medical team leaders are familiar with the formula used in
their facility so that the team can begin fluid infusion immediately the
patient arrives in the resuscitation room.

CHART FOR ESTIMATING SEVERITY OF BURN WOUND

NAME_____WARD_____NUMBER_____DATE____
AGE_____ ADMISSION WEIGHT_____

LUND AND BROWDER CHARTS

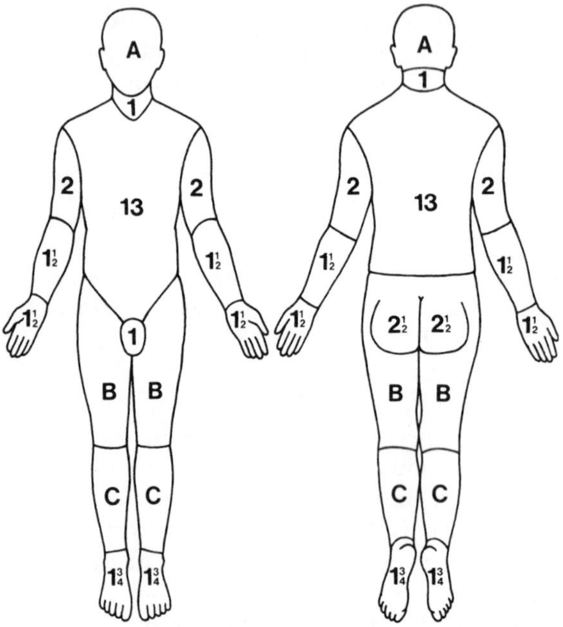

Partial thickness loss (PTL)

Full thickness loss (FTL)

REGION	PTL	FTL
HEAD		
NECK		
ANT.TRUNK		
POST.TRUNK		
RIGHT ARM		
LEFT ARM		
BUTTOCKS		
GENITALIA		
RIGHT LEG		
LEFT LEG		
TOTAL BURN		

RELATIVE PERCENTAGE OF BODY SURFACE AREA
AFFECTED BY GROWTH

AREA	AGE 0	1	5	10	15	ADULT
A=½ OF HEAD	9½	8½	6½	5½	4½	3½
B=½ OF ONE THIGH	2¾	3¼	4	4½	4½	4¾
C=½ OF ONE LEG	2½	2½	2¾	3	3¼	3½

Smith+Nephew

For further supplies of this pad or of Flamazine* Cream for the prevention and treatment of infection in burns contact Ingrebourne (04023) 49333 or your Smith & Nephew Pharmaceutical representative.   *Trade mark

Figure 12.2a Lund and Browder chart: estimating the severity of the burn
Source: © Lund & Browder 1992. Romford, Essex: Smith & Nephew Pharmaceuticals.
Reproduced by kind permission.

TRANSFER INFORMATION CHART

Contact your Regional Burn Centre early for advice.

TIME OF INCIDENT:

TIME OF ARRIVAL:

HOW ACCIDENT HAPPENED

CLOTHING WORN AT TIME

FIRST AID GIVEN

HOW LONG FOR?

I.V. CANNULA SIZE

SITE OF INSERTION

CATHETER PASSED   YES/NO

CATHETER SIZE:

URINE OUTPUT: ml

Time measured:

ANALGESIA/ANTI-EMETICS

AMOUNT	ROUTE	TIME

TETANUS TOXOID (please tick)

UP TO DATE ☐   GIVEN ☐

Transfer form designed with the help of the staff of the
McIndoe Burns Centre, East Grinstead, England.

† Available from Smith & Nephew Pharmaceuticals Ltd

SMOKE INHALATION SUSPECTED? YES / NO

SOOT IN THROAT/NOSE   YES / NO

HOARSE VOICE   YES / NO

INTUBATION REQUIRED   YES / NO

SIZE OF TUBE:

BLOOD GASES:
(if taken)

FLUID REQUIREMENT CALCULATION

(see also "Burns a Plan of Action" wallchart)†

WEIGHT OF PATIENT: Kg

ESTIMATED BURN AREA: %BSA

$$\frac{\text{WT OF PT} \times \% \text{ OF BURN}}{2} = \begin{array}{l} \text{Total colloid} \\ \text{infusion over} \\ \text{four hours} \end{array}$$

$$= \quad \text{ml per period}$$

FLUID REGIME – FIRST 4 HOURS
FROM INJURY

HOUR	FLUID	AMOUNT
1		
2		
3		
4		

COMMENTS:

Figure 12.2b Lund and Browder chart: transfer information
Source: © Lund & Browder 1992. Romford, Essex: Smith & Nephew Pharmaceuticals.
Reproduced by kind permission.

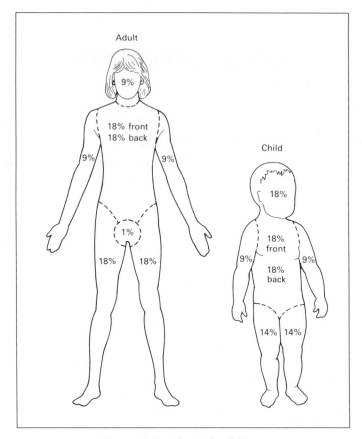

Figure 12.3 The Rule of Nines

It should be understood that all formulae are *guidelines* for fluid administration and, in the case of the Muir and Barclay formula, are in addition to normal daily maintenance requirements, and that successful fluid resuscitation is ultimately determined by the patient's response to the therapy. Using information from all the physiological parameters, adjustments to the formula can be made. Warm intravenous solution should be used so as to prevent heat loss.

Baxter or Parkland formula

This formula is commonly used in the United States and in parts of Europe. It covers the first 48 hours post-injury. The time of starting the treatment is calculated from the time of *injury*, not from the time of admission to hospital.

1   In the first 24 hours:
    • 4 ml of Ringer's lactate (Hartmann's solution)/kg body weight/%
      TBSA burn:
      – one-half in the first 8 hours post-injury;
      – one-quarter in the second 8 hours;
      – one-quarter in the third 8 hours.

2   In the second 24 hours:
    • 5% dextrose, in sufficient quantities to maintain serum sodium be-
      low 140 mEq/l;
    • potassium to maintain normal serum levels;
    • plasma or plasma expander to maintain an adequate circulating
      volume with normal pulse, blood pressure and urine output.

Muir and Barclay formula

This is the most widely used formula for predicting fluid requirements in
the UK. **The first 36 hours are divided into six successive periods of 4, 4, 4,
6, 6 and 12 hours,** *starting from the time of the burn.* A volume of plasma
(in millilitres) is calculated that should be infused by the end of each
time period. Note that the formula is dependent on the type of plasma
available:

•   freeze-dried plasma = % TBSA burns × body weight (kg) × 0.5;
•   human plasma protein fraction (HPPF) = % TBSA burns × body weight
    (kg) × 0.65.

This volume can be checked and modified in the light of the volume
calculated by plasma deficit. This is the volume missing from the circulation. It assumes however, that there is no loss of red cells and that the
patient initially had a normal haematocrit (Hct):

$$\text{plasma deficit} = \text{blood volume} - \frac{\text{blood vol} \times \text{normal Hct}}{\text{patient's Hct}}$$

Normal values of blood volume and haematocrit are given in standard
tables and are usually written on the burn chart.

One unit of blood is required for every 10% TBSA full-thickness burn.
This replaces a similar volume of plasma in the fluid regime and it is usually
given during the final time period. In extensive deep burns, however, blood
should be started during the first time period.

Additional crystalloid, in the form of 5% dextrose, is also required to
replace normal fluid requirements.

The patient must be reassessed at the end of each time block and the
volume given during the next time period adjusted accordingly.

Evaluation of the patient's response to fluid replacement is crucial if he
is to be appropriately resuscitated. Only by monitoring the physiological
response frequently can the team determine how the volumes should be

modified. Signs of appropriate treatment include adequate urine production, a pulse rate within high normal limits, blood pressure normal for age, and an alert, orientated patient.

Fluid requirements following an electrical burn

As the standard burn formulae are based on the percentage of TBSA burned, these formulas do not work for electrical burns. Patients with such injuries should receive intravenous volumes that will restore adequate vital signs and maintain urine production at 2–3 times the normal rate (100–150 ml/hour in adults, 2 ml/kg/hour in children).

Given below is a formula that retrospectively gives a gross estimate of the extent of an electrical burn, based on fluid requirements over the first 24 hours post-injury.

Reverse Parkland formula:

$$\% \text{ TBSA} = \frac{\text{fluid requirement (ml) in 24 hours}}{\text{body weight (kg)} \times 4}$$

Estimation of burn depth

Accuracy in determining the depth of the burn is less important in the initial resuscitative phase than later. The extent may change as oedema and poor perfusion of the burn area increase the tissue injury. As the patient's priority changes from resuscitation to recovery, burn depth information becomes very important because it is needed for planning the definitive care of the wound.

Three depths of burns are described in the literature. It has to be said, however, that there is no totally reliable test that distinguishes them in the resuscitation room.

First-degree (superficial) burns present with erythema, pain and no blisters. This is the typical appearance produced after mild sunburn. Second-degree (deep dermal) and third-degree (full-thickness) burns are described in Figure 12.4.

Pain management in the burned patient

Most patients who have sustained a major burn will require analgesia and perhaps sedation, particularly during treatment. However, these requirements are usually small because full-thickness burns are insensitive.

During the pre-hospital phase analgesia can be provided by administering Entonox (50% oxygen and 50% nitrous oxide), unless there is a coexisting severe chest injury with the risk of a pneumothorax. In the resuscitative phase this can be continued or replaced with an opiate, most commonly morphine. It is important that the opiate is given by the intra-

Depth of Burn	Signs & Symptoms	Severity
Second Degree Second-degree burns are deeper than first-degree burns, and involve partial thickness. They result from a very deep sunburn, contact with hot liquids, or flash burns from gasoline flames. They are usually more painful than third-degree burns.	Red or mottled appearance. Blisters and broken epidermis. Considerable swelling. Weeping, wet surfaces. Painful. Sensitive to cold air.	**Critical:** Burns complicated by respiratory tract injury and fractures. Burns involving 15% to 30% of body surface. **Moderate:** Burns involving 15% to 30% of body surface. **Minor:** Burns of less than 15% of body surface.

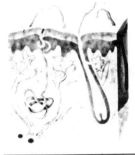

Third Degree Third-degree burns cause damage to all skin layers, sub-cutaneous tissue, and nerve endings. They can be caused by fire, prolonged exposure to hot liquids, contact with hot objects or electricity.	Pale white or charred apearance, leathery. (At first, may resemble second-degree burn.) Broken skin with fat exposed. Dry surface. Painless, insensitive to pinprick. Edema.	**Critical:** Burns complicated by respiratory tract injury and fractures. Burns involving the critical areas of the face, hands, or feet. Burns involving more than 10% of body surface. **Moderate:** Burns of 2% to 10% of body surface, and not involving face, hands, or feet. **Minor:** Burns of less than 2% of body surface.

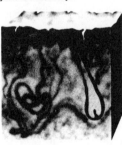

Figure 12.4 Second- and third-degree burns

Source: © 1993. *Advanced Trauma Life Support*™ *Student Manual*. American College of Surgeons. Reproduced by kind permission.

venous route, and titrated to patients' needs. The altered circulation and oedema that accompany major burns makes absorption from intramuscular administration irregular and unpredictable. The administration of an opiate should be accompanied by a suitable antiemetic and other measures, such as positioning and cool compresses, to relieve the burning sensation. When cool compresses are used, care should be taken to prevent hypothermia developing in the burned patient.

Careful monitoring of the patient's temperature and the magnitude of the burn should guide the circulation nurse in the use of cool compresses for pain relief. Evaluation of the patient's pain is important to assist in other clinical evaluations. It is easy to mistake the restlessness and irritability of hypoxia as being due to pain.

Additional requirements in special populations

Burn injuries in certain groups require special consideration. Children have a larger skin surface area in relation to body size than adults; they therefore tend to cool and become hypothermic more easily. Consequently care must be taken to prevent heat loss in children with burns greater than 15 per cent TBSA. Furthermore, the fluid shifts associated with skin injuries make children more likely to develop hypovolaemia. They should therefore be monitored very closely for subtle signs of shock.

The elderly tend to compensate less well than their younger counterparts. They deteriorate more rapidly from the hypovolaemia that accompanies major burns, and tend to become hypothermic as well. Due to decreased acuity in sensory function, they may have suffered burns of greater significance than they feel, and close observation of their recovery is essential. Healing is generally slower with this population, and attention to wound care, range of motion and ambulation presents a nursing care challenge as the patient recovers.

The mortality in females in the second or third trimesters of pregnancy is higher than in the normal population. Though the reasons for this are unclear it is recommended that immediate delivery should be carried out if the maternal TBSA burn exceeds 50 per cent. It follows that experienced obstetric help must be summoned early on in the patient's resuscitation.

If the facilities are immediately available in the resuscitation room, humidified oxygen should be administered to patients who have inhaled smoke. Beta-2-agonists (e.g. salbutamol), administered by an oxygen-powered nebulizer, also have a role to play in relieving bronchospasm.

Myocardial ischaemia, infarction and dysrhythmia can occur in burn victims with known ischaemic heart disease or carbon monoxide levels greater than 15 per cent: these patients require continuous cardiac monitoring and a 12-lead ECG at the end of the primary survey.

☐ Secondary survey

After the patient's cardiovascular status has been restored and other life-threatening injuries and complications have been satisfactorily addressed, the team leader can carry out the detailed head-to-toe assessment of the patient. This is described in detail in Chapter 1.

Full-thickness circumferential burns of the limbs and digits should be detected at this stage. These will require escharotomies, which are carried out in the manner described before. In these cases, however, the incision is along the lateral and/or medial longitudinal axis of the limb and digit.

AMPLE

A good history of the burn event is essential for planning the resuscitation and ultimately the definitive care of the burn victim. The mechanism of injury, the pre-hospital care and response, the patient's previous health status, current medications and the existence of allergies are all essential pieces of information needed for developing an optimal management plan for the patient.

The severity of the burn

By the end of the secondary survey, the team leaders must know the severity of the burn so that a definitive care plan can be developed. The factors determining the severity of a burn are listed in Box 12.2.

BOX 12.2   Factors that determine the severity of a burn

- The patient's physiological response
- The mechanism of injury:
  - scald
  - flame
  - chemical
  - explosive
  - electrical
- The TBSA of the burn
- Complicating factors:
  - smoke inhalation
  - associated injuries
  - toxic chemical inhalation or contamination

As a general rule, burn severity may be classified using the following guidelines.

Major burn

In the adult patient:
- second-degree burn > 25% TBSA;
- third-degree burn > 10% TBSA.

In children:
- second-degree burn > 20% TBSA;
- third-degree burn > 10% TBSA.

In adults or children:
- any burn involving hands, face, feet or perineum;
- all electrical injuries.

Burns complicated by:
- smoke inhalation;
- major associated trauma;
- pre-existing illnesses.

Moderate burns

In adults (not involving face, hands, feet or perineum):
- second-degree burn 15–25% TBSA;
- third-degree burn 3–10% TBSA.

In children (not involving face, hands, feet or perineum):
- second-degree burn 10–20% TBSA;
- third-degree burn 3–10% TBSA.

Minor burns

In adults (not involving face, hands, feet or perineum):
- second-degree burn < 15% TBSA;
- third-degree burn < 3% TBSA.

In children (not involving face, hands, feet, or perineum):
- second-degree burn < 10% TBSA;
- third-degree burn < 3% TBSA.

☐ Definitive care

Following the secondary survey, wound care of the burn area should be carried out. This does not mean that prevention of infection should not be involved in the initial resuscitation of the burn patient: nevertheless, the burn wound has a low priority when the patient's life is at risk. The irrigation of chemical burns referred to earlier in the chapter is the exception to this rule.

Treatment of specific types of burns

Thermal burns

Education of the pre-hospital care providers in transporting patients in dry, sterile (or clean) sheets is very important. If the patient is brought to the hospital by the family, they may have attempted initial burn care with the application of a home remedy or ointment. This must be removed to expose a clean wound.

Cleansing of burn wounds is often one of the most difficult nursing procedures because of the discomfort it causes, not only in the resuscitative phase but also in the recovery of the patient. It is important to inform the patient of details of the procedure, make him as comfortable as possible before beginning the treatment, and give analgesia early enough to be certain of it working before wound care is begun.

The wound should be cleansed with sterile water containing an anti-microbial solution. Debris and loose skin can be removed using soft cloths or gauze. Blisters larger than 3 cm should be cleaned and broken and the skin removed, unless they are located on the soles of the feet or the palms of the hand. Hair should be clipped or shaved away from the burn and the immediately adjacent areas.

As skin bacterial colonies tend to regenerate every 8–12 hours, cleansing of the wound must be repeated two or three times a day to prevent infection. Systemic antibiotics are generally ineffective in skin wound infections, so the value of good topical wound care should not be underestimated.

After the burn wound has been properly cleaned and dried, it should be covered immediately with a light dressing. Wounds to the extremities and face, neck and head should be elevated to facilitate venous drainage and prevent unnecessary oedema.

Chemical burns

Diluting and removing the chemical agent that is causing the burn is a high priority in the event of a chemical burn (see earlier). Further information on this is given in Chapters 15 and 19.

Substances that do not contain much water, such as tar, melted plastics and asphalt, are not affected by dilution, but cooling with water may reduce the amount of heat that is being conducted through the clothing. The diluting solution need not be sterile and rinsing the patient with a hose or in a shower will usually suffice provided any associated injuries do not prevent this being carried out. If the patient's wound is being irrigated in bed, it is important that the diluted chemical is not allowed to pool around his body.

Using antidotes for chemicals is not recommended because mixing solutions often creates a heat-producing reaction that can accelerate the burn.

Once the chemical has positively been removed and the wound is clean, it is treated as a thermal burn.

Tar burns

These injuries are usually caused by a container of tar spilling from a work surface, for example a roof. Although tar is heated to several hundred degrees for roofing purposes, it has usually cooled somewhat by the time it strikes the patient.

Patients with tar burns generally look more frightening upon arrival at the hospital than their injuries actually justify. Nevertheless life-threatening priorities should be addressed before any attempt is made at removing the tar and examining the burn.

Tar removal is often the most challenging part of the patient's emergency care. If the patient arrives with the tar still warm, cool water can be applied to reduce the temperature of the tissues and prevent progressive injury. Removal must *not* include peeling the tar from the skin: instead the tar should be dissolved with petroleum-based ointment (for example, mineral oil or petroleum jelly).

The risk of infection is low because tar is generally superheated. It may therefore be effective simply to apply a heavy coat of petroleum jelly, cover with dry gauze dressings and remove the coarse coverings after several hours.

Once the tar has been removed and the wound is clean, it is treated as any other thermal burn. Generally these are partial-thickness burns and cause very little scarring. Reassurance and psychological support are important, however, as the patient may be very frightened by the pain and the appearance of the sticky wound.

Electrical injuries

Most of the deaths due to electrocution are due to two events. Electricity passing through the body causes sustained tetanic contractions: these can be severe enough to cause a respiratory arrest either from inability to breathe or from laryngeal spasm. The patient may also sustain a cardiac arrest from cardiac muscle dysfunction as a result of the shock.

Treatment at the scene consists of the careful removal of the patient from the hazard. Only then are the appropriate advanced life-support measures carried out. As with other burns, care of the wound itself becomes a low priority when life-threatening complications occur. However, cadaver-like limbs should be treated very gently, and with as little motion as possible, so that further damage is minimized.

As previously discussed, the shocked patient should be treated for circulatory failure with fluid resuscitation in volumes adequate to sustain vital signs and urinary output of 100–150 ml/hour in adults and 2 ml/kg/hour in children.

Later care of the patient includes anticipation of progressive tissue loss and renal damage. Haemoglobin or myoglobin or both are excreted in the urine during the first 24 hours post-injury (port-wine urine). In order to protect the kidneys from renal tubular obstruction and tubular necrosis, a diuresis must be maintained and urine output measured hourly to ensure that an adequate flow rate is maintained.

As part of this phenomenon, a profound metabolic acidosis can occur. Patients may even have a pH of 6.8–7.2 directly after injury. Consequently arterial blood pH must be monitored to evaluate this condition. These patients need to be transferred to an intensive care environment. Intravenous sodium bicarbonate may be required until the acidosis resolves in 24–48 hours, but attempting to do this without careful monitoring of the patient can lead to hypernatraemia.

Emotional support

In addition to the life-threatening and disfiguring characteristics of major burns, the victim who is badly burned must face many other hurdles. Long hospitalization, pain, cosmetic and functional disabilities, expense, and slow and difficult rehabilitation can create incredible stresses for the recovering patient. Furthermore the patient's family may have a difficult time adjusting to the changes in their lifestyles as well as their concern for their relative.

Having the patient describe the pain relative to other pain he has known is helpful and having him score his pain on a scale of 1–10 can help anticipate medication demands. It is important to include the patient in planning a pain-control regime, as the complications of a long recovery may present special problems with analgesia. A good history of the patient's tolerance of pain and any previous problems with habituation or intolerance of medications are essential information.

Early intervention by the rehabilitation counsellor, and guidance for families, can help support the patient throughout the very difficult adjustment. This support should be established initially in the emergency department by the relatives' nurse, as the patient and the family's initial reaction to the crisis may set the stage for their longer-term acceptance of the situation.

Transfer

Consideration for transfer of major and moderately burned patients should be made depending on the resources of the facility and the patient's response to injury. In view of the longevity and complexity of the care required by burn victims, having the patient at the right facility can make significant differences in outcome, length of hospitalization and the cost of care.

Familiarity with burn care facilities and their protocols is helpful in choosing the right location for the patient's treatment and recovery. It also makes his transition from resuscitation to recovery as smooth as possible. It has been demonstrated that recovery in a burn care facility that is equipped to offer good burn nursing, reconstructive surgery, physical therapy, nutritional support and all of the many other facets of burn care is a significant advantage to the patient. Likewise, the strain that a major burn patient puts on the resources of a community hospital not geared to care for patients with such intensive requirements means not only that the burn patient is able to receive less than optimal care, but also that the efficiency of the care of other patients is reduced.

A detailed description of the transfer of injured patients is given in Chapter 1. The same principles apply to the burned victim, however the wounds should be covered with a PVC film (such as clingfilm) or sterile foam dressing (such as a Roehampton dressing) and dressed in a dry sheet. Lotions and creams must not be used as these would have to be removed when the patient arrives at the burn centre.

■ Summary

Patients with burn injuries present with a complicated picture of altered physiology and wound care demands. Appreciation of the physiological response to major burns and the immediate threat to airway and cardiopulmonary function is a priority. Appropriate resuscitation with adequate volumes of isotonic solution and the maintenance of body temperature are crucial for the rapid recovery of the burned individual and the avoidance of complications.

A detailed history is important to determine all of the circumstances of the situation that may have an effect on the patient's condition, particularly the presence of smoke inhalation or entrapment in a closed space. Assisting the patient and family with the very difficult emotional acceptance of the injury and the long recovery that is required with major burns is a significant part of the role of the relatives' nurse in the resuscitation team.

■ References and further reading

American College of Surgeons Committee on Trauma 1993. *Advanced Trauma Life Support for Physicians.* Chicago: American College of Surgeons.
Archambeault-Jones S 1978. Burn nursing is nursing. *Crit. Care Nurs.* 1: 77.
Baxter C 1979. Fluid resuscitation, burn percentage, and physiologic age. *J. Trauma* 19(11 Suppl.): 864.
Baxter C 1981. Guidelines for fluid resuscitation. *J. Burn Care Rehabil.* 2: 279.
Bingham H 1986. Electrical burns. *Clin. Plast. Surg.* 13(1): 75.
Cardona V, Hurn S, Mason S, *et al.* 1988. *Trauma Nursing from Resuscitation through Rehabilitation.* Philadelphia: W B Saunders.

Emergency Nurses Association 1991. *Trauma Nursing Core Course (Provider) Manual*, 3rd edn. Chicago: Emergency Nurses Association.

Kravitz M 1988. Thermal injuries. In Cardona V (ed.): *Trauma Nursing*. Philadelphia: W B Saunders.

Marvin J 1979. Burn nursing as a speciality. *Heart Lung* 8(5): 913.

Marvin J 1992. Burns. In Sheehy S, Marvin J & Jimmerson C (eds): *Emergency Nursing, Principles and Practice*, 3rd edn. St. Louis: C V Mosby.

Robertson C & Fenton O 1991. Management of severe burns. In Skinner D, Driscoll P & Earlam R (eds): *ABC of Major Trauma*. London: BMJ Publications.

Settle J 1986. *Burns – The First Five Days*. Romford: Smith & Nephew Pharmaceuticals Ltd.

Sheehy S, Marvin J & Jimmerson C 1992. Burn injuries. In Sheehy S, Marvin J & Jimmerson C (eds): *Clinical Trauma Nursing: the first hour*. St. Louis: C V Mosby.

Shuck S & Moncrief S 1986. Burns. In Schwartz G, Safer P & Stone S (eds): *Principles and Practice of Emergency Medicine*. Philadelphia: W B Saunders.

Chapter 13

Hypothermia

Peter Driscoll and Terry Brown

Objectives

The objectives of this chapter are for members of the trauma team to understand:

- how the body regulates its core temperature;

- how thermoregulation is disrupted in the trauma victim;

- how to manage a patient suffering from hypothermia.

■ Introduction

Hypothermia is a state in which the body's core temperature is less than 35 °C. The severity of this condition can also be graded according to the core temperature. Though various temperature ranges have been suggested, the ATLS system will be used in this chapter:

- mild = 32–35 °C;
- moderate = 30–32 °C;
- severe = < 30 °C.

■ Physiology

The skin, great vessels and viscera all have special nerve endings which detect the temperature of their environment. This information is then transmitted, by the spino-thalamic tracts in the spinal column, to the hypothalamus (see Chapter 8). The latter regulates the body's response such that there is a balance between heat loss, from the skin surface and mucous membranes, and heat production by metabolism.

If this balance is upset and there is a net heat loss, then the core temperature will fall. To prevent this the body has several protective mechanisms.

Reducing heat loss from the skin surface

Vasoconstriction is a very effective method of limiting the degree of heat loss from the surface of the body. However, it can be blocked by various drugs, for example alcohol. Furthermore, at core temperatures below 24 °C, vasoconstriction fails and relative vasodilatation begins.

Behavioural responses, such as putting on protective clothing, moving to a warmer place and taking up certain postures (e.g. curling up) are also very important in reducing heat loss.

Increasing heat production

Shivering can enhance the metabolic rate by 2–5 times. This protective mechanism is lost at core temperatures below 30–32 °C, however. Other causes of increased metabolic rate, including eating, are also capable of elevating the body's heat production.

■ Pathophysiology

If the environmental conditions are too severe, or the patient is unable to carry out these protective actions, the core temperature will fall. The causes for this are as follows.

□ An increase in heat loss

Conduction

This is the transfer of heat by direct contact between the body and the environment. It can be an important source of heat loss in certain situations, for example water immersion can increase the normal loss of body heat by 25 times.

Convection

When cooling currents of air or water pass over a structure, heat is lost by convection. Thus a trauma patient exposed in a wet or windy environment can quickly lose his body heat. This loss is increased if dermal diseases or major burns coexist.

Radiation

A significant amount of heat is lost by radiation from the warm body to the cooler environment. In the normal situation, 60 per cent of the body heat is lost in this way.

Evaporation

Sweating and insensible water loss can be a significant source of heat loss in certain hot environmental situations.

Children, with their relatively large surface areas, will have a higher rate of heat loss by all of these mechanisms. Furthermore, vasodilatation, from whatever cause – including alcohol, drugs, infection, old age, dermal diseases and major burns – will increase the heat loss by convection and radiation.

☐ A decrease in heat production

Many conditions can inhibit the body's ability to produce heat. Metabolism can be depressed by the patient being unconscious or there being a co-existing endocrine defect (e.g. hypothyroidism, hypopituitarism or hypo-adrenalism).

Both children and the elderly have only a limited ability to increase their heat production. With the elderly, this is commonly aggravated by nutritional deficiencies and immobility.

☐ CNS dysfunction

Hypothalamic defects from whatever cause – such as trauma, tumour, cerebrovascular accident, drugs, sepsis or Wernicke's disease – can limit the patient's ability to regulate his core temperature.

☐ Unknown mechanism

Severe underlying diseases, such as pancreatitis, bowel perforation, hypoglycaemia, pneumonia and acute renal failure all inhibit the body's ability to regulate its response to temperature changes. Various suggestions have been made but the actual cause for this inhibition is unknown.

Hypothermia can also occur from any combination of these factors. For example, the drunk trauma victim, trapped in a car for several hours, on a rainy cold night, has a very high chance of being hypothermic when he reaches the emergency department.

It is important to realize that the trauma victim can develop this condition even in temperate climates, for example the injured patient who is unable to move from an exposed place may become hypothermic. Elderly people, especially if they are living in substandard accommodation, may have a persistently low core temperature. The mildest change in their health or mobility can be enough to produce hypothermia.

■ Signs and symptoms of hypothermia

Once the core temperature falls, the patient will begin to demonstrate signs and symptoms which are a combination of both the low temperature and the protective mechanism (Box 13.1).

As the core temperature falls below 32 °C, the anatomical and physiological dead space increases and sinus bradycardia develops. The latter is resistant to atropine and eventually gives way to atrial fibrillation with a slow ventricular response.

In those patients with a core temperature below 28 °C, the myocardium can became very sensitive to the mildest of stimuli, including simply moving the patient. This can lead to ventricular fibrillation which is resistant to electrical therapy until the core temperature is elevated to over 30 °C. As the core temperature falls there is a leftward shift in the oxyhaemoglobin dissociation curve, making oxygen release to tissues more difficult (see Chapter 4). There is also an impairment of renal concentration leading to a 'cold diuresis' and hypovolaemia. The latter is aggravated by a plasma shift into the extravascular space and by any associated haemorrhage. Intravascular thrombosis can also occur, with subsequent embolic complications.

The reduction in cerebral blood flow and metabolism which occurs with the fall in temperature leads to a reduction in conscious level. This impairs the cough and gag reflexes, so making aspiration pneumonia a common complication. The immobile, hypothermic patient is also liable to develop rhabdomyolysis and acute tubular necrosis from the myoglobinuria and renal hypoperfusion. Hyperkalaemia can therefore be found in the hypothermic patient due to the presence of renal failure, metabolic acidosis and rhabdomyolysis.

In cases of immersion, the external water pressure can increase the central venous volume and also enhance the diuretic effect of hypothermia. The resulting hypovolaemia usually becomes evident when the outside pressure is removed as the patient is lifted out of the water. The fall in

---

BOX 13.1   Signs and symptoms of hypothermia

Mild hypothermia
- Pale and cold skin (vasoconstriction)
- Shivering
- Increased metabolism:
  - raised heart rate
  - raised blood pressure
  - raised respiratory rate
- Conscious

Moderate hypothermia
- Pale and cold skin
- No shivering
- Fall in
  - respiratory rate
  - heart rate
  - blood pressure
- Confusion or combative
- Lethargy

Severe hypothermia
- Pale and cold skin
- No shivering
- Hypoventilation
- Slow heart rate
- Dysrhythmias
  - sinus bradycardia
  - atrial fibrillation/flutter
  - nodal rhythms/block
  - ventricular ectopics
  - ventricular fibrillation
  - asystole
- Fall in blood pressure
- Stupor, coma, areflexia
- Dilated pupils
- Oliguria

---

venous return can cause the patient to lose consciousness, a phenomenon known as 'post-immersion syndrome'.

☐ **Hypothermia in the trauma victim**

Several studies have now shown that many trauma victims have lower than normal core temperatures. This is particularly the case in patients with severe injury. Though many causes are probably responsible, it is not yet clear whether this temperature fall is mainly due to environmental conditions, metabolic changes, blood loss or the injury itself. It is well recognized, however, that trauma patients with a low core temperature have the worst prognosis. Efforts should therefore be made to help prevent further falls in core temperature, for example by not infusing cold intravenous solutions.

■ Assessment and management

☐ Primary survey and resuscitation

The same management principles described throughout this book apply equally well for the hypothermic patient. In addition, the team must ensure that the resuscitation room is warm (over 25 °C) and that all temperature recordings are taken by a low-reading thermometer. The new infra-red tympanic temperature probes are ideal for this. They are easy to use and hygienic, and give quick and accurate readings.

Mild hypothermia

The previously discussed life-support measures (see Chapter 1), in conjunction with passive rewarming techniques listed below, are usually all that is required. Caution is needed with regard to the rate of fluid administered because the cold myocardium does not tolerate an excessive fluid load.

Moderate hypothermia

The same measures as described above are required. These patients will also benefit from active external rewarming using top- and bottom-heated blankets.

Severe hypothermia

Patients who have a palpable output but are severely hypothermic must be handled as gently as possible. This is to try to prevent spontaneous dysrhythmias developing. Basic and advanced life support should be maintained as active rewarming techniques are used. Dysrhythmias, other than ventricular fibrillation, tend to correct themselves as the core temperature rises, and require no specific treatment.

. In cases of severe hypothermia it maybe difficult to diagnose death because all the life-support systems are either markedly slowed or difficult to measure. To overcome this problem the team must follow this rule:

The patient is not dead until she or he is *warm* and dead.

☐ **Investigations**

The plasma electrolytes, alcohol level, thyroid function, blood cultures, glucose level and arterial blood gases (ABG) should be measured. Blood should also be taken for a toxicology screen. It is important to remember that the ABG analysis will need to be corrected for the low core temperature. A chest x-ray and a 12-lead ECG are also essential. The latter may show 'J' waves, which are best seen in the V leads. They can occur at any subnormal temperature and so have no prognostic power.

☐ **Rewarming**

This is an essential part of the management of the hypothermic patient. However, it is important to remember that the moderately or severely hypothermic patient can develop coagulation problems and hypoglycaemia whilst the core temperature is rising. These parameters must therefore be monitored whilst the patient is being rewarmed.

Intravenous fluid

In all cases intravenous fluids must be warmed before use. A simple and quick method of warming crystalloids is to use a microwave. Depending on the machine, 2 minutes at high heat will bring a 1 litre bag to 38.8 °C. It is important thoroughly to mix the contents of the bag before they are administered so that there is an even temperature throughout the fluid. Blood cannot be heated in a microwave as this causes haemolysis of the red cells. A blood warmer is therefore used instead.

Passive rewarming

This approach allows the patient to rewarm himself using his own metabolism. It consists of moving the patient away from the hostile environment, removing any wet clothes, and drying the patient's skin. He is then covered in warm blankets. Warm (42–46 °C), humidified oxygen is very good at preventing heat loss by respiration but does little, by itself, to elevate the core temperature. Passive rewarming, on its own, is inappropriate if there is a cardiovascular compromise.

Continuous monitoring of the vital signs, including the core temperature, is essential: the aim should be to elevate the temperature by 0.5 ° per hour.

Active external rewarming

This is required until the core temperature is above 30 °C. The procedure usually consists of placing the patient in a warm bath; obviously this is not possible if there are associated injuries – in these cases heated blankets are used. Another disadvantage of the procedure is that the resulting peripheral vasodilatation leads to cold blood returning to the core from the periphery. This aggravates the hypothermia and possibly increases the incidence of dysrhythmia production. Vasodilatation can also result in hypotension, as well as acidosis from the washout of peripheral-tissue lactic acid. Once the core temperature is over 30 °C, passive rewarming can be used.

To prevent the stimulation of ventricular fibrillation in the sensitive myocardium, the pulse is felt for 60 seconds. Only if no pulse is detected should external cardiac massage be started. Obviously this time delay is not required if a monitor is available and demonstrates ventricular fibrillation or asystole.

The basic and advanced life-support techniques taught in this book must be continued by the team until the core temperature is at least in the range of 30–32 °C. Only then can a definitive diagnosis of death be made.

Active internal warming

Ventricular fibrillation may be resistant to cardioversion if the core temperature is less than 30 °C. In this event a rapid rise in the core temperature is required (1–2 °C/hour) and so active internal rewarming is used. This entails irrigation of the patient's core with warm (40 °C) fluid by gastric lavage, peritoneal lavage, central venous line, pleural lavage, a thoracic heat cradle or, in extreme situations, blood warming by haemodialysis or cardiopulmonary bypass. These techniques require varying degrees of expertise and equipment but all are better carried out in the intensive care unit. The more extreme measures should be reserved for persistent ventricular fibrillation or asystole.

☐ Prognosis

Neurological recovery is still possible after prolonged arrest, as hypothermia reduces cerebral oxygen requirements. The prognosis is usually determined by the severity of the underlying illness and injury. However, marked hyperkalaemia and disseminated intravascular coagulation have been implicated as indicators of a poor outcome.

■ Summary

Even though the trauma victim may be hypothermic for many reasons, the same principles of trauma care apply. Resuscitation is more difficult in these patients as the low temperature itself can produce signs and symptoms as well as disguise internal injuries. It is therefore vital that the patient is continuously monitored, both clinically and physiologically, so that any deterioration is detected early and treated.

■ References and further reading

Advanced Life Support Group 1993. *Advanced Cardiac Life Support: the practical approach*, ed. Driscoll P, Gwinnutt C, Mackway-Jones K, *et al.* London: Chapman Hall.

American College of Surgeons Committee on Trauma 1993. Injuries due to burns and cold. In *Advanced Trauma Life Support for Physicians*. Chicago: American College of Surgeons.

Andrews R 1987. Cold injury complicating trauma in subfreezing environment. *Military Med.* **152**: 42.

Carden D, Doan L, Sweeney P, *et al.* 1982. Hypothermia (clinical conference). *Ann. Emerg. Med.* **11**(9): 497.

Hauty M, Esring B, Hill J, *et al.* 1987. Prognostic factors in severe accidental hypothermia: experience from the Mt. Hood tragedy. *J. Trauma* **27**: 1107.

Jimmerson C 1992. Environmental emergencies. In Sheehy S, Marvin J & Jimmerson C (eds): *Emergency Nursing, Principles and Practice*, 3rd edn. St. Louis: C V Mosby.

Kalant H & Le A 1983. Effects of ethanol on thermoregulation. *Pharmac. Ther.* **23**(3): 313.

Keatinge W 1991. Hypothermia: dead or alive. *Br. Med. J.* **302**: 3.

Kumar K & Ahmed R 1991. Hypothermia. *Br. Med. J.* **302**: 352.

Miller J, Danzl D & Thomas D 1980. Urban accidental hypothermia: 135 cases. *Ann. Emerg. Med.* **9**(9): 456.

Myers R, Britten J & Cowley R 1979. Hypothermia: quantitative aspects of therapy. *JACEP* **8**(12): 523.

Schneider S 1992. Hypothermia: from recognition to rewarming. *Em. Med. Repts* **13**: 1.

Stoneham M & Squires S 1992. Prolonged resuscitation in acute deep hypothermia. *Anaesthesia* **47**: 784.

Woodhouse P, Keatinge W & Coleshaw S 1989. Factors associated with hypothermia in patients admitted to a group of inner city hospitals. *Lancet* **18**(2): 1201.

Zell S & Kurtz K 1985. Severe exposure hypothermia: a resuscitation protocol. *Ann. Emerg. Med.* **14**(4): 339.

Chapter 14

Near-drowning

Peter Driscoll and Terry Brown

Objectives

The objectives of this chapter are for members of the trauma team to understand:

- the causes of near-drowning;

- the basic pathophysiology of near-drowning;

- management at the scene and in the resuscitation room.

■ Introduction

The term 'near-drowning' refers to an episode of suffocation by submersion following which there is at least transient survival.

There are 50 000 cases of near-drowning each year in the USA and 4500 drownings. Unfortunately there are no records of how many cases of near-drownings there are in the UK, but there are 700 drowning episodes each year, 10 per cent of whom are of children under 1 year. Near-drowning affects all ages, but a significant number are in their second decade or are children under 4.

☐ Causes

In many cases of adult near-drowning there are underlying conditions which increase the patient's difficulty in water (Box 14.1). However with children the most important factors are lack of supervision or protective barriers.

BOX 14.1   Factors that predispose to near-drowning

- Hypothermia
- Exhaustion
- Trauma – especially to the cervical spine
- Medical conditions:
  - epilepsy
  - hypoglycaemia
  - air emboli (scuba diving)
- Drugs/alcohol
- Accidental and non-accidental submersion (children)

■ Pathophysiology

The main causes of late death in near-drowning episodes are respiratory failure and ischaemic brain damage.

Initially, water enters the airway and breathing stops, but the heart continues to beat and maintain cerebral perfusion for some time. This, in conjunction with the hypothermia, may explain why some patients (especially children) can survive neurologically intact after long periods of submersion. Eventually the circulatory system fails when the patient has a cardiac arrest.

If the victim survives, the water will have entered some of the alveoli and washed out surfactant. This is a naturally produced chemical agent which helps to keep the alveoli open. When it is removed, sections of the lung collapse during expiration and do not re-expand in inspiration. Adding to this problem are areas of the lung which have a marked ventilation-perfusion mismatch, or damage to the alveolar-capillary membrane (see Chapter 3), or both. Furthermore, pulmonary oedema occurs in 75 per cent of cases as a consequence of the surfactant loss as well as direct pulmonary injury, inflammatory contaminants in the water, gastric aspiration and cerebral hypoxia.

The end result of all these pathological processes is a decrease in oxygen delivery to the tissues of the body and an inhibition of carbon dioxide elimination from the lungs. Thus hypoxia and acidosis from a respiratory source (increased carbon dioxide) and from a metabolic source (anaerobic metabolism) are the major consequences of near-drowning. By the time the patient reaches the emergency department spontaneous respiration may already have been started. If this is adequate only the lactic acidosis will remain.

■ Assessment and management

□ Primary survey and resuscitation

The same principles described throughout this book should be used in managing a victim of a near-drowning episode.

At the scene

The first priority is to protect oneself and others so that no risks are taken during the rescue.

Mouth-to-nose or mouth-to-mouth resuscitation can be started immediately but all effort should be made to get the patient quickly from the water. The ABCs of basic life support (BLS) can then be carried out more effectively. Simultaneously, care must be taken to prevent any cervical injury, by maintaining inline stabilization of the neck. This must be continued even when the patient is being turned to clear away any vomitus.

Time should not be wasted in attempting to drain water from the lungs. This makes little difference to the oxygen uptake but it does delay BLS and potentially jeopardizes an unstable neck. If the equipment is to hand, a high flow of oxygen by a reservoir bag-valve-mask system should be given as early as possible (see Chapter 2).

In hypothermia cases central pulses may not be felt (see Chapter 13), even though there is a cardiac output. If external cardiac massage (ECM) is started in patients with a core temperature of less than 28 °C then this may precipitate ventricular fibrillation. The recommended guidelines are to administer oxygen and examine the patient for 1 minute before commencing ECM if the central pulses are still not felt.

Death cannot be declared until basic and advanced life support have been continued without success for 45 minutes and the core temperature is over 32 °C. A longer time should be allowed for children.

BLS may be difficult to maintain in transit, so the rescue team should try to stabilize the patient as much as possible before transporting him to hospital.

Pre-hospital information

The same information as is described in Chapter 1 needs to be collected and sent to the trauma team as early as possible so that preparations can be made. As a similar clinical picture is produced from near-drowning episodes in salt- or freshwater, this should not affect the patient's immediate management. It has been reported, however, that shock lung (see Chapter 3) occurs in 10–15 per cent of freshwater near-drownings whereas none were found with saltwater near-drownings.

In the emergency department

The airway nurse and doctor must reassess and secure the patient's airway while maintaining inline cervical stabilization. It is important to remember that there can be an associated neck injury following trauma, for example following a diving injury. In many cases the patient will be conscious and able to control his own airway, but occasionally intubation will be required.

The adequacy of spontaneous ventilation is determined by the clinical judgement of the team leader, augmented by the arterial blood-gas results. Artificial ventilation will be required if the PaO_2 is less than 60 mmHg while the patient is receiving an inspired oxygen concentration of 40–50% (see page 50).

A search for the six immediately life-threatening thoracic conditions must be carried out (see pages 77–87) because associated chest injuries do occur in near-drowning episodes (e.g. a pneumothorax and air emboli in divers).

A chest radiograph is needed in all cases for the detection of thoracic trauma as well as for predicting future ventilatory problems. Almost 50 per cent of the patients with an abnormal chest x-ray will require intubation and ventilation. The film may also show perihilar infiltrates or pulmonary oedema.

As in all trauma resuscitations, the 'circulation' personnel should commence two intravenous lines and draw blood for laboratory analysis. At the same time, the remaining circulation nurse should record the patient's vital signs (BP, pulse, respiratory rate and core temperature) and attach him to a monitor. A low-reading thermometer will be required. Any dysrhythmias should be noted and a 12-lead ECG performed to help detect myocardial injury or disease. Dysrhythmias usually disappear once the hypoxia, hypothermia and acidosis have been corrected.

A nasogastric tube and urinary catheter should be inserted if the patient is not fully conscious, and efforts should also be made to warm him. The techniques used to manage hypothermia are described in Chapter 13.

☐ **Secondary survey**

Once the primary survey and resuscitation have been completed the detailed examination of the secondary survey is carried out. This is described in detail in Chapter 1.

☐ **Definitive care**

Long-term care is dependent on the associative injuries and the chances of the trauma victim developing pulmonary insufficiency. The latter can be determined from the clinical findings and accounts from witnesses, relatives and ambulance personnel (Box 14.2).

BOX 14.2 Features of a near-drowning incident

- Severe hypoxia – transient or prolonged
- Aspirated
- Underlying cardiopulmonary disease
- Loss of consciousness in the water
- Symptoms such as coughing, dyspnoea and tachypnoea

Using these features, patients who have nearly drowned can be divided in the emergency department into four groups.

Group 1

These patients are fully conscious, have no respiratory distress and have an insignificant history of immersion. They can be discharged home from the emergency department after six hours if there are no associative injuries, if no abnormalities are found on examination of the chest, and if there are both a normal chest radiograph and a normal arterial blood-gas result when the patient is breathing room air.

Group 2

These patients are conscious but have mild or moderate respiratory distress. Provided there is no spinal injury, these patients should be managed on their sides because there is a significant chance of their vomiting. Even if there is no other injury, these patients will require overnight observation in hospital.

Group 3

These patients are apnoeic but have a palpable pulse. They will therefore require intubation, mechanical ventilation, central venous pressure monitoring and plasma expansion, irrespective of any associative injuries.

Group 4

These patients are apnoeic and pulseless. They will therefore require the advanced support measures described in this book. Active rewarming techniques may also be needed.

Further management of Groups 3 and 4

These patients will require prolonged intensive monitoring and management. Pulmonary oedema develops gradually over hours, resulting in progressive hypoxia, lung crackles on auscultation, and increased shadowing on the chest-ray. This has been called 'secondary drowning'. Some form of mechanical ventilation is needed in almost all cases until this resolves. These patients should therefore be transferred to an intensive care unit following the resuscitation and stabilization.

Sedation, pharmacological paralysis and hyperventilation are commonly used to minimize secondary neurological injury. Certain centres also add mannitol, barbiturate coma and hypothermia, but the value of these techniques remain in doubt.

The electrolyte disturbance following the water absorption is usually minor and rarely clinically significant. Occasionally, freshwater absorption can lead to anaemia due to haemolysis.

Renal failure can appear as a late consequence of hypoxia, hypotension, lactic acidosis and myoglobinuria. Pulmonary infections can also occur in victims of near-drowning, but incidental pyrexia is common in the first few hours. However, if the temperature rise develops after 24 hours, systemic infection should be suspected. After blood cultures have been taken, intravenous antibiotics can then be started. The chosen agent must be effective against gram-negative organisms.

Prophylactic antibiotics and steroids are not required, but regular tracheal swabs should be taken, as should blood for cultures, electrolyte measurement and white cell counts.

Prognosis

The prognosis depends on the degree of hypoxia and neurological damage. Patients may be categorized as A (awake), B (blunted) or C (comatosed) following successful resuscitation. In one study, of the patients in group A, 100 per cent survived with excellent neurological result. Only 55 per cent of the patients in group C survived normally; 35 per cent died and 10 per cent had significant brain damage.

Further studies concentrating on childhood near-drownings have shown that survival without neurological damage is unlikely:

- if immersion lasted longer than 5–9 minutes;
- if the child is pulseless when he arrives at the hospital;
- if the child presents in ventricular fibrillation or ventricular tachycardia;
- if the child presents with dilated pupils or a low Glasgow Coma Scale score or is suffering from fits;
- if prolonged resuscitation was required.

■ Summary

The management of the near-drowned victim can present the trauma team with many problems. In addition to the hypoxia and acidosis resulting from the episode of immersion, there may also be injuries and hypothermia. Nevertheless, the team must still manage these patients using the principles described throughout this book.

■ References and further reading

Allman F, Nelson W, Pacentine G, *et al.* 1986. Outcome following cardiopulmonary resuscitation in severe pediatric near-drowning. *Am. J. Dis. Child* 140(6): 571.

Conn A, Montes J, Baker G, *et al.* 1980. Cerebral salvage in near-drowning following neurological classification by triage. *Can. Anaesth. Soc. J.* 27(3): 201.

Haynes B 1988. Near-drowning. In Tintinalli J, Drome R & Ruiz E (eds): *Emergency Medicine*, 2nd edn. New York: McGraw-Hill.

Jimmerson C 1992. Environmental emergencies. In Sheehy S, Marvin J & Jimmerson C (eds): *Emergency Nursing, Principles and Practice*, 3rd edn. St. Louis: C V Mosby.

Kemp A & Sibert J 1992. Drowning and near-drowning in children in the United Kingdom: lessons for prevention. *Br. Med. J.* 304: 1143.

Modell J, Calderwood H, Ruiz B, *et al.* 1974. Effects of ventilatory patterns on arterial oxygenation after near-drowning in sea water. *Anaesthesiology* 40: 376.

Pearn J 1980. Secondary drowning in children. *Br. Med. J.* 281: 1103.

Peterson B 1977. Morbidity of childhood near-drownings. *Paediatrics* 59: 364.

Pratt F & Haynes B 1986. Incidence of 'secondary drowning' after saltwater submersion. *Ann. Emerg. Med.* 15(9): 1084.

Russell R & Ross S 1992. Drowning and near-drowning in children. *Int. Care* Vol 2(3) April: 135.

Chapter 15

Radiation

Steven Walker and Tim Hodgetts

Objectives

The objectives of this chapter are for the trauma team to understand:

- that in dealing with radiation incidents the standard principles of trauma care remain the same;

- how the department and personnel can be protected whilst dealing with a contaminated trauma victim.

■ Introduction

In April 1986 we were reminded of the consequences of a nuclear accident. An explosion and fire at Chernobyl No. 4 plant in the USSR caused the worst nuclear power plant disaster in history. Not since the bombing of Hiroshima and Nagasaki has there been a more damaging nuclear event.

Radiological emergencies are not all so large, indeed they can occur after any situation which gives rise to an abnormal or unexpected leak of radioactive material. This may involve anything from a minor laboratory spillage, involving a small amount of radioactive solution, to a major reactor accident in which many thousands of radioactive products are released.

■ The NAIR scheme

In the UK the Regional Health Authority (RHA) must designate specific hospitals to be responsible for the treatment of contaminated casualties.

These centres should also be available to give advice following any radiological incident. This is called the NAIR scheme (National Arrangements for Incidents Involving Radiation).

The features of a hospital capable of handling severely contaminated individuals are listed in Box 15.1.

BOX 15.1   Features of a NAIR scheme hospital department

- The facilities of an A/E department manned on a 24-hour basis
- The necessary clothing, floor covering, and physical barriers available for immediate use in the A/E department
- The presence of a medical physics department able to measure and monitor the extent and distribution of the contamination
- Simple facilities for changing, washing or showering
- Experienced medical and nursing care available for patients with severe damage to haemopoietic systems, and gastrointestinal and lung-function problems
- Ability to treat severe burns
- Isolation facilities for protection against infection

■ Pre-hospital communication

The RHA must also ensure that the ambulance service is familiar with the designated hospitals capable of treating severely contaminated casualties. The paramedic personnel at the scene can then inform the receiving hospital in advance:

- that a radioactive substance has been involved;
- of the nature of the substance;
- how many patients have been exposed and/or injured.

This advance warning enables the A/E department to prepare for the incoming contaminated patients. Different countries have different methods of communicating this vital information, therefore it is important that the local system is well known by the nursing and medical trauma team leaders.

■ Pre-planning and preparation

It should be emphasized that low-level contamination presents no immediate hazard to the patient, or those with whom he comes into contact.

Attention to specific guidelines and precautions listed here will ensure that any long-term risk is also greatly minimized.

In the A/E department, an area should be designated as the Radiation Emergency Area, preferably with a separate entry and exit point. Upon warning of the arrival of a contaminated casualty, the floor from the ambulance bay to the Radiation Emergency Area must be covered either with plastic sheeting, or, if this is not available, a heavy-duty paper (Figure 15.1).

All non-essential equipment must be removed from the Radiation Emergency Area. It should then remain out of bounds both to the general public and to hospital personnel not directly involved in the resuscitation process. If possible, a physical barrier should be erected to deter entry. This allocated area too can be protected by covering the floor with a heavy-duty paper. Plastic sheeting will suffice, but care should be taken as this may become slippery.

Similar arrangements must be made for other areas of the hospital which could become involved in dealing with contaminated patients. Examples of such places include theatre and intensive care.

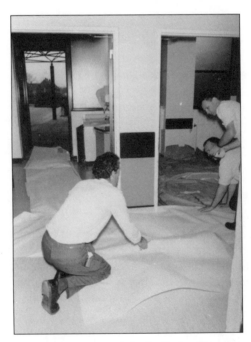

Figure 15.1 Preparation of the Radiation Emergency Area

☐ **Task allocation and team organization**

The principles described in Chapter 1 still apply even if the trauma victim has been contaminated with radioactive waste. However, certain adaptations need to be made to the tasks allocated and the team organization.

The nursing team leader must allocate a member of staff to remain outside the Radiation Emergency Area. This person's responsibilities are to act as liaison between the trauma team and other members of staff or departments, to pass into the room any items of equipment that may be required and, finally, to log the movement of any staff who have to leave the room. There should also be facilities for staff to change their footwear and protective clothing if leaving the area is deemed absolutely necessary. This is to minimize the contamination of the rest of the department.

The team leaders must limit the number of staff who come into contact with the patient, but they should ensure that the team is sufficient to meet the needs described in Chapter 1.

A medical physicist is an essential member of the team. It is his or her responsibility to measure and monitor the level of contamination; to arrange for the collection, monitoring and disposal of contaminated waste; and to declare the patient, staff and room free of radioactive particles.

Members of staff who are pregnant or who have dermatitis or eczema should be excluded from the team.

All enquiries from the Press and the news media should be dealt with by a member of staff from the administration department (see Chapter 18).

☐ **Protection of the trauma team**

Personnel treating the patient must be gowned and wear hair caps, masks, foot covers, double gloves and waterproof aprons (Figure 15.2). It is also useful for staff to wear personal monitoring devices, such as film badges, thermoluminescent dosimeter badges or pocket dosimeters. These must be clearly labelled for monitoring later.

☐ **Special equipment**

In addition to the standard equipment described in Chapter 20, a 'radiation incident pack' should be in the designated area so that essential items are immediately available should the need arise (Box 15.2).

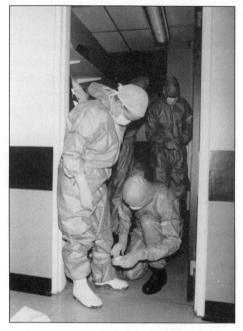

Figure 15.2   Protective clothing worn by the trauma team

BOX 15.2   Contents of a radiation incident pack

- Cottonwool swabs
- Post-operative pads
- Gauze swabs
- Large paper tissues
- Blank sticky labels and a pen
- Small plastic specimen bags
- Large plastic waste bags and tape
- Receivers for collecting water
- Waterproof tape (Sleek™)
- Povidone-iodine
- Sterile dressings
- Boxes of disposable gloves (all sizes)

The large plastic bags are required for the collection of the patient's clothing, and contaminated waste. These must be clearly labelled for monitoring later.

■ Management of the contaminated patient

☐ Primary survey and resuscitation

The initial treatment of radiation-exposed patients must be directed to the immediately life-threatening conditions. Upon arrival, therefore, the team should manage the patient in the way described in Chapter 1.

Whilst undressing the patient, the clothing is rolled inside out as this reduces the risk of spreading surface contamination to unaffected areas of the body. Later, when the patient has been completely exposed, he can be washed with warm soapy water. This will effectively remove most of the contaminated material from the patient's skin.

Open wounds should have dry swabs taken for accurate estimations of contamination, then be covered with sterile dressings and sealed with waterproof tape (Figure 15.3). This will prevent any subsequent recontamination. Contaminated wounds should be left open for 24 hours and then sutured, or débrided as necessary. This time delay allows most of the remaining contamination to be removed both by bleeding and the formation of an exudate.

If the patient's condition allows, ask him to blow his nose and to refrain from swallowing. The mouth can be effectively decontaminated by giving the patient a mouthwash which is then expelled into a receiver. Ears should be gently syringed with warm water, and when the fluid runs clear, the external auditory canals can be plugged with cottonwool. Hair can be gently back-washed if necessary.

It is essential that the outer pair of gloves is changed frequently throughout this decontamination procedure and that the used water is collected and

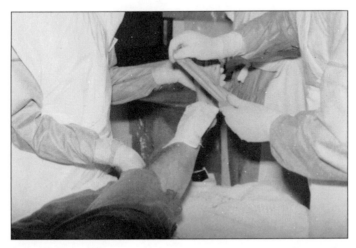

Figure 15.3   Sealing an open wound with a waterproof tape after decontamination

placed in a sealed container and appropriately labelled. This should not be emptied into the hospital drains, unless a special licence has been previously obtained.

Once the primary survey and resuscitation phase have been completed, the patient must be checked with a Geiger counter for remaining surface contamination. Particular attention should be paid to any open wounds (Figure 15.4). A member of the medical physics department is the most appropriate person to do this. In the UK, however, if a hospital physicist is not available the police should be contacted so that a NAIR physicist can be notified.

An irradiated person can receive local or total body exposure. The team should therefore determine whether any radioactive material has been ingested or inhaled or has contaminated an open wound. In these uncommon situations, material may irradiate internal tissues and subsequently lead to extensive cellular damage. Indeed some radioactive elements may become permanently incorporated into the body's molecular structure. It is imperative in these cases that immediate treatment with a chelating agent is started.

A commonly used chelating agent is diethylenetriaminepenta-acetic acid (DTPA). This provides an ion exchange that results in the formation of an excretable stable complex containing the radioactive substance. This may be used locally or by intravenous infusion.

☐ **Secondary survey**

The detailed head-to-toe assessment of the patient must be carried out in the

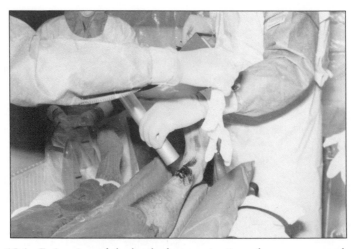

Figure 15.4   Estimation of the level of contamination of an open wound using a Geiger counter

manner described in Chapter 1. The subsequent management of the patient will depend on his associated injuries (see appropriate chapters).

Radiation burns are similar to electrical burns in that physical findings might be quite minimal initially, but excision followed by full-thickness skin grafting may be necessary later (see Chapter 12).

The patient may also have been exposed to chemical hazards when he was being contaminated with radioactivity. Berylium, for example, is present in a number of nuclear weapons, and so can be released as fumes or smoke. This may lead to respiratory distress, anxiety, agitation and fever. A suitable chelating agent in this case is ethylenediaminetetra-acetic acid (EDTA). Other hazards may also be present at the site of a nuclear accident. Lead used for shielding, when burnt, produces toxic fumes which can cause a number of complications including pneumonitis. Delayed-onset pneumonitis may also be caused by inhaling fumes from the combustion of plastic which is common to most nuclear devices.

Antibiotic therapy is indicated if there is evidence of infection, or prophylactically against fungal infections. Tetanus immunization must not be overlooked.

☐ Clearing up

Upon completion of all necessary treatment, the patient and team members must be monitored and decontaminated. Following this the patient can be moved out of the Radiation Emergency Area. This is achieved by means of a scoop stretcher placed under the patient. He can then be lifted out, onto a clean trolley, with the stretcher being brought back into the Radiation Emergency Area.

The protective clothing worn by the team must be placed in sealed plastic bags and labelled before leaving the Radiation Emergency Area, and all staff should have had a Geiger counter reading taken. The team should then shower and put on freshly laundered clothing. Ambulance personnel should also be monitored and their vehicle taken out of service until it has been fully checked and cleared of any residual contamination. The contaminated waste is removed by the medical physics department for monitoring and then safe disposal.

■ Summary

Whatever the reason for a radiation accident or disaster, prior communication, instruction and staff training are the best preparation. It should be pointed out that in the absence of a major nuclear disaster, it is very unlikely that most hospitals will receive any patients who have been involved in life-threatening radiation accidents. Patients are much more likely to die from the underlying traumatic injuries. We are in a changing world, however, with the ever-increasing production and use of radiation-producing machines, radioactive products, nuclear plants and nuclear weapons. Forewarned is forearmed.

■ References and further reading

Department of Health 1989. Hc (89) 8 HN (FP) (89)8. *Health Service Arrangements for Dealing with Accidents Involving Radioactivity.* March 1989.
Foreman H 1970. *Nuclear Power and the Public.* University of Minnesota Press.
Martin A & Harbison S 1979. *An Introduction to Radiation Protection,* 2nd edn. London: Chapman & Hall.
Muller A 1990. Radiation injuries. *Journal of Environmental Injuries* 4: 107.

Chapter 16

Social and psychological issues in major trauma and sudden death

Gill Ellison, Olive Goodall and Terry Brown

Objectives

The objectives of this chapter are for the members of the trauma team to understand:

- the role of the relatives' nurse in the trauma team;

- how to communicate with the patient's relatives;

- the trauma team's response to death.

■ Introduction

Every year in the UK 5000 people are killed and another 63 500 are seriously injured on the roads. No one knows how many more are traumatized emotionally by being involved either as a witness or as an uninjured participant.

In trauma situations, relatives and friends of the deceased are usually totally unprepared. This death also presents the team with emotional burdens at a time when they are clinically stretched and emotionally vulnerable. Following a major incident all these problems are magnified.

It is often difficult to manage the emotional aspects of critical incidents in the A/E department because the situation develops in an unstructured way, over a short period of time. Therefore a trained member of the trauma team must take charge of communication to the relatives and of their emotional support. This role is filled by the 'relatives' nurse' (see Chapter 1).

■ The critically ill patient

□ Emotional crisis: nurse intervention

Crisis is an unusual experience which most people will go through at some time in their life. It is an urgent and stressful situation which seems over-whelming at the time. However, with the right support, *from the beginning*, most people will come to terms with the experience.

The care of the relatives and friends of the critically ill or dying patient should be seen as being as important as the other tasks in the trauma team. The support for distressed relatives begins with their arrival in the A/E department. A trained member of the nursing trauma team must therefore be allocated to this task before the patient arrives.

During a crisis, family and friends often gather in the A/E department. The care they receive may well determine their mental state during the course of their grief. In the case of sudden death these 'helpers' are often just as devastated as the immediate next-of-kin. The relatives' nurse needs to be able to act and intervene, being informative as well as compassionate.

The relatives' nurse should accompany the relatives and friends to a private room with suitable facilities available – a telephone, tea-making equipment and toilets. Here information useful to the resuscitation team may be gathered from them. This act also gives the relatives the opportunity to express or learn how the patient was injured. Likewise, the nurse can inform the relatives of the severity of the patient's present state. By giving them time, a rapport is begun which will be maintained throughout their time in the department.

Explanatory terms such as 'poorly' or 'critical' are meaningless unless accompanied by honest explanation. For example 'cardiac arrest' could be explained as, 'Your husband's heart has stopped beating and he is not breathing. He may die.' This gives a better account than 'Your husband is very ill.' Of course, being with already distressed relatives and giving such information is not easy; this may explain why hospital staff tend to give limited information early on in any resuscitative situation. Nonetheless, if relatives are told exactly what is going on they usually cope much better than if given a modified explanation or, worse still, no explanation at all.

It is an assumption on the part of many hospital staff that relatives may not cope with bad news. Experience has shown that given the *facts*, most people, though distressed, will deal successfully with the situation. It is when facts are vague that extreme reactions such as anger and abuse occur, because the relatives feel excluded from the situation and no longer in control. A nurse assigned to the relatives in this time of crisis for them can build up a relationship of trust so that she can act as a link between them and the resuscitation team. This link is very important should the patient die.

The relatives' nurse should also allow a continuous appraisal of the patient's condition to be relayed to the relatives in a structured way. Honest answers to questions can be given, with gentle explanations of what the resuscitation team is attempting. This nurse can also facilitate arrangements for the family, for example the distressed wife who remembers she has to collect the children from school. She can also be of further help when other relatives arrive in the department.

☐ Seeing is believing

Should the relatives be allowed to see the patient? This is totally acceptable provided they are accompanied by the relatives' nurse and have been prepared for what they might experience – equipment, tubing and noise, and maybe a badly injured patient. Seeing with their own eyes helps them to come to terms with the event as it is happening. This may be the last time they will see their loved one alive, so the encounter should not be prevented.

This type of policy can create personal issues for the team members. Nonetheless, these views should not be forced onto others: what is right for one person may be completely wrong for another. Each set of relatives must be allowed to respond in their own way whilst being guided and supported by the nurse.

☐ The philosophy of caring for relatives – cultural and religious aspects

The A/E department must have a philosophy for caring for the distressed relatives which is acceptable to their own locality with its various religious and cultural communities. There is no right or wrong way to proceed. Each family is different, but in each case their views and customs must always be respected.

■ When the patient dies

☐ Communication – breaking bad news

There is no standard way of breaking bad news. However, if the relatives are dealt with sensitively and honestly from the very beginning this can lessen the impact when death has to be announced.

Among the trauma team, the nurse providing support is possibly in the best position to break the news should the patient die. After all, it is she who has built up the relationship with the relatives. It is therefore inappropriate always to expect a doctor to break the bad news. When this does happen, the medical team leader should first pause to collect his thoughts and to be clear about the events in the resuscitation room. Finally it is important to make sure that he is not spattered with blood nor looks dishevelled. He should also be prepared to stay with the relatives for a while and to answer all their questions to the best of his ability.

It is at the point of breaking the bad news that medical and nursing staff often feel inadequate. All that can be done is to listen and share the grief as it unfolds.

Words spoken at the time of death will often remain with the relatives forever: choosing the correct words is important. When breaking the news, care should be taken to avoid using indirect or ambiguous statements. For example, ' . . . I'm sorry we lost him' does not describe accurately that someone has died, even if that is what is being communicated.

☐ **Saying 'goodbye' – viewing the dead person**

Following the death, the relatives must be given time to absorb the information. Every conceivable emotional response is possible in any relative. The relatives' nurse must stay with them to guide them through the next stage of their stay in the A/E department.

Shocked and numbed by the news, relatives may leave the A/E department without saying their 'goodbyes'. Some will regret this in the future, so all relatives should be offered the opportunity to see their loved one.

They may never have seen a dead person before and consequently they may experience a great deal of fear. The nurse can help displace these anxieties by active encouragement. It is important, especially when death has just occurred, to go with the relatives and to let them touch and hold their loved one. If the deceased is a baby then a Moses basket should be available with suggestions given by the nurse as to the holding of their baby.

The relatives must be assured of plenty of time in which to say their 'goodbyes'. There can be no fixed rules and procedures; each family is different and the response must be geared to the particular situation. Their wishes must be respected. If a chaplain is required he should be notified.

If a particularly horrific trauma has occurred the team may wish to protect the relatives from viewing the body. Unfortunately, though well meant these actions can lead to problems in the future. The family's fantasy of what the victim *might* look like may ultimately prove far worse then the real thing. They have to come to terms with reality. Furthermore, a formal identification of the deceased often has to take place by law. It is better to explain the circumstances and let the relatives decide rather than impose your own perceptions on the family.

It is important that each A/E department should be conversant with the local arrangements and have a good working relationship with the local coroner's officer. In cases of major trauma the deceased person will be deemed to 'belong' to the coroner until the cause of death has been established (see Appendix 16.1). This should not interfere with relatives saying their 'goodbyes' and holding and touching their loved ones. Where possible, the coroner's officer should be informed by one of the team leaders so that arrangements can be made for formal identification while the relatives are in the hospital. This will save them from having to return to the mortuary the following day and perhaps compounding their distress.

It is important for the nursing team leader to remember that the deceased person's clothing should not be destroyed. This is not only from the point of view of the relatives, but also for legal reasons as the clothing may be required for forensic evidence.

☐ Further support

Ongoing support is needed for relatives once they leave the A/E department. Written information may be required and should be readily available (see Appendix 16.2). A useful leaflet is the DSS one entitled, *What to do after a death* (Leaflet D49).

The medical and nursing teams in the community should be informed of the death, and clergy may need to be notified. A major asset in this follow-up care is to have a grief support nurse working from the A/E department. This person can act as a link between the hospital and the community it serves.

☐ Staff response to death

Following major trauma or death in the department it is important to be able to acknowledge the distress amongst the staff. When actively involved in the resuscitation the team are often performing at their peak. Once the resuscitation has finished, especially if the outcome is death, then time must be taken to unwind. It is the practice in some A/E departments to have an operational debriefing to determine whether the trauma team did everything that was required. It follows that an emotional debriefing also should take place, albeit informally, with the more experienced members being able to share their feelings with the less experienced. In this way no one person should feel ashamed of feeling sad or inadequate. It is far better to be able to share these feelings rather than 'bottling them up': the latter can lead to days off duty from sickness or, ultimately, 'burnout'. It takes great courage to say one feels upset, and it takes a non-judgmental team to share these feelings openly together so that they are ready to cope with the next critically ill person.

■ Summary

Developing a philosophy of care for the distressed relative and carrying out preventive emotional debriefing for all staff members reduces the future need for counselling, therapy and psychiatric intervention. Prevention is better than cure, and more cost-effective!

■ Appendix 16.1: Legal aspects of death

☐ The role of the coroner

In most cases of death resulting from trauma, the coroner will make arrangements for the deceased to be removed for formal examination. Following this, he is obliged by law to hold an inquest if death cannot be attributed to natural causes. A post-mortem (PM) may or may not precede an inquest, but if one is ordered by the coroner, the person in possession of the body has no choice but to agree. The PM is usually carried out by an independent pathologist appointed by the coroner, but interested parties have a right to be represented by a medical practitioner at this examination.

☐ Inquests

These meetings allow the interested parties to ask questions of the witnesses called by the coroner. They are also open to the public and the press.

It is the coroner's officer who is responsible for preparing the evidence and organizing the inquest proceedings, and to this end he or she has to assemble all the statements and evidence.

Nurses and doctors involved in the trauma team are likely to be involved in an inquest at some stage in their career. Evidence is usually given orally, with the coroner initially taking witnesses through their statements (Box 16.1) before cross-examination. It is therefore important that they have looked through their statements with their legal representatives, before these are signed.

BOX 16.1 Statements to the coroner

- Give name, qualifications, occupation, place of work
- Be as detailed as possible
- List relevant facts in chronological order
- Avoid abbreviations

Before attending the inquest, nurses and doctors should again seek legal advice with regard to their presentation. Remember to speak slowly, clearly and in everyday language. If medical terms are used, the team members must be able to explain them in everyday terms. It is important to remember that there is no such thing as privileged information at an inquest, so patients' confidentiality (see Chapter 17) does not apply.

■ Appendix 16.2: Organizations that offer support

All of the help groups listed below have local contacts. The national offices will provide helpful leaflets and further information.

CRUSE (bereavement care)
126 Sheen Road, Richmond, Surrey TW9 1UR (*Tel.* 081–940 4818).

The Compassionate Friends (an international organization of bereaved parents)
6 Denmark Street, Bristol BS1 5DQ (*Tel.* 0272 292778).

The Foundation for the Study of Infant Deaths
35 Belgrave Square, London SW1X 8PS (*Tel.* 071–235 0965).

Stillbirth and Neonatal Death Society (SANDS)
28 Portland Place, London W1N 4DE (*Tel.* 071–436 5881).

The Samaritans (24-hour support for the despairing)
Local branches in most towns in the UK.

■ References and further reading

Awooner-Renner S 1991. I desperately need to see my son. *Br. Med. J.* **302**: 356.
Bell S 1990. Ethical dilemmas in trauma nursing. *Nurs. Clin. N. Am.* **25**: 143.
Doyle C, Post H, Burney R, *et al.* 1987. Family participation during resuscitation: an option. *Ann. Emerg. Med.* **16**: 673.
Finlay I & Dallimore D 1991. Your child is dead. *Br. Med. J.* **302**: 1524.
Hanson C & Strawser D 1992. Family presence during cardiopulmonary

resuscitation: Foote Hospital emergency department's nine-year perspective. *J. Emerg. Nursing* **18**: 104.

Lake A 1987. *Living with Grief*. London: Heinemann Press.

MaLauchlan C 1991. Handling distressed relatives and breaking bad news. In Skinner D, Driscoll P & Earlam R (eds): *ABC of Major Trauma*. London: BMJ Publications.

Phipps L 1988. Stress among doctors and nurses in the emergency department of a general hospital. *Can. Med. Assoc. J.* **139**(5): 375.

Solursh D 1990. The family of the trauma victim. *Nurs. Clin. N. Am.* **25**(1): 155.

Steele T & Grover N 1992. Psychosocial and mental health assessment. In Sheehy S, Marvin J & Jimmerson C (eds): *Emergency Nursing, Principles and Practice*, 3rd edn. St. Louis: C V Mosby.

Woodward S, Pope A, Robson W J, *et al.* 1985. Bereavement counselling after sudden infant death. *Br. Med. J.* **290**: 363.

Yates D W, Ellison G & McGuiness S 1990. Care of the suddenly bereaved. *Br. Med. J.* **301**: 29.

Chapter 17

Medico-legal problems in trauma care

Olive Goodall and Peter Driscoll

Objectives

The objectives of this chapter are for the members of the trauma team to understand the medico-legal aspects of:

- confidentiality;

- data protection;

- the media;

- consent;

- professional accountability;

- negligence;

- criminal law.

■ Introduction

In caring for the trauma victim, the team is led through a minefield of ethical, legal and moral decisions. Increased awareness by the public of new technology and the expectations of a high standard of care can also subject the team to many aspects of the legal system. Additional difficulties arise when there is a conflict between ethics and the law.

This is obviously a vast subject, but the aim of this chapter is to cover those areas most likely to be encountered when dealing with the trauma victim.

■ Confidentiality

The personnel involved in treating trauma patients include the professionals working in the pre-hospital setting. Consequently close co-operation with all the emergency services is essential and in the best interest of the patient and relatives. This relationship should not however cloud one's judgement when making decisions as to whether to disclose confidential information: the patient has the right to expect that information he has given will not be passed on to any other party without his consent.

Consider these real-life situations:

1   A policeman investigating a robbery has reason to believe that the perpetrator has sustained a laceration to his hand and may have attended the emergency department for treatment. A member of the nursing or medical staff is approached by the policeman, who asks for the names of patients who have attended the department within the past 24 hours having sustained such an injury.

2   A patient is admitted to the emergency department, unconscious, having been involved in a road traffic accident. A policeman asks a member of the nursing or medical staff for the name of the patient.

3   In the course of undressing a patient, the nurse discovers a sawn-off shotgun.

What should the nurse or doctor do? To help in such situations there are three sources of information and guidance.

UKCC and GMC guidelines

It is stated in these guidelines that the nurse or doctor is permitted to disclose confidential information in the following cases:

1   With the patient's consent.

2   Without the patient's consent when disclosure is considered in the public interest.

3   By accident.

4   Without the patient's consent when required by law.

5   Without the patient's consent to other health-care professionals who need the information if they are to care for the patient.

Local policies

It is recognized by Health Authorities and directly managed Units and Trusts that the patient has the right to confidentiality. However, there may be instances when a public moral duty to give information to the police may override the duty to maintain confidentiality.

The request for disclosure is usually in relation to a serious arrestable offence (see Appendix 17.1). It is essential that Health Authorities or directly managed Units and Trusts have written guidelines to assist staff in making appropriate decisions in these cases.

The law

There are a number of Acts relating to disclosure of confidential information. For example, the 1982 Road Traffic Act requires Authorities to divulge certain information so that the police can identify the driver of a vehicle which has been involved in an accident. It is important to note that the information is in relation to the *driver* and does not necessarily include other occupants of the vehicle.

The Prevention of Terrorism Act Prov. 1984 Sec. II is covered, to a certain extent, under serious arrestable offences (see Appendix 17.1).

Public Health Acts

These cover the disclosure of information under the section dealing with public interest.

☐ Examples

Let us now consider the questions posed on page 366. In Example 1 the police are not automatically entitled to be given information unless the offence is deemed to be of a serious nature. Even under these circumstances, the chief constable must formally apply to the consultant in charge of the department.

Example 2 invokes the use of the Road Traffic Act 1982 which requires Authorities or Trusts to divulge information to enable the police to identify the driver of the vehicle involved. However, this does not apply to information dealing with the other occupants.

If, as in Example 3, the nurse discovers her patient to be in possession of a firearm, then the team's duty to other patients, colleagues and the public at large overrides the confidentiality due to that particular patient (see Appendix 16.1 regarding serious arrestable offences). However, the Department of Health guidelines advise that it must be clear that the task of preventing or detecting the crime would otherwise be seriously prejudiced or delayed. Furthermore, there should be a formal agreement that the information will not be used for any other purpose and will be destroyed if the subject is not successfully prosecuted.

Before choosing to disclose confidential information for whatever reason, the nurse or doctor must consider the matter thoroughly and then document it along with their reasons for disclosure. They also need to be aware of actions which may be taken against them if they reveal confidential information inappropriately. These are:

1   The UKCC or GMC may find them guilty of professional misconduct.

2   The employer may dismiss them for breach of contract.

3   The patient may sue in a court of law.

☐ **The media**

The media have *no* right to information without the patient's consent. Any requests for information should be referred to the administration department who must obtain the patient's or relatives' consent before any statement can be made.

■ **The Data Protection Act 1984**

The Data Protection Act 1984 gives a patient the right to see his medical records if these are held on computer and provided there is no exemption. Patients have had the right of access to any health records held on computer since November 1987. This includes both medical and nursing records. However, the information can be withheld from the subject if it is felt that in consequence of seeing the records he is likely to suffer serious physical or mental harm. Access can also be refused if, by such a disclosure, another party who has not given consent could be identified. If the patient wishes to see computerized records, an application must be made to the Health Authority and a fee paid. The information should be provided within 40 days or an explanation given for withholding the information.

The Health Records Act 1990 also gives patients access from 1 November 1991 to written information recorded about themselves. The effect of the Act is essentially the same as that of the Data Protection Act mentioned above.

The need to write clear, legible, accurate and detailed notes has always been important, but never more so in the light of these changes.

■ **Consent**

The trauma team may occasionally face problems with consent when dealing with patients who are members of religious sects or who have relatives who are members of such sects. A common problem is the refusal of blood transfusion by Jehovah's Witnesses.

The patient has the right under common law to give or withhold consent for examination or treatment. This consent can be withdrawn at any time or at any stage of a procedure or treatment. Indeed, an action for damages can be sought by patients against health-care professionals if they treat patients without their consent. This action includes trespass to the person, battery where the person is touched, and assault when he fears he may be touched. If a patient is able to give consent he needs to be told about the procedure, any alternatives and possible side-effects so that he can make an informed decision whether to accept the treatment or not. It is important that he understands the nature of the treatment or procedure and that he is not pressurized into making a decision.

In many cases the consent will be implied, as in the case of a patient attending the Accident & Emergency department having been bitten by a dog, who requires a tetanus toxoid injection. If, when the nurse has informed the patient of the procedure, the patient rolls up his sleeve and offers his arm, this is implied consent.

It is advisable, however, to obtain written consent for procedures where some risk is contemplated, for example where an operation under anaesthetic is required. In an emergency, it is not always possible to gain consent and often treatment is carried out in the best interest of the patient. The substantive law is that the proposed treatment is lawful if it is in the best interest of the patient, and unlawful if it is not. The trauma team may assume consent to enable them to save life or limb, and to relieve pain when the patient is unable to give consent. This is most likely to occur when the trauma victim is unconscious or semiconscious. In some cases a relative is asked to give consent, but if she or he refuses the doctor can still proceed on the grounds of acting in an emergency. In such cases the courts would not recognize the relatives' right to give or withhold consent.

In some situations the patient's injuries may be the result of a criminal act, as in the case of sexual abuse. It is essential that intimate samples are obtained as soon as possible, but the patient's consent must be obtained. In the case of the unconscious patient, these samples may still be obtained and then stored and the patient's consent sought at a later stage. In case law it is presumed that 'the reasonable man' – that is, the patient – would want those involved with his care to take such measures as would enable his assailants to be brought to justice.

☐ Children

The legal age of majority in the UK is 18 years of age, but by statute a 16-year-old should be treated as an adult for the purposes of consent. A child over the age of 16 years can give consent to treatment and it is not necessary to obtain a separate consent from the parents. If the child is not competent to give consent, then the parents' consent is required, but only up to the age of 18 years. A child under the age of 16 can give consent, if he has reached maturity and has sufficient understanding of the treatment proposed. However, in all cases the consent of the parent should be sought, if there is time to do so.

☐ Withheld consent

What if a patient or relative refuses to give consent? The mentally competent adult has the right to refuse treatment and to take his own discharge. The patient should still receive a detailed explanation of the illness and the need for treatment. He also needs a clear explanation of the consequences if the treatment is not carried out and this should be given in the presence of another member of staff. If he still refuses the treatment then he must be asked to sign a release form, stating that he is refusing treatment against medical advice. If he refuses to sign the form, then a member of staff must act as a witness and this must be documented in his notes.

As mentioned above, a parent cannot veto treatment a 16- or 17-year-old is willing to accept. Under this age, the law gives parents the right to custody, but it also lays down a duty to provide medical aid. Therefore, the parents' rights can be overridden, if care is required to save the life of the child or to prevent some marked disability. If there is time, a court order can be obtained. In the case where the parents are separated or divorced, it may be difficult to ascertain who has legal custody; the consent of one parent is sufficient. If a doctor decides to proceed without the parents' consent, and there is time, it should be after a full discussion with them and after obtaining a supporting opinion from a medical colleague. The discussion with the parents should be witnessed by another member of staff and documented in the child's records.

☐ Patients suffering from a mental disorder

The fact that a patient may have a mental disorder does not in itself imply an incapacity to give consent. This is also the case with those held under the Mental Health Act. The decision must still be based on information about the treatment's nature, purpose and likely side-effects. The patient must obviously be allowed to make the decision freely and without any pressure from the staff.

The team needs to take into account the importance of the decision required as well as the patient's mental state during the resuscitation.

■ Professional accountability

The registered nurse is accountable for her actions to a number of people, and, morally, it can be argued that she is accountable to herself. Her primary concern is to her patients and to ensure that their interests are respected. The UKCC has produced a document to clarify the extent of the accountability of the nurse in order for her to achieve high standards.

The nurse is accountable for her actions at work and also when she is off-duty. Her employer will expect her to provide the service that she is employed to provide, and to make proper use of the resources which are available. In relation to the UKCC, she is accountable for any failure to satisfy the introductory paragraph of the Code of Professional Conduct, which reads:

> Each registered nurse, midwife and health visitor shall act at all times in such a manner as to justify public trust and confidence, to uphold and enhance the good standing and reputation of the profession, to serve the interests of society, and above all to safeguard the interests of individual patients and clients.   UKCC 1984

It is essential that the public has trust and confidence in the nursing profession, especially in the light of the many changes taking place in the NHS, and, to this end, the nurse must exercise her accountability in a reasonable manner.

■ Negligence

In the course of their work, team members may be involved with the law of tort, which relates to civil wrongs and can permit common-law actions for damages. One of the most important torts deals with negligence to patients. Three points have to be shown to exist before negligence can be proved:

1   The nurse, or doctor, has a duty to care for the patient.

2   There was a breach of that duty.

3   As a result of (2), the patient suffered damage.

The patient bringing the action has to prove that a duty of care was owed to him. This can be said to exist if the team member can see that her or his actions are reasonably likely to cause harm to the trauma victim. If it can be reasonably foreseen that an act or omission may cause injury or harm to a patient, she or he must take reasonable care to avoid it.

The professional person must be able to attain a higher standard of care than that of the ordinary person. Therefore, he or she would be expected to exhibit the expertise normally demonstrated by an ordinary nurse or doctor who has had his or her particular training and experience.

As well as being sued for negligent acts or omissions, the team member could also be sued for misstatements. This can happen when false information is given to patients or relatives. It is therefore important that what is said is accurate.

As each individual is responsible for her or his own actions, there is no concept of team negligence in law. Consequently, in trauma resuscitation, each member of the team is individually responsible for her or his own negligence.

The importance of documentation cannot be overemphasized. The times of patient registration, nurse assessment and medical examination should all be recorded in the patient's notes. These are all vital pieces of evidence in alleged cases of negligence where a delay in treatment has been claimed.

■ Criminal law

Criminal law deals with crimes against the state, the person or property:

- offences against the state include homicide, perjury and contempt of court;
- offences against the person include homicide (murder or manslaughter), assault, wounding and sexual offences;
- offences against property include arson, robbery and burglary.

Nurses and doctors are not above breaking the law and can be prosecuted like anyone else. In the past, they have committed crimes ranging from assaults to manslaughter, where their recklessness resulted in a patient's death.

The Crown Prosecution Service usually brings prosecutions under the criminal law; private prosecutions are possible, but rare. The prosecution must, in criminal cases, prove the case beyond a reasonable doubt.

A summons or warrant is issued when an individual is brought to trial in a criminal court. In more serious cases the Justice of the Peace issues a warrant to a police officer ordering the accused to be brought to court; in the case of a minor crime, a summons is used to order the accused to appear in court.

The punishment of these crimes is either by fine or imprisonment. The state presumes that a person acted voluntarily and was sane at the time he committed the crime, until it is proved otherwise.

Nurses and doctors can also use the law to protect themselves against patients, for example prosecuting trauma victims who have assaulted members of the trauma team. They can also take out private summonses but in such cases it is advisable for them to consult their employer before proceeding.

□ Criminal evidence

The definition of evidence is anything that furnishes or leads to the furnishing of truth.

Often it is the nurse who is the first to assess a patient, when she may be given vital information that may later be useful as evidence. When undressing the patient it is also important to consider physical evidence: where possible, clothes should be carefully removed and folded before being put into a property bag, with the minimum of handling by staff.

Nurses and doctors do not have absolute privilege and can be asked to give evidence about a patient in court. They do, however, have the unique privilege of being allowed to repeat what a patient actually said – from other witnesses this would be considered as hearsay and not admissible as evidence. Furthermore, they might be asked to comment on the demeanour of a patient and so during assessment they should consider that this is information for documentation.

Both with civil and with criminal injury, there may be a long delay in the case being brought to court. The nurse and doctor may therefore be required to give evidence months or even years after the event. Consequently, it is important that they document all information legibly and accurately at the time, as the patient may change his account by either adding to or omitting details.

Cases of sexual assault are difficult and traumatic for both the patient and the team involved in the care. It is often worth consulting the local forensic department for advice in such cases to ensure that the patient's best interests are upheld.

■ Summary

The trauma team must be aware of the medico-legal aspects of trauma care. It is therefore important that they know their responsibilities in relation to the patient, colleagues, themselves and the community. Although it is easy to forget the legal implications when dealing with life-or-death situations, the team leaders must remain conscious of these issues. Where there is any doubt, it is important to seek advice as early as possible so that the team can make informed decisions based on accurate information.

■ Appendix 17.1: The term 'serious arrestable offence'

Section 116 and Schedule 5 Parts I and II of the 1984 Police and Criminal Evidence Act contain the definition of 'serious arrestable offence'. Schedule 5 of the Act Parts I and II lists offences that are always serious:

Part I

1 Treason.

2 Murder.

3 Manslaughter.

4 Rape.

5 Kidnapping.

6 Incest with a girl under 13 years of age.

7 Buggery with a boy under the age of 16 years or a person who has not consented.

8 Indecent assault which constitutes an act of gross indecency.

Part II

1 Causing an explosion likely to endanger life or property.

2 Intercourse with a girl under the age of 13 years.

3 Possession of firearms with intent to injure.

4 Use of firearms and imitation firearms to resist arrest.

5 Carrying firearms with criminal intent.

6 Hostage taking.

7 Hijacking.

8 Offences under Sections 1, 9 and 10 of the Prevention of Terrorism (Temporary Provisions) Act 1984.

Section 116, subsections 3, 4, 7 and 8 have the effect that any other arrestable offence is 'serious' only if its commission has led to or is intended or is likely to lead to the consequences listed below; or, if the arrestable offence consists of making a threat, if carrying out the threat would be likely to lead to any of these consequences:

1 Serious harm to the security of the state or to public order.

2 Serious interference with the administration of justice or with the investigation of offences or of a particular offence.

3 The death of any person.

4   Serious injury to any person, which includes any disease and any impairment of a person's physical or mental state.

■ References and further reading

Benjamin M & Curtis J 1986. *Ethics in Nursing.* Oxford: Oxford University Press.
Bloch S & Chodolt P (eds) 1981. *Psychiatric Ethics.* Oxford: Oxford University Press.
Boyd K, Melia K & Thompson I 1988. *Nursing Ethics.* Edinburgh: Churchill Livingstone.
Burnard P & Chapman C 1990. *Professional and Ethical Issues in Nursing.* Chichester: John Wiley.
Cardona V 1985. *Trauma Nursing.* Bristol: John Wright.
Carson D & Montgomery J 1989. *Nursing and the Law.* Basingstoke: Macmillan.
Creighton H 1981. *Law Every Nurse Should Know.* W B Saunders.
Dimond B 1990. *Legal Aspects of Nursing.* New York: Prentice Hall.
Dyer C 1992. Court says doctors were right to treat Jehovah's Witness. *Br. Med. J.* 305: 272.
Finch J 1984. *Aspects of Law Affecting the Paramedical Profession.* London: Faber & Faber.
Hargreaves M 1979. *Practical Law for Nurses.* London: Pitman Medical.
Johnson A 1990. *Pathways in Medical Ethics.* London: Edward Arnold.
Marsden A 1989. Legal aspects. In Rutherford W, Illingworth R, Marsden A, *et al.* (eds): *Accident and Emergency Medicine*, 2nd edn. Edinburgh: Churchill Livingstone.
Melia K 1989. *Everyday Nursing Ethics.* London: Macmillan.
NHS Management Executive 1990. *A Guide to Consent for Examination and Treatment.* London: NHS Publications.
Padfield C F (revd Barker D L) 1990. *Law.* London: Heinemann.
Quinn C & Smith M 1987. *Professional Commitment: issues and ethics in nursing.* Philadelphia: W B Saunders.
Rumbold G 1989. *Ethics in Nursing Practice.* London: Baillière Tindall.
Speller S 1986. *Law Notes for Nurses.* London: Royal College of Nursing.
Tate B 1971. *The Nurse's Dilemma.* New York: International Council for Nurses, Florence Nightingale International Foundation.
Tschudin V 1989. *Ethics in Nursing.* London: Heinemann.
United Kingdom Central Council of Nursing, Midwifery and Health Visiting 1984. *Code of Professional Conduct*, 2nd edn. London: UKCC.
Veatch R & Fry S 1987. *Cast Studies in Nursing Ethics.* Philadelphia: J P Lippincott.
Wail A 1989. *Ethics and the Health Service Manager.* London: King's Fund Publishing Office.
Williams J 1990. *The Law of Mental Health.*
Young A 1989. *Legal Problems in Nursing Practice.* London: Harper & Row.

Chapter 18

Major incidents

Tim Hodgetts, Kevin Mackway-Jones and Gabby Lomas

Objectives

The objectives of this chapter are for the trauma team:

*   to understand the principles of major incident planning;
*   to understand the principles of medical management during a major incident.

■ Introduction

A major incident for the fire or police service may not constitute a major incident for the health services, and vice versa. Understandably, therefore, each emergency service has developed its own definition. For the health services a major incident exists when:

> . . . the number and severity of *live* casualties, or its location, requires special arrangements by the Health Service.
>
> Ambulance Officers Group 1990 (Section 2, Para. 2)

This definition deliberately specifies neither the cause of the incident nor the particular number of victims involved.

Recent events have demonstrated an alarming frequency of major incidents. Some hazards are predictable (for example, the kinds seen at the Chernobyl nuclear works and at the Bhopal chemical works), but most are not; a number result from deliberate acts of terrorism (Table 18.1).

Table 18.1 Major terrorist incidents, 1987–1993

Date	Incident	Injured	Dead
8/11/87	Enniskillin	60	11
18/2/91	Victoria station, London: bombing	38	1
10/4/92	City of London: bombing	93	3
20/3/93	Warrington town centre: bombing	55	2

Each incident is likely to produce a disproportionate number of specific injuries, for instance burns (Bradford City fire), hypothermia and drowning (*Herald of Free Enterprise*, Zeebrugge), or blast effect (terrorist bombs). Transportation systems are particularly vulnerable to mass casualty incidents (Table 18.2), and there is a disturbing potential for a major disaster at any event involving a large crowd (Bradford City football stadium fire, 1985; Hillsborough football stadium crushing of crowd, 1989).

Table 18.2 Transportation system disasters, 1987–1991

Type	Incident	Date	Injured	Dead
Sea	*Herald of Free Enterprise*	6/3/87	402	137
Rail	King's Cross underground fire	18/11/87	60	31
Air	Pan Am bombing, Lockerbie	20/12/87	5	270
Rail	Clapham Junction	12/12/88	123	35
River	*Marchioness* pleasure-boat sinking	20/8/89	80	51
Rail	Cannon Street station	8/1/91	265	2

Every hospital that is equipped to receive casualties must have a major incident plan: this should include the provision of a medical team to the scene of the incident, and the plans for any internal hospital disaster (for example, Musgrave Park Hospital bombing, 1991, when there were 2 dead and 7 injured).

At the scene, one doctor will assume control of the health resources, and the role of Medical Incident Officer (MIO). Where the scale of the incident requires on-scene co-ordination of nursing activities, a Nursing Incident Officer (NIO) will also be appointed: this may be necessary when more than one hospital mobile medical team is involved.

A structured approach by the MIO to the management of the incident is essential, and can be considered under the headings shown in Box 18.1. Without such an approach, the Medical and Nursing Incident Officers will not function to their maximum capability.

BOX 18.1   The essential features of major incident management

---

- Command and control
- Safety
- Communications
- Assessment
- Triage
- Treatment
- Evacuation

These fundamental steps can be remembered by means of the mnemonic: *C*ontrol *S*pells *C*alm *A*nd *T*ime to *T*reat *E*veryone.

There are two further important prerequisites to successful major incident management:

- planning;
- training.

As has been said, 'To fail to plan is to plan to fail'; this aphorism cannot be more true than in the case of a major incident. Training will be discussed later in the chapter.

■ Planning

> Proper planning and preparation prevents poor performance.
>
> Army alliteration

The aim of a major incident plan is to mobilize the appropriate personnel to the right place (the incident or the hospital) in the optimum time, and to provide them with the equipment they need and a degree of guidance on their tasks. It should not try to dictate clinical practice, but should concentrate on the extraordinary organizational requirements of the situation. The key elements in effective planning (Box 18.2) will be discussed.

BOX 18.2   Key elements in major incident planning

---

1. Activation of the plan
2. Call-in of key personnel
3. Departmental call-in
4. Lines of responsibility
5. Action Card production
6. Equipment preparation

☐ 1: Activation of the plan

Hospitals are usually notified of a major incident by ambulance control. There may be an advanced warning that allows time for limited preparation, or a message to activate the full plan with immediate effect. In either case, a specified form of words will be used to reduce the chances of misunderstanding. The messages used in the UK are:

- MAJOR INCIDENT – STANDBY;
- MAJOR INCIDENT DECLARED – ACTIVATE PLAN.

A standby alert may be rescinded at any time with the phrase:

- MAJOR INCIDENT – CANCELLED.

Ambulance control will provide the hospital with as much detail as possible, but at the outset little may be known. Certain specific points should be actively sought by the member of hospital staff receiving the call (Box 18.3).

BOX 18.3 Key initial information on receiving a major incident alert

- The nature of the incident (explosion; rail; air crash?)
- The site of the incident (including grid reference)
- The number of casualties
- Special considerations (chemical or radiation spillage?)
- Requirement for a mobile medical team

Some hospitals may have arrangements for direct notification from the site of known hazards (such as at airports and large chemical works): in these cases activation procedures must be agreed and understood by both parties. Occasionally, however, the first indication that a major incident has occurred may be the arrival of large numbers of casualties directly from the scene, particularly if the hospital is in close proximity to the incident, when the 'walking wounded' may arrive within a few minutes. To anticipate this, there must be a facility within the plan to allow the emergency department itself to initiate the plan's activation.

If notification comes from a source other than those indicated above, there should be urgent discussion with ambulance control before the major incident plan is implemented.

☐ 2 & 3: Call-in of key personnel and departmental call-in

The responsibility for calling in key personnel usually rests with the hospital switchboard. Since the plan will identify these key staff by title rather than name, it is important that the list is updated daily. A template to facilitate this can be included in the plan (Figure 18.1).

Once key personnel have been alerted, many of them will then be responsible for continuing the departmental call-in. They may do this themselves, or delegate the task to a more junior member of staff. It is important that such calls are not made via the hospital switchboard, which will still be busy contacting key personnel. Direct-dial lines or public payphones within the department should be used. Some departments will operate a cascade system, whereby the call-in is achieved by staff members telephoning each other from home.

☐ 4: Lines of responsibility

One of the problems during a major incident is that many key staff and their juniors will have to carry out tasks that are not part of their daily routine. Furthermore, the command structure will not be one they are used to. It is essential that the plan includes clear guidelines on lines of responsibility. An example of such guidance is shown in Figure 18.1.

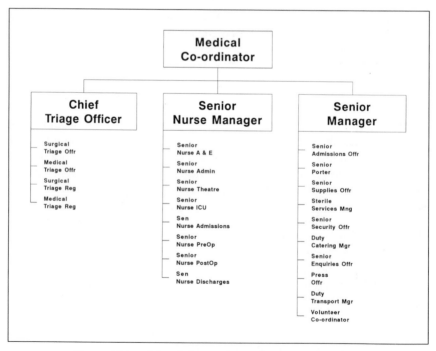

Figure 18.1a Hospital organization: organization chart

Hospital Call-In List	Standby	Activate

Use the exact phraseology shown on relevant Action Sheets and record the time contacted in the space provided.

Give full details to the following:

		Standby	Activate
1	Senior Nurse on duty A & E	....	....
2	Senior Doctor on duty A & E	....	....
3	Medical Incident Officer	....	....
4	Site Nurse Manager	....	....
5	Designated Medical Officer	....	....
6	Duty Consultant A & E	....	....
7	On-call Manager	....	....

Then inform the following that Major Incident procedure is activated:

		Activate
8	Duty Consultant Surgeon	....
9	Duty ICU Consultant	....
10	Senior Porter	....
11	Duty MLSO Haematology	....
12	On-Call Radiographer	....
13	Duty Security Officer	....
14	Duty Consultant Anaesthetist	....
15	Duty Consultant Physician	....
16	Duty Orthopaedic Registrar	....
17	Duty Medical Registrar	....
18	Additional Telephonists	....
19	Tannoy Message	....
20	Duty JHO Medicine	....
21	Duty JHO Surgery	....
22	Duty JHO Orthopaedics	....
23	On-Call Radiologist	....
24	Duty Consultant Pathologist	....
25	General Manager	....
26	Director of Nursing Services	....
27	On-Call Pharmacist	....
28	Social Worker	....
29	Sterile Sevices Manager	....
30	Hospital Chaplain	....
31	Senior Supplies Officer	....
32	Volunteer Co-ordinator	....
33	Duty Engineer	....
34	On-Call Photographer	....
35	Duty Catering Manager	....
36	Duty Linen Services Manager	....
37	Duty Transport Manager	....

Figure 18.1b Hospital organization: call-in list

Senior Nurse A & E

Responsibilities

1. Preparation of reception areas.

2. A & E staff call-in.

3. Control of nursing in the reception areas.

4. Monitoring of clinical stores in the reception areas.

5. Provision of hourly casualty statements (MajIn Form 2) to the Medical Co-ordinator.

6. Operational debriefing of A & E nursing staff involved in the Major Incident Response.

Immediate Action

1. Ensure that the reception areas are being prepared.

2. Ensure that A & E staff call-in has been instituted.

3. Arrange for existing patients in the department to be cleared as follows:

Minor Cases(seen by Dr)	Minimum dressing and review
Minor Cases(waiting)	Advised to attend another A & E
Major Cases	Admitted with minimum documentation

4. Appoint senior A & E Nurses to act as Senior Nurses in the Priority 1, 2, and 3 areas.

5. Brief these senior nurses as regards staffing, equipment supply, and documentation in their areas.

6. Contact the Senior Porter as soon as Major Incident casualties begin to arrive.

7. Liaise with the Chief Triage Officer and assist him in the triage area.

Priorities during the Incident

1. Preparation of the reception areas.

2. Senior nurse staffing in the reception areas.

3. Control of nursing in the reception areas.

4. Monitoring of clinical stores in the reception areas.

5. Provision of accurate hourly casualty statements from the reception areas.

Figure 18.1c   Hospital organization: responsibilities of the senior nurse in A/E

☐ **5: Action Card production**

Senior key personnel involved in a major incident must be familiar with the whole major incident plan in detail. Others do not need to know the whole plan, but clearly they should be aware of their individual roles and responsibilities. To this effect, Action Cards should be produced which contain concise instructions under the following headings:

- immediate actions;
- responsibilities;
- priority of tasks.

The cards for key personnel will be reproduced in the hospital plan, while those for more junior members of staff should be written and kept by individual departments. The instructions are derived from the overall major incident plan, and the cards should therefore be reviewed and updated whenever the plan is changed. An example is given in Figure 18.1.

☐ **6: Equipment preparation**

Additional equipment will be required both for the hospital response and for the response to the scene.

Hospital equipment

Within the hospital, three key areas will require reserve stocks of equipment to cope with a major incident. These are:

- the emergency department;
- the operating theatres;
- the wards (pre- and post-operative).

Arrangements for additional stock must be in place at the *planning* stage – there will be no time to organize this once the major incident plan has been activated. The plans may incorporate special arrangements with manufacturers and automatic arrangements with suppliers, as well as holding a stock designated for major incident use. Problems may be anticipated at the planning stage (see 'Training', page 392), and their solutions already determined (Box 18.4).

On-scene equipment

Clothing

A doctor in sandals and a white coat, or a nurse in uniform, would not be appropriately dressed at the scene of a major incident. In such clothing they

---

BOX 18.4 Problems anticipated in major incident planning, and their solutions

---

Problem A ward that usually deals with low-dependency patients is used for the immediate reception of pre-operative casualties.
Solution Extra stock should be bought and held in the hospital.

Problem There is a predictable shortfall in emergency department equipment occurring 1–2 hours after the casualties start to arrive.
Solution A list of predicted requirements should be prepared and given to bulk suppliers. Agreement should be reached that in the exceptional circumstances of a major incident, all items will be delivered within 2 hours. The supplier should be added to the hospital call-in list.

Problem There will be a large number of patients requiring external fixation of fractures.
Solution Emergency delivery should be arranged directly from the manufacturer. Contact is assured from a list of telephone numbers held in the operating theatres for this purpose.

BOX 18.5 Protective clothing for the mobile medical team

- High-visibility waterproof jacket with identifying panel (DOCTOR or NURSE)
- High-visibility waterproof trousers
- Fire-retardant suit (e.g. Proban®)
- Safety helmet
- Eye protection (visor, or safety glasses)
- Ear protection
- Oil- and acid-resistant boots
- Heavy-duty gloves

---

would be a liability to themselves, and a safety concern to others: they should be refused entry to the scene by the MIO or Ambulance Safety Officer. It is unfortunate that such representations of ill-prepared hospital staff still occur. Box 18.5 lists the minimum clothing requirements for all members of the mobile medical team (MMT).

Medical equipment

The medical equipment carried by the MMT will be considered in terms of the containers and their contents.

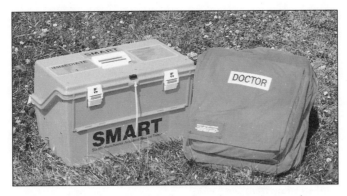

Figure 18.2 A medical rucksack and an equipment box

The containers

The equipment containers should be light, portable, highly visible, and secure. They should not be so small that they become overpacked, nor so large that they are heavy to carry and awkward to open in confined spaces. When opened, all the equipment should be easily identifiable – in a rucksack, items may be packed together in labelled 'snatch' bags, such as SIMPLE AIRWAY, INTUBATION, or INFUSION. Rigid boxes also may be used. Examples are shown in Figure 18.2.

The contents

Often very little initial information is available on the number and type of casualties. The equipment taken must therefore be versatile, because it is during this phase of uncertainty that the medical team will be mobilized. An excessive amount of equipment need not be carried, as resupply from the hospital can be established as soon as ambulances start leaving the scene. Everything that is carried, however, must be carefully selected.

Appendices 18.1 and 18.2 give suggested packing lists for the two types of container shown in Figure 18.2. The rucksack is designed to carry non-disposable items (e.g. laryngoscope and stethoscope), and enough disposable items (e.g. dressings) to treat two multiply injured patients; the box is designed to carry enough disposable items to treat a further four multiply injured. Several of each type of container should be stored in the emergency department. The advantage of this system is that the rucksack can also be used in routine pre-hospital work (as in the case of road traffic accident entrapments), allowing the staff to become familiar with the equipment before there is a major incident crisis.

When the MMT is activated, a designated nurse must check the equipment and any drugs that are to be taken out to the scene. A thorough check is not possible; nor should it be necessary, as the contents of the containers should have been checked on a regular basis. The call-out check is best done by working through a prepared list. Keys must always be available for the locked items (controlled drugs), and be taken to the scene.

■ Medical management

The medical management of a major incident will be considered under two headings:

- on-scene management;
- hospital management.

□ On-scene management

Casualties need to receive optimum medical care as soon as possible, starting with advanced pre-hospital immediate care. But it is naive to presume that a hospital doctor or nurse may simply go to the scene of a major incident and begin to treat patients as they would in the emergency department. A structured approach to the medical management of a major incident is required.

Command

Medical care at the scene of a major incident is provided primarily by the ambulance service, under the direction of the Ambulance Incident Officer (AIO). Medical support in the form of a Medical Incident Officer (a doctor) and a mobile medical team (one or more doctors and one or more nurses) may be requested by the AIO. Once in attendance, the MIO has responsibility for the management of all the medical resources at the scene. All mobile medical teams and independent doctors must report to the MIO on arrival for allocation of tasks – they must accept the overall authority of the MIO.

The MIO should not be part of any mobile medical team, and *must not* be involved in the direct treatment of any casualties: command and control would be lost. The MIO may be a hospital doctor (e.g. an Accident & Emergency consultant), or a general practitioner member of BASICS (the British Association for Immediate Care) – the exact background of the doctor does not matter, so long as he or she is adequately trained. In particular the MIO will liaise closely with the AIO and with incident officers from the other emergency services, in regular briefings. The MIO will maintain close contact with the receiving hospitals, initially to determine the number of intensive-care and general beds available, and the number of manned operating theatres.

A Nursing Incident Officer (NIO) is appointed if the number of nurses at the scene necessitates their separate coordination: this is often the case when two or more mobile medical teams are deployed. The NIO should not be a member of any MMT, and must maintain close contact with the MIO.

Safety

The MIO is responsible for the safety of all medical personnel, which includes recognizing individual fatigue. It is likely that team members will be relieved after about 4 hours, even if they wish to continue. The individual must ensure that she or he wears adequate, approved protective clothing (see Box 18.5), as she or he might otherwise be refused entry to the site for failing to comply with safety standards.

Communications

The ambulance service will issue UHF radios (with a short range) to the MIO and NIO. A knowledge of correct radio voice procedure is essential, and will be presumed, including how to structure a message, key words (e.g. 'over', 'out', 'roger'), and the phonetic alphabet ('alpha, bravo, charlie, delta . . . '). Do not wait until there is a major incident to learn how to use a radio!

VHF radios (with a long range) may also be carried; these allow direct communication with central ambulance control and the receiving hospitals. However, whenever possible all messages should be passed through the ambulance emergency control vehicle (ECV) on the UHF net, to maintain control at the scene and to prevent duplication of efforts.

Cellnet telephones can be useful, but if large numbers of the Press are in attendance it is common for all the available cells to be occupied: access to the system is then denied to the emergency services. To overcome this problem the police may then authorize the activation of ACCOLC (ACCess OverLoad Control), whereby only those telephones with 'protected' cells will continue to function. This is a privilege extended to the emergency services via the Home Office (but you must apply individually for each departmental Cellphone).

Assessment

The MIO will make an assessment of the scene, often in conjunction with the AIO. This is to obtain an idea of any hazards, as well as the number and severity of the casualties. This information is used to decide on the primary medical response that is needed, and to relay casualty estimates to the receiving hospitals.

Triage

'Triage' means to sift, sort or classify. Its first use is attributed to Baron

Dominique Jean Larrey, Napoleon's Surgeon-Marshal, who developed the principle of sorting casualties for treatment on the battlefield. Triage has continued to be developed within a military framework, but also has many applications in civilian medicine. Triage is a dynamic process, with reassessment and changing priorities reflecting each patient's changing condition. It is carried out repeatedly both at the scene and in the hospital, and is used to define the urgency of treatment and transport. The classification used is shown in Box 18.6.

BOX 18.6   Triage categories

Priority 1 – Immediate – RED
- Patients with immediately life-threatening injuries

Priority 2 – Urgent – YELLOW
- Patients with serious injuries that will require treatment, but which are not immediately life-threatening

Priority 3 – Delayed – GREEN
- Patients with only minor injuries who can tolerate a significant delay before treatment

Priority 4 – Expectant – BLUE
- Patients who have such serious injuries that to treat them with limited resources would reduce the chance of survival of others with less serious injury

Deceased – WHITE/BLACK

Triage at the scene is carried out where the casualties lie, principally by the ambulance personnel; and again at the central treatment point (Casualty Clearing Station), when experienced nurses may be involved as well as the doctors. After initial treatment the priority for evacuation may change, and there must be continuing alertness to any deterioration in the patient's condition that would increase their priority.

Initially any patients who have problems with airway, breathing and circulation should be sifted from the rest: these require immediate treatment and early evacuation. Those casualties who are walking will, by and large, be allocated to the 'delayed' category. The remaining patients can be sorted by fuller examination.

Once a triage decision has been made it is important to display this on the patient. To do this a triage label will be attached around the wrist, or to the clothing. One of the most popular is the *Cambridge Cruciform Casualty Card* (Figure 18.3) – note, however, that this label does not include identification of 'expectant' category patients. As well as this card, there are some 120 other designs to choose from.

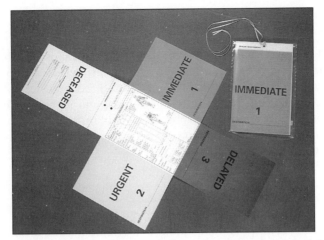

Figure 18.3 The *Cambridge Cruciform Casualty Card* triage label

The *Cambridge Card* opens out into a cross shape, allowing the displayed priority to be altered simply by refolding the card. Most modern labels also allow a destination hospital to be indicated, which may assist in the efficient spreading of the casualty load among a number of hospitals. It has been recognized that it is undesirable to flood a single hospital with the majority of the casualties.

The dead also should be labelled: if they are not there will inevitably be repeated unnecessary examinations as they are rediscovered. Death is confirmed by a doctor, ideally in the presence of a police officer, who is the coroner's representative. Forensic examination usually plays an important part in the investigation of a major incident and the dead should therefore not be moved unless they are preventing access to the living.

Treatment

Treatment at the scene is provided by the ambulance service, supported by a number of mobile medical teams and independent doctors (e.g. members of BASICS). The MIO will decide how many doctors and nurses are needed at the scene, but the AIO will decide from where they come. The MIO will concentrate the medical teams at the Casualty Clearing Station, but allow personnel forward to attend to individuals with specific problems (e.g. those requiring analgesia to effect their release); paramedics will otherwise provide the medical support at the scene itself.

The precise composition of a mobile medical team is variable, but often consists of two doctors and two nurses, who may be from any specialty. At the planning stage it is important to balance the clinical usefulness at the scene of a certain combination of experience with the need not to deplete the receiving hospital of essential personnel.

Evacuation

Priorities for evacuation will be decided using the triage principles already described. The AIO is responsible for determining the most suitable form of transport. Although on the whole this will involve wheeled ambulances, it may be appropriate to use a helicopter for direct transfer to a distant specialist centre (e.g. a burns centre, or a spinal injuries centre), or convenient to commandeer public transport, especially for the minor injured (e.g. a bus could be used to take thirty minor injured to a hospital outside the immediate receiving hospital area).

☐ In-hospital management

At each receiving hospital there should be a single entry triage point through which all patients pass (irrespective of whether or not they were involved in the major incident). This point is manned by the Chief Triage Officer, who is usually the duty A/E consultant. Patients are rapidly reassessed and re-categorized depending on their condition, and then moved to different areas depending on their priority. Subsequently, admitting teams will make triage decisions concerning the urgency of further resuscitation and definitive treatment.

Other patients, who have not been involved in the major incident, may arrive at the department. These patients must also be triaged and treated appropriately, but identified as separate from those arriving from the incident scene by using a different form of documentation. This assists the police, who will set up a casualty bureau to collate the names of the injured.

For immediate hospital care to be efficient, two things must happen quickly: first, the areas designated for the response must be prepared; second, adequate staff must be assembled, formed into teams, and dispatched to the appropriate clinical areas. Resuscitation and clinical care of individual patients should follow the principles outlined elsewhere in this book.

Preparation

As soon as the plan has been activated, each department involved in the response should begin their preparations for the incident. For the duration of the major incident other services should be restricted to those required for urgent cases. However, existing in-patients must be cared for, and junior house staff (interns) should continue to take responsibility for their management.

Initially the brunt of the work will be in the receiving area – that is, the emergency department. Priority should therefore be given to the preparation of this area. The senior nurse on duty should carry out or delegate the tasks shown in Box 18.7.

BOX 18.7 Tasks in preparing the receiving area

1 Inform all staff
2 Initiate departmental call-in
3 Set up the triage point
4 Staff the clinical areas
5 Equip the clinical areas
6 Clear existing patients from the department

During the incident it is useful if staff who usually work in the receiving area can be distinguished from other hospital personnel by coloured tabards: these people will be familiar with the equipment and communication system in the A/E department, and will be able to assist those who are not.

Team formation

Staffing is always a problem during a major incident, and this is particularly so in the reception phase. The A/E personnel will provide the infrastructure to which doctors and nurses from other departments can be added: those not specifically tasked in the plan should be given a reporting point, which should be under the control of a senior member of staff whose job it is to form the teams necessary to deliver clinical care.

Two types of team are required:

- casualty treatment teams;
- casualty transfer teams.

A casualty treatment team consists of two doctors and two nurses, who are tasked with the clinical care of the casualties. As a rule each team will be capable of looking after one Priority 1 patient, or two or three Priority 2 patients. The Priority 3 area may require only two teams in all, but this should be judged according to circumstances. Other areas, such as pre- and post-operative wards and other wards used for admission, will require teams at a later stage.

A casualty transfer team consists of one doctor (usually an anaesthetist) and one nurse, with portering staff. Such teams are used to supervise the movement of critical patients from the receiving areas to the admitting areas. In a major incident this may involve secondary inter-hospital transfer. The movement of all patients in and out of the department must be recorded.

Definitive care

Definitive care involves treatment other than resuscitation. Casualties may require an operation (which can be considered 'life-saving', 'urgent' or 'elective') or admission to a high-dependency area; or they may need admission simply for a period of observation. The decisions about what care is needed, and how urgently it is required, can have a critical effect on the casualty's outcome – they must be taken by senior members of staff.

A senior surgeon should assess all surgical priorities, and a senior physician or intensivist must assess all medical priorities. To be sure that they maintain the correct perspective on priorities, they must be kept continually informed of the casualty status. Team leaders should discuss their patients with these key personnel before making decisions about disposal.

■ Training

Training is fundamental if the plan is to work effectively. For the hospital response to run smoothly, key personnel must be made aware of their tasks and other staff must know their duties and reporting areas. Staff likely to be sent to the scene must train with their equipment, be practised in field triage and pre-hospital care, and be made aware of the dangers they may face. These objectives can be achieved in the following ways:

- lectures and workshops;
- paper exercises;
- table-top exercises;
- small-scale practical exercises;
- large-scale inter-service exercises.

☐ Lectures and workshops

These can be used to enable staff to become familiar with the overall major incident plan, and their own particular roles in it. Given the high turnover of staff it is important that a simple introduction to the major incident plan, with specific mention of activation procedures and reporting areas, be given during induction.

Key personnel can be briefed about their duties, and discussion groups held to highlight any difficulties.

☐ Paper exercises

A paper exercise consists of a written scenario followed by a series of questions. Further information with accompanying questions is given as the exercise progresses. These exercises are particularly useful as an introduction to the principles of triage, and can be written specifically to test other aspects of the plan such as equipment resupply.

☐ Table-top exercises

All or part of the major incident plan can be rehearsed using a game board or computer program. This is a cheap and effective way of testing aspects of the plan, and is particularly useful in testing the organizational side.

☐ Small-scale practical exercises

These involve the practical testing of individual aspects of the plan. Examples include activation exercises, during which the call-in is tested (with staff availability and response time being recorded), and exercises involving specific areas within the hospital such as the operating theatres or the emergency department.

☐ Large-scale inter-service exercises

In a large exercise the whole hospital plan, and the plans of the emergency services, can be tested. A mock incident is arranged with realistically made-up casualties, and each emergency service is expected to act out its part in full. With sufficient planning and preparation this can be a very effective test.

There are, however, significant limitations – such exercises can be very expensive, and they often disrupt normal services. This is balanced by their value in promoting inter-service co-operation, and in rehearsing pre-hospital immediate care skills.

■ Other matters

☐ Utilization of staff

For a long time the attendance of a large number of staff at the beginning of a major incident was seen as the hallmark of a successful hospital response. Although it is true that the reception phase is the most intensive, it should not be forgotten that there will be an increased workload for a number of days. It is therefore essential that sufficient staff are rested, and capable of working over this period. To anticipate this, only those staff required should be called immediately, and any in excess of requirements should be sent home to rest. Specific instructions about when to return should be given.

☐ Identification of patients and staff in hospital

Patients

Each patient should be given a unique number at the hospital triage point, usually in the form of an identification wristband (some triage labels used at the scene have unique numbers, and this identification may be retained in hospital). In the early stages this reference number may be the only means of identification, and it is therefore crucial that it is not removed.

Staff

Key personnel must be easily identifiable during the incident; this will help in maintaining adequate command and control. Coloured tabards marked clearly with job titles are one possible solution.

For security reasons it is helpful if other staff wear hospital identification badges. Similarly, only volunteers identified by an official hospital badge should be allowed into clinical areas.

☐ Staff debriefing

All the staff involved should receive an immediate debriefing when the order to 'stand down' has been given. An operational debriefing (to identify any problems with the plan) should be undertaken by heads of departments.

The emotional debriefing of staff is also necessary. This is best done by means of small-group discussions. These should be compulsory and must take place as soon as possible after the incident.

Formal post-traumatic counselling can be offered to any staff who are identified as being at particular risk during the informal debriefing: this can take the form of individual or group counselling, as indicated.

☐ Audit

A medical audit, to look at the standard of care delivered during the incident, should be held within one month. A separate audit should be held to discuss the major incident plan. All key personnel involved in the management of the incident should attend this meeting. The problems encountered can be discussed and the plan amended appropriately.

■ Summary

The cornerstone of successful major incident management is planning. The plan should not dictate clinical matters, but should concentrate on the extraordinary organizational requirements of the situation.

Hospital staff may be required to provide care at the site of the incident, as well as within the hospital itself. For those who have to work at the scene, proper clothing and adequate training are essential. In hospital, the team concept can be successfully extended to major incident management. At each location triage is the fundamental principle behind effective medical care – do the most, for the most!

Appendices 18.1 – 18.3 and 'References and further reading follow'.

■ Appendix 18.1: The accident rescue rusksack

Intravenous 1

Gelofusine®: 500 ml × 2

0.9% Saline: 500 ml × 2

Blood-giving sets × 4

Airway 1

Bandage 1"	Lignocaine jelly
Catheter mount	Magill forceps
Chest drain bags (2)	Mini-Trach™ set
Endotracheal tubes:	
7, 8(2), 9	Sleek™
Guedel airways:	Spare batteries/bulb
2, 3, 4	Suction catheters
Introducer (ETT)	Yankauer/soft-tipped
Laryngoscope	Syringe (20 ml)

Desilets(2) – Chest drains(2) – Cervi VII collars

Airway 2	Intravenous 2	
Laerdal™ pocket mask	Blood sample kits	
	U&E, FBC, CXM	Syringes: 20 ml × 4
	Elastoplast™ 7.5	3-way taps × 2
Nasopharyngeal airways: 6, 7, 8	Gauze squares	Tourniquet
	Gloves: 4 prs	Transpore™ 2.5
	ID bands × 2	Venflons™: 16 g × 4
Oxygen masks (high conc.) × 2	Needles: 21 g × 8	Venflons™: 18 g × 2
	Sharps pad underneath	

Drugs 1 – Black	Instruments	Dressings
Ketamine	Clips × 3	
Lignocaine	Mosquitos × 3	
Naloxone	Needle holder	
	Pen torch	
	Pens	Ambulance
Drugs 2 – Yellow	Scalpel 23 × 4	dressings
Kept in CD safe	Scissor: large	× 4
Morphine	Scissor: small	
Prochlorperazine	Silk W 791 × 4	
Phone card/10p's	Tooth forceps	

CALL THE SMART NURSE VIA 962 9101

FRONT POUCH

SMO tabard
Triage cards × 20

FORMS ON CLIPBOARD
Equipment used × 5
Incident report × 5

MAPS
Manchester A–Z
MA Crash
Predicted sites

AIDE MEMOIRES
Phone numbers
Equipment
Triage

ACTION CARDS
Emergency Standby
Co-ordinator
SMART
Major Accident
Co-ordinator
SMART
MIO

REMEMBER THE AIRWAY BOX

OTHER EQUIPMENT
Propaq
– ECG
– NIBP
– Temp.
– Inv. BP
Oximeter
Head immobilizer
Spinal board
Donway splints
Vacuum splints
MAST
Oxylog™
Portable radio
Major accident equipment

CLOTHING
Fire-resistant suit
Yellow jacket
Helmet
Visor
Belt
Light
Radio holster
Equip. pouch
'Doctor' label for jacket
Name badge

**CALL A/E 447 3744
AND TELL THE SMART NURSE
WHAT YOU NEED**

■ Appendix 18.2: The major accident box

(Contents list inside lid; sharps pad on flap)

Top compartment

10 ml syringe × 2	23 g scalpels × 4	W791 × 4	Scissors	18 g Venflon™ × 1	18 g Venflon™ × 1	21 g needles × 10	
		Pens × 4	Batteries × 4				
Tape 2.5 cm	10 ml syringe × 2	Marking pen	Tourniquet	16 g Venflon™ × 5	16 g Venflon™ × 5		
		Pen torch	*DRUGS in 2 only (in CD)* Laryng. bulb			Sterets™	

Middle shelf

Endotracheal tubes 9 × 1 8 × 2 7 × 1	Nasopharyngeal airways 8 × 1 7 × 1 6 × 1
Guedel airways 4 × 2 3 × 2 2 × 2	Gauze squares × 10 20 ml syringes × 2 Lignocaine gel Mini-Trach™ set
Oxygen masks (high) × 4	

Bottom compartment

0.9% Saline 500 ml × 4	CXM sets × 4
Gelofusine™ 500 ml × 4	Gloves × 10
Giving sets × 4	Chest drains × 2
Chest drain bags × 2	

■ Appendix 18.3: The drugs box

Anaesthetic agents

- Etomidate: 20 mg/10 ml × 10 ampoules
- Midazolam: 10 mg/5 ml × 10 ampoules
- Suxamethonium*: 100 mg/2 ml × 5 ampoules
- Atracurium*: 50 mg/5 ml × 5 ampoules

Analgesics

- Morphine *Mini-jets*: 20 mg/2 ml × 10 ampoules

Antiemetic agents

- Metoclopramide: 10 mg/2 ml × 10 ampoules

Cardiac arrest drugs

- Adrenaline 1: 10 000 in 10 ml × 3 *Mini-jets*
- Atropine: 1 mg/10 ml × 3 *Mini-jets*
- Lignocaine: 2% 100 mg/5 ml × 2

Other

- Naloxone: 0.4 mg × 10 ampoules
- Dextrose: 50%/50 ml × 1
- Glucagon: 1 mg × 1 set
- Water for injection: 10 ml × 10 ampoules
- Sticky labels
- Marker pen

* To be stored in a fridge

■ References and further reading

Key document
NHS Management Executive 1990. *Emergency Planning in the NHS: Health Services arrangements for dealing with major incidents.* Health Circular (90)25, October 1990. London: HMSO.

Baskett P & Weller R (eds) 1988. *Medicine for Disasters.* London: Wright.
Blythine P 1988. *Triage – A Nursing Care System: management and practice in emergency nursing.* London: Chapman & Hall.

Hines K & Robertson B (eds) 1985. *Guide to Major Incident Management* Ipswich: BASICS Publications.

Hodgetts T 1993. Lessons from the Musgrave Park Hospital bombing. *Injury* **24**(4): 219.

Jones G 1988. *Provision of Pre-hospital Care*. London: Chapman & Hall.

Neal W 1992. *With Disastrous Consequences: London disasters 1830–1917* Enfield Lock: Hisarlik Press.

New B 1992. *Too Many Cooks? The response of the health-related services to major incidents in London*. London: King's Fund Institute.

Miles S 1991. Major accidents. In Skinner D, Driscoll P, Earlam R (eds): *ABC of Major Trauma*. London: BMJ Publications.

Savage P 1979. *Disasters – Hospital Planning*. Oxford: Pergamon Maxwell.

Regional Ambulance Officers Group 1990. *Ambulance Service Operational Arrangements: civil emergencies*. London: HMSO.

Chapter 19

Trauma team protection from infective contamination

Joanne Walker and Peter Driscoll

Objectives

The objectives of this chapter are for members of the trauma team:

- to recognize the high-risk areas in which they work;

- to understand how they can obtain maximum protection against bodily fluids during the resuscitation of a trauma victim.

■ Introduction

'The risk of the health care worker contracting the disease is proportional to the prevalence of AIDS and hepatitis within the population served.'

Expert advisory group on AIDS

In 1988, the incidence of hepatitis B carriers was estimated to be 200 million worldwide, with 6–10 per cent of the population in the UK having antibodies, and 5 per cent being in a carrier status. Other studies have shown that an average UK Accident & Emergency department, seeing 30 000–40 000 patients per annum, would be exposed to 30–250 carriers of hepatitis B annually. In the majority of these cases the patient will asymptomatic and unaware of his condition. It is therefore unlikely that the team will receive reliable prior warning about the carrier status of a trauma patient.

In addition to the hepatitis problem, there is also now the risk of HIV contamination. WHO estimates that there are 1.5 million people with fully developed AIDS in the world, and an additional 10 million individuals who are HIV-positive. In the USA, 107 308 cases of AIDS had been reported to the Center of Disease Control by October 1989. In the UK, the Department of Health estimated that up to 46 000 individuals were HIV-positive by September 1991.

A disproportionately high number of these patients attend A/E departments. In the USA, The John Hopkins University found that over 7 per cent
of the patients attending their emergency departments were positive on HIV
testing, with victims of penetrating trauma being at a particularly high risk
(19 per cent HIV-positive). Further data from Florida supports these findings and shows that 24 per cent of the people dying from violent or
unexpected means were HIV-positive.

It follows that trauma teams tend to deal with 'high risk' patients – that
is, those who have a higher than average chance of carrying one of the HIV
or hepatitis viruses. The risk of hepatitis B virus transmission by innoculation
is 3–16 per cent, and that for HIV is 0.4 per cent.

During the initial resuscitation there is no time for members of the
trauma team to assess the degree of risk to which they will be exposed.
Instead protective clothing must be in place before the patient arrives.

■ Methods of protection

There are two standard methods of protecting the team from the risk of
contamination and infection.

First, each member should be routinely immunized against hepatitis B
and later checked for sero-conversion.

Secondly, universal precautions should be taken (Box 19.1; Figure
19.1).

BOX 19.1   Universal precautions against contamination

- Gloves
- Water-repellent gowns and apron
- Protective headwear
- Masks
- Protective eyewear
- Protective footwear

☐ Compliance

Even with the known risks and recommendations, medical personnel are
notorious for being lax about protecting themselves during emergency
procedures. Recent research from the UK showed that during emergency
settings only 42 per cent of nurses wore protective aprons and 75 per cent
wore gloves. A/E doctors were more likely to protect themselves, with a

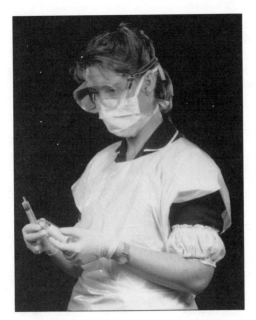

Figure 19.1   Universal precautions

compliance rate of 66 per cent and 90 per cent respectively. This compared with non-A/E medical and ambulance personnel wearing gloves in 46 per cent and 16 per cent of cases, respectively (Figure 19.2). A similar study in the USA found that while gloves were nearly always worn, protective eyewear, ankle and foot protection, and body protection such as gowns or aprons, were commonly ignored. Even when invasive procedures were undertaken, the compliance rate was less than 40 per cent.

To overcome this problem, **the nursing and medical team leaders must take the responsibility of ensuring that *all* persons present are wearing *full* protection *before* the patient arrives.**

A recurring problem is when a patient's condition suddenly deteriorates whilst protective measures are not being taken. There are two possible solutions: either all staff routinely take universal precautions, or the team leaders coordinate the donning of protective clothing once the situation arises. In the latter case they will have to instruct each member, in turn, to take up universal precautions while the rest of the team manage the patient.

☐   **Effectiveness**

For universal precautions to be effective, the protective barriers have to remain intact whilst the nursing and medical personnel are in contact with

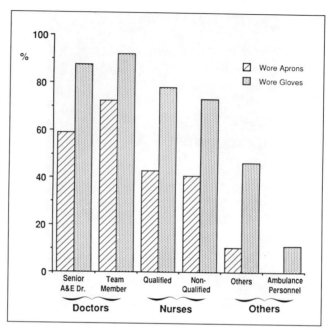

Figure 19.2   Incidence of team members wearing protective clothing

the trauma victim. A watertight test has shown that after clinical use latex gloves have macroscopic and microscopic defects of 2.7 per cent and 14 per cent respectively. Unpublished work, from a study conducted in the University Department of A/E Medicine in Manchester, has demonstrated that 13 per cent of gloves develop defects during a resuscitation. The commonest site was over the lateral aspect of the hand, with the index finger showing the highest incidence. It is suspected that in most cases the defects were caused by the team members having to handle tape, glass and sharp metal objects during the resuscitation.

It is therefore important that nursing and medical staff either wear robust gloves whilst clearing away debris, or 'double-glove' throughout the resuscitation. They must also change their gloves immediately if they notice any defects.

☐ **Additional protection**

All team members must follow the basic principles of hygiene and decontamination. These standard tenets of good nursing care will not be discussed further here, but the interested reader should consult the 'further reading' list given at the end of this chapter.

☐ Needle-stick injuries

The risk of contracting hepatitis B following a needle-stick injury has been estimated to be as high as 16 per cent. This is in contrast to the 0.5 per cent chance of contracting HIV. In 1991 13 cases of occupationally contracted AIDS had been documented worldwide following needle-stick injuries.

Four basic rules should therefore be followed by each team member (Box 19.2).

BOX 19.2   Precautions against needle-stick injuries

1 Never resheathe a needle after use. Up to 40 per cent of self-inoculation accidents have been reported to occur whilst this procedure was attempted.
2 Dispose of all sharp objects in a metal bin which will be incinerated later.
3 Always dispose of 'sharps bins' when they are three-quarters full. *Never* put your hand in one!
4 Do not put your colleagues at risk by the careless use of sharp objects or their disposal.

■ Summary

There is a higher than average chance that trauma patients will be HIV-positive or infected with one of the hepatitis viruses. The team leaders must therefore recognize that their first priority is the protection of all the team members, even if the patient arrives unexpectedly. Consequently, they should ensure that all personnel are protected at all times and that precautions are taken to prevent needle-stick injuries.

■ References and further reading

Anderson D C, Blower A L, Packer J M, *et al.* 1991. Preventing needlestick injuries. *Br. Med. J.* 302: 769.

Anon 1992. Needlesticks: preaching to the seroconverted? *Lancet* 340: 640.

Boxall E 1993. Risk to surgeons and patients from HIV and hepatitis. *Br. Med. J.* 306: 653.

Buck B E, Malinin T I & Brown M D 1989. Bone transplantation and human immunodeficiency virus. An estimate of risk of acquired immunodeficiency syndrome (AIDS). *Clin. Orthop.* 240: 129.

Centres for Disease Control: update 1988. Universal precautions for the prevention of human immunodeficiency virus, hepatitis B virus, and other blood-borne pathogens in health care settings. *MMWR* **37**: 378.

Dubay E & Grubb R 1978. *Infection prevention and control*. St. Louis: C V Mosby.

Fosse E, Svennevig J, Pillgram J, *et al.* 1989. Human immunodeficiency virus and hepatitis B virus in injured patients and victims of violence. *Injury* **20**: 13.

Genberding J 1989. Risk of health care workers from exposure to hepatitis B virus, human immunodeficiency virus and cytomegalovirus. In Moellering R, Weber D, Rutala W, *et al* (eds): Nosocomial infections: new issues and strategies for prevention: *Infect. Dis. Clin. N. Am.* **3**: 735.

Hammond J, Eckes J, Gomez G, *et al.* 1990. HIV, trauma, and infection control: universal precautions are universally ignored. *J. Trauma* **30**(5): 555.

Helen G, Fritz S, Qaquish B, *et al.* 1989. Substantial increase in human immunodeficiency virus (HIV-1) infection in critically ill emergency patients: 1986 and 1987 compared. *Ann. Emerg. Med.* **18**(4): 378.

Heywood J 1988. Hepatitis B vaccination in UK A/E departments. *Arch. Emerg. Med.* **5**: 59.

Kennedy D 1988. Needlestick injuries: mechanisms and control. *J. Hosp. Infec.* **12**(4): 315.

Korniewicz D, Laughon B, Butz A, *et al.* 1989. Integrity of vinyl and latex procedure gloves. *Nursing Research* **38**: 144.

Kuykendall J 1992. Rebels at risk. *Nursing Times* **88**: 26.

Maurer I 1978. *Hospital Hygiene*. London: Edward Arnold.

Recommendations of the expert advisory group on AIDS 1990. *Guidance for Health Care Workers: protection against infection with HIV and hepatitis viruses*. London: HMSO.

Sheehy S, Marvin J & Jimmerson C 1992. Infection control. In Sheehy S, Marvin J & Jimmerson C (eds): *Emergency Nursing, Principles and Practice*, 3rd edn. St. Louis: C V Mosby.

Chapter 20

Resuscitation room layout and equipment

Mark Doyle, Olive Goodall, Peter Driscoll and Terry Brown

Objectives

The objectives of this chapter are to describe:

- the structure and layout of the resuscitation area;

- the equipment necessary for resuscitation of the injured patient along the guidelines delineated in other chapters.

■ Introduction

There must be a dedicated room for the reception, stabilization and resuscitation of seriously injured patients. It should be fully equipped and should stand in readiness at all times; ideally it should be reserved for patients with life- or limb-threatening problems.

■ The resuscitation area

It needs to be a large room, or part of a larger high-care area, sited close to the ambulance bay (Figure 20.1). As is self-evident, the doors to this room must be wide enough to permit the rapid and unhindered access of the ambulance trolley and personnel. The walls, doors and floor should have coverings which can easily and effectively be cleaned. Lead shielding of these surfaces is also required so that staff in nearby rooms can be protected from x-ray exposure.

It is essential that communication with the rest of the emergency department and the hospital be smooth, rapid and uncluttered. An intercom,

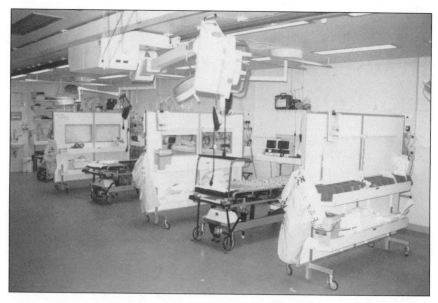

Figure 20.1   Overall view of a resuscitation room, showing resuscitation bays and a ceiling-mounted x-ray gantry

backed up by an alarm system, can be used to summon staff from the department. Communication with the rest of the hospital should be via one or more dedicated phones in the area.

The larger resuscitation rooms are usually divided into a series of bays each of which is fully equipped to handle any single trauma case (Figure 20.1). These bays are separated by screens for the sake of the injured patient's privacy. Commonly curtains on rails are used because these are easily placed and removed and cannot be knocked over. However, they do not protect medical personnel in adjacent bays from radiation, so in busy units solid, x-ray blocking screens are used to separate resuscitation bays: this enables multiple resuscitations to continue whilst radiographs are taken in different parts of the room.

If a resuscitation area is being purpose-built, it is preferable to install a ceiling-mounted x-ray gantry (Figure 20.1). This saves space and improves the quality of the radiographs. However, it is very expensive!

□ The resuscitation bay

There must be enough room for an ambulance trolley to come alongside the resuscitation trolley so that a smooth transfer of the patient can be carried out. Additionally, in the absence of an overhead x-ray gantry, there must also be space for both access and manoeuvring of portable x-ray equipment.

As good illumination is necessary, fluorescent lighting, supplemented with directable spotlights, is required. Each bay must also have wall points for oxygen and suction and, ideally, an anaesthetic gas supply. Several mains electricity sockets are necessary, to run the various monitoring instruments and portable x-ray machines. A wall-mounted x-ray viewing box is required in each bay so that the three essential radiographs can be checked without the medical team leader having to leave the patient.

A wall-mounted whiteboard helps the nursing team leader to rapidly document the patient's initial vital signs and pre-hospital findings before the permanent notes can be written. Wall charts showing protocols for major emergencies should also be prominently displayed, as should nomograms for rapid calculation of paediatric drug doses, fluid requirements and endotracheal tube sizes. Local factors may dictate the possibility of providing a specific paediatric resuscitation bay (Figure 20.2).

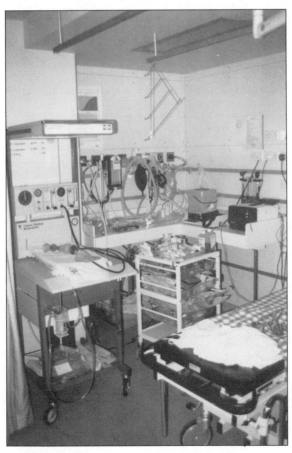

Figure 20.2   A paediatric resuscitation bay

☐ Storing equipment in the resuscitation bay

Shelving needs to be deep and securely mounted to take large equipment trays and monitoring instruments (Figure 20.3). However, these should not obstruct members of the trauma team – especially those dealing with the patient's airway. Wall rails provide extra capacity for siting instruments (Figure 20.4). Mobile equipment trolleys also facilitate patient transfer and access for portable x-ray equipment, because they allow some of the equipment to be temporarily displaced.

■ Equipment

In describing the equipment needed in the resuscitation of the multiply injured patient, it is important to adhere to the ABC format used in the management of these patients. Therefore the equipment will be described in the following order:

* equipment required for the primary survey;
* equipment required for the secondary survey;
* monitoring equipment used during a trauma resuscitation;
* drugs required for trauma resuscitation.

All staff should be aware of what equipment is available and where it is. It must also be checked regularly by designated personnel so that missing or

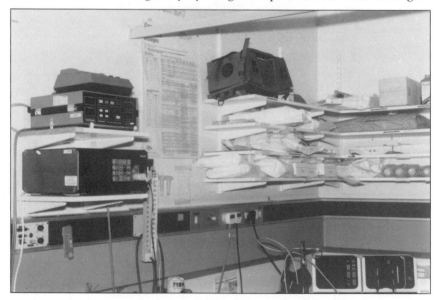

Figure 20.3 Shelving in the resuscitation bay

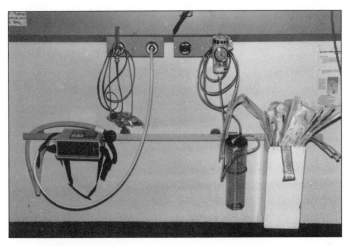

Figure 20.4 Wall rails in the resuscitation bay

out-of-date items can be replaced and regular servicing of particular items carried out.

Occasionally, resuscitation incorporates the definitive management of the underlying problem. For example, a massive haemorrhage may require a laparotomy for it to be controlled. The resuscitation area must therefore have some anaesthetic and surgical capability.

All monitoring and supportive equipment needs to be light, portable and able to run on batteries as well as mains electricity. These features enable the use of the equipment to be continued during the patient's transfer from the resuscitation room.

☐ Equipment required for the primary survey

Transferring a patient between trolleys

In the UK, many patients are transported on a scoop stretcher in the pre-hospital phase. This device also expedites the transfer of patients with a suspected spinal injury from the ambulance to a hospital trolley. However, it is important to remember that the cervical spine must still be independently immobilized.

In cases where the trauma victim has been brought in prone, a 'scoop sandwich' enables the patient to be safely and simultaneously transferred and turned supine. This method utilizes two scoop stretchers. One is placed under the patient and the other one put on his back; they are then tied together. A second scoop stretcher should therefore be available in the resuscitation room for this purpose.

(A) Airway

Facemask

All trauma patients need high inspired oxygen concentrations. This is achieved, in the conscious spontaneously breathing patient, by using a tight-fitting facemask with a reservoir bag attached. A high flow of oxygen is always required in trauma patients (over 12 l/min).

Airways

A range of sizes of oropharyngeal (000–5) and nasopharyngeal (5–7) airways should be available (see Chapter 2). These can be used in the spontaneously breathing patient or in association with positive ventilation using a bag-valve-mask technique.

Bag-valve-mask

This is a self-inflating bag, with a system of inlet and outlet one-way valves which ensure that the patient's expired air is vented and not rebreathed. The inlet end of the self-inflating bag should be connected to an oxygen reservoir bag, thereby providing the mask with nearly 100% oxygen (see Chapter 2). The outlet valve directs flow to the patient from the bag and prevents the patient's expired gas re-entering the bag.

A facemask is connected to this valve, and fitted over the patient's mouth and nose. There is a range of paediatric and adult sizes which can achieve a tight seal by means of a soft rubber ring. Self-inflating bags also come in different sizes but the adult 2L bag can generally be used with only slight modification of technique.

The self-inflating bag and valve can be connected to an endotracheal tube. This can be either by a direct attachment between valve and ET tube adaptor (in children) or with a catheter mount.

Endotracheal intubation

Securing and isolating the airway by endotracheal intubation may be needed as part of the resuscitation of a trauma patient. A range of cuffed endotracheal tubes (5.5–9.0 mm) is needed to allow for various ages and sizes of patient. The cuffs should ideally be self-sealing when inflated. A supply of 2.5–5.0 mm uncuffed tubes for children should also be available, together with their appropriate connectors or adaptors. The adult tubes must be pre-cut at 25 cm and connected to the 15 mm connector, as this saves vital time during the resuscitation.

Introducers and gum elastic bougies are required to help with difficult intubations.

For the laryngoscopes, four types of blades are required:

- short, straight (Wisconsin 0) – for under 1 year;
- short, curved (Robertshaw 0, 1; or Macintosh) – for children;
- curved (Macintosh 3, 4) – for standard adults;
- long, straight (Macintosh) – for adults who are difficult to intubate.

Personnel must ensure that batteries and bulbs are replaced regularly and that there are back-up laryngoscopes in case of failure.

Other items necessary for intubation are listed in Box 2.6 (page 53).

Surgical airway

In the event of severe upper-airway trauma, approach to the airway via the mouth or nose may be impossible. In these situations the airway is usually entered and secured via the cricothyroid membrane.

Needle cricothyroidotomy

A large IV cannula (14 g or 12 g) can be inserted through the cricothyroid membrane and then connected to standard ventilatory equipment by means of a 3.5 mm paediatric ET tube adaptor. This method is the only emergency surgical airway recommended in children under 12 years.

Surgical cricothyroidotomy

A number of self-contained packs are available, for example the Portex Mini-Trach™ II and the Cook Critical Care's Melker emergency cricothyroidotomy catheter set. These involve insertion of a tracheostomy tube through the cricothyroid membrane. The ones mentioned are the most suitable types because they utilize a Seldinger technique (Figure 20.5).

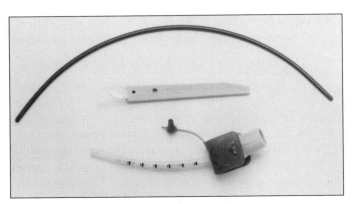

Figure 20.5   A Portex Mini-Trach™ II

Cervical stabilization

This is provided by manual inline stabilization. However, it should be rapidly replaced by a rigid collar, sandbags and tape or by a proprietary stabilization system (see Figure 1.5). Soft collars are used only for symptomatic relief in patients with common neck sprains and have no place in the trauma setting as they are ineffective as neck stabilizers.

Hard collars are of value only if they are moulded about the chin to form a rigid strut anteriorly between chin and chest and postero-laterally between occiput and shoulders. Recommended types of collars are the vertebrace, Zimmer™ extrication collar or the Ambu® Stifneck™. A selection of sizes from 'paediatric' to 'tall adult' must be available.

A local decision should be made whether to have a skull traction set available in the emergency department.

(B) Breathing

Chest drainage

A 16 g IV cannula, attached to a 20 ml syringe and a three-way tap, enables air to be aspirated and vented from a pleural cavity. This can provide temporary improvement in the clinical state of a patient with a tension pneumothorax so that a chest drain can be inserted (see Chapter 3).

A complete, pre-packed intercostal drainage set should be ready at all times, along with a variety of chest drains. The contents of this pack are described in detail in Chapter 3. The largest possible drain size should be used to prevent the drain being obstructed with blood clot. In the adult patient, therefore, a 36–40 F is required.

Either an underwater-seal drainage system or a Portex™ emergency drainage bag is also needed. In the former case, sterile water must be poured into the bottle prior to its use. The advantage of the Portex™ system is that water is not required because there is a mechanical one-way valve at its neck. As the bag is plastic and water is not necessary, the Portex™ system is strongly recommended when the patient has to be transported by land or air.

Ventilation

Ventilation can be achieved with a bag-valve-mask system as described in the 'Airway' section above. However, if it is to be prolonged the patient should be connected to a mechanical ventilator. Many types exist but for the purposes of emergency resuscitation they should be small, light, portable, robust and volume-cycled, with variable minute volume and rate settings for use in children and adults. They also need to be able to run on either wall or cylinder oxygen. Dials should be straightforward to use and visual cues built in, for example colour bands for different ages of patient. Both the

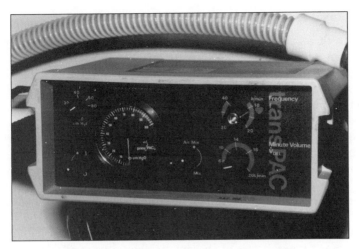

Figure 20.6 A Pneupac Transpac 2™ ventilator

Oxylog Ventilator™ and the Pneupac Transpac 2™ (Figure 20.6) fulfil all of these requirements.

An open pneumothorax can cause respiratory embarrassment. A dressing that can create an airtight seal is therefore necessary. This usually involves Vaseline™ gauze and airtight plastic adhesive tape. When it is secured on three sides, a one-way flap valve is created, releasing pleural air on expiration but preventing indrawing of air through the wound on inspiration. **This must be followed as soon as possible by the insertion of an intercostal drain.**

(C) Circulation

Circulatory support requires any haemorrhage to be stopped and lost circulatory volume to be replaced. External haemorrhage can usually be controlled by local pressure administered by the application of packs and bandages. The splintage of unstable fractures will also reduce blood loss. A particular example of this is the emergency external fixation of a pelvic fracture. As this can be life-saving for the severely injured patient, a local policy should be made whereby this equipment is kept in the emergency department, or stored in a place from where it can be brought rapidly when required.

Pneumatic anti-shock garment (PASG)

The use of a PASG is controversial but one of its functions is to stabilize pelvic fractures and prevent further blood loss. The cardiovascular system is temporarily supported also by autotransfusion from the compressed areas. If this device is available, familiarization with its safe application and removal is essential.

Circulatory access

Access to the circulation for administration of fluid (crystalloids, colloids, blood) can be achieved by various routes. The most common way is by insertion of large-bore cannulae (16 g or 14 g) in large peripheral veins. When this is not possible either central vein cannulation or a cutdown is carried out. In the former case, large-bore central venous cannulae should be used. These may be standard intravenous cannulae using an 'over-needle' technique (e.g. Vygon Intraflon™). However, those which utilize a Seldinger technique are less likely to cause complications (e.g. Vygon LeaderCath™). This procedure involves the prior insertion of a guide wire over which the cannula is threaded.

Surgical cutdown to a peripheral vein in the antecubital fossa, inguinal region or ankle requires a prepared pack containing scalpel, artery and dissecting forceps, ties, sutures and drapes.

A whole range of sizes of IV cannula should be available (24 g–14 g), with T-connectors to interpose between small paediatric cannulae (22 g and 24 g) and the giving set. This reduces the risk of dislodgement.

In a child in whom venous access proves impossible, consideration is given to intraosseous infusion. This involves insertion of a trocar/cannula percutaneously in the subcutaneous aspect of the upper tibia. The Cook™ intraosseous needles are recommended, but a variety of other intraosseous cannulae is available.

Once in place, fluid can be administered by connecting the cannulae either to a standard giving set, or to a large syringe.

Essential IV fluids are:

- normal saline;
- Hartmann's solution (Ringer's lactate);
- colloid;
- blood.

1 litre of crystalloid should be run through a giving set and be available immediately should a trauma patient arrive unannounced. To prevent infection, however, this fluid must be used within 12 hours.

The blood bank needs to be able to provide group O-negative blood immediately, and grouped but uncrossmatched blood within 15 minutes. Crossmatched blood should be available as soon as practically possible (usually within 45 minutes). If blood is needed then a blood warmer must be available, along with a pressure-infusion device for rapid transfusion.

Thoracotomy

In certain situations of penetrating chest trauma it may be necessary to perform a thoracotomy in the resuscitation room (see Chapter 3). A full thoracotomy set should therefore be kept available in the resuscitation room.

(D) Dysfunction

The only equipment needed to assess the patient neurologically in the primary survey is a bright pen torch so that the pupillary reaction can be accurately assessed. It is important to remember that bright room lights will drown out the illumination of a simple pen torch: the overhead lights will need to be turned off whilst the pupillary response is being assessed.

(E) Exposure

A variety of implements is available for cutting rapidly through clothes, including various scissors, shears, and guarded blades. Implements least likely to inflict inadvertent wounds on the patient or staff should be chosen, so either guarded blades or blunt-tipped heavy-duty scissors are recommended.

☐ Equipment required for the secondary survey

Peritoneal lavage

Diagnostic peritoneal lavage is performed in the resuscitation area to detect intra-peritoneal injury when clinical signs are unreliable (e.g. when the patient is unconscious). A peritoneal dialysis set must contain sterile drapes, a scalpel, skin retractors, a peritoneal dialysis catheter, saline, a giving set, sutures, and lignocaine with adrenaline.

Extremities

Fractured limbs should be splintered initially in the position in which they are found. Plastic limb splints or plaster-of-Paris slabs are preferable. However, immediate reduction is required when there is vascular compromise or when the skin is endangered by pressure. Femoral fractures must be splinted in a traction device, with the choice varying between a modern pneumatic splint (e.g. the Donway™ traction splint), the Hare™ traction splint or the Trac3™ splint, or skin traction in the traditional Thomas splint.

Bladder and stomach drainage

A variety of sizes of naso- or orogastric tubes is required, along with a 50 ml syringe for aspiration.

Prior to urinary bladder catheterization, a rectal examination is performed; for this disposable gloves and lubricating jelly are needed. Bladder catheterization sets comprise antiseptic skin wash, drapes, sterile lubrication jelly, self-retaining urinary catheters (14–18 F), a syringe of sterile water (10 ml) to inflate the balloon, and a drainage bag, preferably connected to a urometer to measure urine output.

Neurological examination

An auroscope is used to examine the external auditory canal and tympanic membranes for signs suggestive of basal skull fracture (see Chapter 6). A bright ophthalmoscope is also required to assess integrity of the globe and to examine the ocular fundi. Finally a tendon hammer is needed to check tendon reflexes.

□ Monitoring equipment used for trauma resuscitation

The major trauma patient requires close and frequent monitoring of all vital functions.

The pulse oximeter measures the percentage oxygen saturation of haemoglobin ($\%SaO_2$) in the periphery and is a very useful piece of monitoring equipment. There are various models on the market; the machine chosen must be portable, able to work from mains or battery, produce a clear display, have inbuilt alarms and sensors for fingers, ears and children. The Physio Control Lifestat 1600™ is one model that fulfils all these requirements.

Other essential monitors are:

- an ECG monitor/defibrillator;
- a non-invasive blood-pressure monitor (NIBP);
- a central venous pressure measurement set;
- an ECG machine to record a 12-lead ECG;
- blood-gas analysis.

The ECG/defibrillator, NIBP and pulse oximeter should be light, robust and both mains and battery operated to allow uninterrupted transfer of the patient from the resuscitation area. An automatic NIBP machine is desirable as this can record the BP at prefixed time intervals with an audible warning if the BP is outside predetermined limits.

Very rapid access to a laboratory blood-gas analyser is less satisfactory than having a machine in the emergency department.

□ Drugs required for trauma resuscitation

Note: Drugs marked * must be stored in a refrigerator or a secure cabinet.

Oxygen

- Piped wall supply
- Trolley cylinder (checked and replaced both routinely and after use)

Cardiovascular

- Adrenaline
- Atropine
- Dobutamine and dopamine
- Lignocaine
- Sodium bicarbonate

Anaesthetic

- Atracurium
- Etomidate
- Midazolam
- Suxamethonium*

Analgesic

- Morphine (or diamorphine)*
- Antiemetics (e.g. prochlorperazine, metoclopramide)
- Bupivacaine HCl
- Lignocaine

Antibiotics

- Penicillin
- Flucloxacillin
- Cephalexin
- Metronidazole

Anticonvulsant

- Phenytoin
- Diazepam

Respiratory

- Aminophylline
- Salbutamol
  - Nebulizer solution
  - Intravenous preparation
- Naloxone

Tetanus toxoid and tetanus immunoglobulin

☐ **Miscellaneous**

- Syringes:
  - 2 ml, 5 ml, 10 ml, 20 ml, 50 ml
  - blood-gas samplers
- Hypodermic needles
- Three-way taps
- Sample bottles for:
  - blood count, electrolytes, crossmatch
  - blood culture
  - urine and other fluids (e.g. peritoneal fluid)
- Alcohol swabs, cleansing solutions
  - chlorhexidine
  - povidone-iodine
- Dressings
  - Vaseline™ gauze
  - dry gauze
  - gauze pads
  - clingfilm
  - wool
  - crepe bandages
  - tape:
    plastic watertight/airtight
    non-allergenic fixing
    Elastoplast™
- Sutures: a selection of sizes and types (e.g. absorbable)
- Blood-sugar testing sticks; urine dipsticks
- Fluorescein for corneal staining in eye injury
- Sterile and non-sterile disposable rubber gloves in all sizes
- Plastic aprons for infection control
- Visors/glasses for infection control
- Facemasks for infection control
- Trauma sheets and pens for documentation
- Laboratory and x-ray forms
- Lead gowns for staff during x-ray procedures
- Sharps boxes

■ **Summary**

The effective and orderly resuscitation of the patient who has sustained major injuries requires the 24-hour availability of a well-organized and well-equipped resuscitation area. In addition, all members of the trauma team must be familiar with the room and its contents. Certain personnel must also be responsible for the regular renewal of supplies and the maintenance of equipment.

Senior nursing and medical staff should regularly review and update materials and equipment as technological advances are made, and ensure that all team members are trained appropriately.

■ References and further reading

Marsden A & McGowan A 1990. Resuscitation in the accident and emergency department. In Evans T (ed.): *ABC of Resuscitation*. London: BMJ Publications.

Chapter 21

Trauma scoring

Marilyn Woodford

Objectives

The objectives of this chapter are to understand:

- why trauma needs to be scored;

- how trauma scoring should be carried out.

◼ Introduction

It is essential to investigate whether injured patients are currently being treated as well as they should be. In order to assess systems of trauma care, meaningful statistical analysis must be employed to give useful information to clinicians and health care managers. This chapter outlines the most recent work on trauma scoring systems.

Currently trauma scoring is based on two scales. Firstly, the Revised Trauma Score (Table 21.1), which is a physiological scale, is recorded on arrival of the injured patient at the hospital; and secondly, the Injury Severity Score, an anatomical scale derived from all recorded injuries, is recorded at discharge or death. Since the eventual outcome of an injured patient is also affected by age and the method of injury – blunt or penetrating – both these variables are also taken into account during the scoring process.

■ Physiological scoring system

□ The Revised Trauma Score (RTS)

The physiological response of an injured patient is assessed by the Revised Trauma Score (RTS). The physiological parameters that make up the RTS are respiratory rate (RR), systolic blood pressure (BP), and the Glasgow Coma Scale (see Chapter 6). It has been found that these three observations can be aggregated to yield a reliable indicator of the likely clinical outcome. The selection of these particular parameters is influenced also by their ease of measurement and clinical opinion. RTS is measured, by convention, on arrival of the patient at hospital.

In practice the RTS is a complex calculation combining coded measurements of the three physiological variables. Addition of the coded values has been used for triage purposes both at the scene of the injury and on arrival of the patient at hospital. Further calculations involve the coded values being multiplied by a number (a weighting factor) derived from statistical (regression) analysis of the large North American database (Champion *et al.* 1989). This number reflects the relative value of the particular variable (RR, BP or GCS) in determining survival. The methodology is shown in Table 21.1; an example of the RTS is shown in Table 21.2.

Table 21.1   The Revised Trauma Score methodology

Parameter	Coded value (*a*)	Weight (*b*)	Score: (*a*) × (*b*)
Respiratory rate (/min)			
10–29	4		
>29	3		
6–9	2	0.2908	....
1–5	1		
0	0		
Systolic blood pressure (mmHg)			
>89	4		
76–89	3		
50–75	2	0.7326	....
1–49	1		
0	0		
Glasgow Coma Scale			
13–15	4		
9–12	3		
6–8	2	0.9368	....
4–5	1		
3	0		

Total = Revised Trauma Score   ....

Table 21.2   An example of a Revised Trauma Score

Parameter	Actual values	Coded value (*a*)	Weight (*b*)	Score: (*a*) × (*b*)
Glasgow Coma Scale	9	3	0.9368	2.8104
Systolic pressure	80 mmHg	3	0.7326	2.1978
Respiratory rate	35/min	3	0.2908	0.8724
			Total = Revised Trauma Score	5.8806

■ Anatomical scoring systems

☐ The Abbreviated Injury Scale (AIS)

The Abbreviated Injury Scale (AIS) was first published in 1969 and the fourth edition is now available. The AIS is based on anatomical injury and there is a single AIS score for each injury a patient may sustain. In the present edition more than 1200 injuries are listed. Scores range from 1 (minor) to 6 (fatal) – the higher the score, the more severe the injury. The intervals between the scores are not always consistent, however – for example, the difference between AIS3 and AIS4 is not necessarily the same as the difference between AIS1 and AIS2.

Here are some examples of Abbreviated Injury Scale (AIS) scores:

Injury	*Score*
Fracture 1 rib	1 (minor)
Fractured sternum	2 (moderate)
Ruptured diaphragm	3 (serious)
Bilateral lung lacerations	4 (severe)
Severe flail chest	5 (critical)
Massive chest crush	6 (fatal)

☐ The Injury Severity Score (ISS)

The Injury Severity Score (ISS) is based on the AIS and is calculated at discharge or death when all the injuries have been documented by operative findings, radiology or autopsy. The score obtained has been shown to be closely related to the outcome of patients with multiple injuries (Baker *et al.* 1974, 1976). The ISS is calculated as follows:

1   All injuries are scored using the AIS booklet.

2   The injuries are then assigned to one of the following body regions:
    - head or neck, including cervical spine;
    - face;
    - chest, including thoracic spine;
    - abdomen or pelvic contents, including lumbar spine;
    - extremities or bony pelvis;
    - external.

3   The ISS is derived by adding the sum of the squares of the highest AIS scores in each of the *three most severely injured* body regions.

The example in Table 21.3 should help in understanding the ISS calculation.

Table 21.3   An example of an Injury Severity Score

Region	Injury	AIS	AIS²
Head	Temporal fracture	2	–
	Subdural haematoma (small)	4	16
Face	–	–	–
Chest	3 rib fractures	2	–
Abdomen	Liver laceration (major)	4	16
Extremities	Tibia fracture (displaced)	3	9
External	Abrasions	1	–
		Total = ISS	41

ISS scores range from 1 to 75, a score of 75 resulting in one of two ways. Three AIS5 injuries ($5^2 + 5^2 + 5^2 = 75$) will produce this value; but also injuries coded AIS6 are, by convention, given an injury severity score of 75. There is variation in the frequency of different scores – for example, 9 and 16 are common, 14 and 22 are unusual, and 7 and 15 are unobtainable.

Most importantly, detailed injury descriptions are necessary for accurate coding. Injury Scaling Courses are held regularly to teach nurses, doctors and audit staff how to use the AIS book and assign accurate ISS scores.*

---

* Copies of the Abbreviated Injury Scale booklet, and information about MTOS (UK) and the Injury Scaling Courses, may be obtained from The North Western Injury Research Centre, Hope Hospital, Salford M6 8HD.

☐ **The TRISS methodology**

The next step in trauma scoring has been to combine the physiological score (RTS), the anatomical score (ISS), the age of the patient and the method of injury (blunt or penetrating) to provide a measure of the probability of survival (Ps). This methodology is designated TRISS (Trauma Score and ISS; Boyd *et al.* 1987). An example of the calculation is shown in Appendix 21.1. It should be noted that several computer programs are available for these calculations.

It is important to realize that Ps is merely a calculation used to highlight patients for clinical audit and, as discussed later, to measure the overall performance of different units in the care of injured patients: it is not an absolute measure of mortality. If a patient has a Ps of 70 per cent, this means that 7 out of 10 patients with similar injuries would be expected to survive. The patient may nevertheless die as he could be one of the 3 others.

It is the TRISS methodology that is used in the Major Trauma Outcome Study (MTOS), a system for the auditing of the overall management of injured patients. MTOS was developed in the USA and is now well established in the UK at the North Western Injury Research Centre, although the data-collection form in current use allows assessment of many more parameters of care than those originally used in the USA. This form of data collection is being extended throughout Europe, Australia and South Africa. The study is generally accepted as the definitive system for auditing trauma care in support of hospital analyses and trauma research. Appropriate forms have been designed to facilitate the collection of information on the patient's physiological and anatomical status after injury, and these have been distributed to 80 hospitals which have shown an interest in this initiative. More than 25 000 patients had been entered onto the database by the end of 1992. Data collection includes all aspects of care from time of the injury through to discharge or death. Injury severity scoring is done centrally so that comparisons are based on uniform data sets.

Regular reports and feedback allow hospitals both to analyse overall performance and to look into cases which have an unexpected outcome. Regular audit meetings are helpful in identifying deficiencies and any necessary future improvements in the way that trauma services are provided.

Whilst the concept of characterizing the severity of injury by the use of anatomical and physiologically scales is of proven value on both sides of the Atlantic, there remain some problems with the integration of the scores. Future work is aimed at developing more sensitive statistical techniques, particularly with regard to the weighting for age and for head injuries, to improve further the usefulness of TRISS and its applicability in the UK.

■ Summary

This chapter has described the scoring systems in use at the present time. Mortality is the only outcome predicted by the combination of the RTS, the ISS, the age and the type of injury. For each *death* that occurs, however, more than twenty patients are left with some *disability* after trauma. As yet there is no accepted scoring system to evaluate this.

Further research is necessary to evaluate the TRISS methodology and to provide accurate and clinically acceptable methods of evaluating systems of care for patients with major injuries. The Major Trauma Outcome Study is invaluable for this purpose. It is increasingly being recognized as a procedure that can highlight patients for interdisciplinary trauma audit and thereby identify the areas for improvement in the system of care.

■ Appendix 21.1: Probability of survival

☐ Glasgow Coma Scale

For details see Chapter 6 (page 184).
Modifications of GCS are necessary for use with small children (Simpson & Reilly 1982):

Best verbal response	Score
Appropriate words or social smiles, fixes on and follows objects	5
Cries but is consolable	4
Persistently irritable	3
Restless, agitated	2
Silent	1

Eye and motor responses are scored as in the scale for adults.

☐ Probability of survival

Once RTS, ISS, age and type of injury have been determined, the probability of survival (Ps) for the patient can be estimated from the following formula:

$$Ps = \frac{1}{1 + e^{-b}}$$

where $b = b0 + b1(\text{RTS}) + b2(\text{ISS}) + b3(A)$. The coefficients $b0 \ldots b3$ have been derived from Walker-Duncan regression analysis applied to data from the initial 25 000 patients entered onto MTOS at the Washington Hospital Centre, USA. As improvements in trauma care result in decreased mortality, these coefficients will change. A is the symbol for age: $A = 0$ when age is 54 years or less; $A = 1$ when age is 55 years or more. The constant e is equal to 2.718282, the base of Napierian logs.

Table 21.4 shows an example of this calculation.

Table 21.4   An example of a 'probability of survival' calculation

Using RTS = 5.8806 and ISS = 41:

b = b0   + b1 (RTS)   + b2 (ISS)   + b3 (A)

= −1.2470 + (0.9544) (5.8806)   + (−0.0768) (41)   + (−1.9052)(1)

= −0.6886

Ps = $1/(1 + e^{-b})$ = 0.33

Therefore the patient's probability of survival is 33%.

☐ Group comparisons

The M statistic

Comparisons of groups of patients are made with the MTOS database in North America. Before comparisons can be made it is necessary to ascertain whether the patients in your dataset are similar to those in the US database. The similarity in the mix of severity of injured patients can be examined using the M statistic. This yields a value between 0 and 1: values close to 1 indicate a close similarity of severities; values less than 0.88 are considered unacceptable and further analysis of your dataset would not be valid.

If the M statistic for your dataset indicates a close match in severity to the US database, then further comparisons on the standard of trauma care can be made.

The W statistic

W is the number of excess survivors per 100 patients compared with that predicted by the TRISS methodology.

$$W = \frac{\text{number of survivors} - \text{predicted number of survivors}}{\text{number of patients}/100}$$

Predicted number of survivors = sum of Ps for all patients.

A high positive value of W is desirable as this indicates that more of your patients are surviving than would be predicted from the TRISS methodology. Conversely, a negative value of W signifies that your hospital has fewer survivors than would be expected from the TRISS predictions. Negative W values are evidence that the trauma care in your particular hospital is below the average defined by the North American database.

However, it is necessary to question whether the W statistic could be reasonably expected to be achieved in practice. The variability of the W statistic is therefore examined.

$$\text{Variance of W} = \frac{\text{sum of } [Ps \times (1-Ps)]}{(\text{number of patients}/100)^2}$$

$$\text{Standard error of W} = \frac{\sqrt{(\text{sum of } [Ps \times (1-Ps)])}}{\text{number of patients}/100}$$

Rather more simply, the W score can be looked at with its 95% confidence limits. This is calculated using W and its standard error:

95% CI for W = W ± 1.96 × standard error of W

The 95% confidence interval for W (CI in the above equation) indicates the range of values within which it is 95% certain that W lies. Hence a narrow range would show that there is a good deal of confidence in the value of W.

The Z statistic

The Z value is often quoted when comparisons of trauma care are made between hospitals. This statistic is difficult to interpret; it is included here merely for completeness.

$$Z = \frac{\text{number of survivors} - \text{predicted number of survivors}}{\sqrt{(\text{sum of } [Ps \times (1-Ps)])}}$$

It is often said that Z scores greater than 1.96 indicate that the hospital is significantly better than the US average, and that Z scores less than 1.96 indicate that the hospital is significantly worse than the US average.

■ References and further reading

Baker S & O'Neill B 1976. The Injury Severity Score: an update. *J. Trauma* 16(11): 882.
Baker S, O'Neill B, Haddon W, *et al.* 1974. Injury Severity Score: a method for describing patients with multiple injuries and evaluating emergency care. *J. Trauma* 14: 187.

Boyd C, Tolson M & Copes W 1987. Evaluating trauma care: the TRISS
    method. Trauma Score and the Injury Severity Score. *J. Trauma* **27**(4): 370.
Champion H, Sacco W, Copes W, *et al.* 1989. A revision of the Trauma Score.
    J. Trauma **29**(5): 623.
Simpson D & Reilly P 1982. Paediatric coma scale. *Lancet* **2**: 450.

Chapter 22

Trauma care in areas of limited resources

Alison Brown, Joahre Niener and Peter Driscoll

Objective

The objective of this chapter is to emphasize the many positive actions which can be and are being carried out by trauma teams working in areas with limited resources.

■ Introduction

In developing countries equipment, facilities and back-up support systems are much more limited than those available in parts of Europe, North America, Australia and New Zealand. Sophisticated monitoring apparatus, CT scanners and sometimes even basic blood-analysis equipment are rarely available. Therefore basic nursing skills and clinical expertise must be relied upon.

The principles of trauma care already outlined in this book remain the same. There is no reason why the initial assessment and management of a trauma victim should not be adapted to any particular country or situation.

■ Epidemiology

Road traffic accidents are an important source of major trauma in all countries of the world, including developing ones. Alcohol is a major contributor to these accidents, but other factors, such as poor road conditions, also have their effect.

Physical violence varies from country to country depending upon the cultural aspects of particular population groups. In several areas of Southern Africa, stabbings and gunshot wounds are a daily occurrence, with particular trends developing in certain areas. For example, during the 1980s in South Africa, penetrating trauma of the spinal cord with a bicycle spoke was common. Today this has been replaced by the infamous 'necklacing' technique, in which the victim has a burning tyre placed around his neck.

Burns are a common problem in developing countries because of the abundance of unprotected fires. These are used for cooking all year round as well as for warmth during the winter months. Children are at particular risk.

Endemic to these areas of the world is trauma caused by large animal bites. The management of such injuries is the same as for all major trauma, but in addition meticulous attention to wound toilet and antibiotic cover is required (see Chapter 10).

■ Pre-hospital care

Unfortunately this usually consists of a 'scoop and run' policy, carried out in a poorly equipped vehicle. Invariably a foam mattress is the only piece of equipment carried by the ambulances. Fewer trained personnel are available, with the driver usually having to double up as the 'paramedic'.

In many cases the personnel involved in pre-hospital care will have little or no basic first-aid training. Radio communication is therefore of limited use when it comes to relaying patient information, instigating immediate treatment, or giving an early warning to the hospital. Consequently, the trauma nurse must use her powers of anticipation and insight and always have the resuscitation room adequately prepared for any eventuality.

■ Preparation

□ The resuscitation room

It is advisable, for staff training and the maintenance of standards of care, to have the Glasgow Coma Scale, the Trauma Score and AMPLE (see Chapter 1) prominently displayed on the walls of the area that has been designated for the immediate treatment of trauma victims.

The principles of resuscitation room design and equipment availability are described in detail in Chapter 20. However, these will have to adapted to the resources available in each particular hospital or medical receiving centre.

☐ Protection of personnel

This is of the utmost importance because of the high incidence of blood-borne infection. Gloves, gowns, masks and eye protection should *always* be used (see Chapter 19).

■ Reception

The actual mechanism of injury is extremely important: often it will dictate the management programme for the trauma patient (see Chapter 1). This information should therefore be ascertained from the pre-hospital personnel, relatives or witnesses as soon as they arrive at the hospital.

■ Primary survey and resuscitation

☐ (A) Airway with cervical spine stabilization

An airway can be maintained by the various techniques discussed in Chapter 2. Problems arise when there is no ventilator available, and a spontaneously breathing patient requires either intermittent positive-pressure ventilation or an endotracheal tube to secure his airway.

A possible solution is to use the self-inflating bag-valve-mask system described in detail in Chapter 2. This can then be connected to an oxygen cylinder, via oxygen tubing, with the flow set at 12–15 l/min depending on lung resistance. The ventilation rate should be between 12–15 per minute. The drawback of this system is that it requires an extra member of staff to squeeze the bag.

An alternative method can be tried after naso- or endotracheal intubation. It is possible to use corrugated elephant tubing as a T-piece with a hole cut out of the centre. A connector at the inspiratory end can be attached, via oxygen tubing, to an oxygen cylinder with the flow meter set at 10–15 l/min. Elephant tubing can be acquired from a Ventimask™ oxygen system, as can the connector to the oxygen tubing (Figure 22.1).

Depending on the reason for naso- or endotracheal intubation, some form of sedation and analgesic cover will be required. Whatever drug is used, administration must be via intravenous injections and titrated against the patient's symptoms. Following this, the respiratory rate should be monitored and charted accurately every 15 minutes. Any drop in the patient's respiratory rate, below 10 breaths per minute, requires artificial ventilation and an IV narcotic reversal agent such as naloxone.

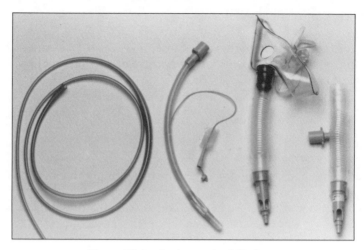

Figure 22.1   An improvised T-piece

Another form of airway management is the passing of a suture through the tongue and anterior chest wall. This is particularly useful in patients with bilateral parasymphyseal fractures of the mandible. In this condition the airway can be obstructed because the middle aspect of the mandible moves posteriorly, taking with it the attached tongue.

Once the airway has been cleared and secured, the patient must receive oxygen therapy.

Cervical spine stabilization must be carried out in conjunction with the airway management (see Chapter 2). If no cervical collar is available, cardboard or newspaper can be used by folding it to a width of 10 cm. It is then wrapped in a triangular bandage (Figure 22.2) and shaped, by bending it over one's thigh, before placing the centre of the 'collar' at the front of the casualty's neck, below the chin. The collar is then folded around the patient's neck. Before tying it in position at the front, the nurse must ensure that there is no obstruction to the airway. Finally, the neck can be secured using sandbags and tape, as described in Chapters 1 and 8.

□   **(B) Breathing**

The chest must be inspected and assessed in the manner described in Chapter 3. An intercostal (IC) drain must be inserted if there is a high index of suspicion of a pneumothorax, even if radiological confirmation is not possible. If no IC drain equipment is available, a substitute can be inserted by utilization of the equipment listed in Box 22.1.

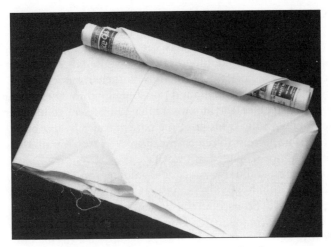

Figure 22.2 An improvised cervical collar

BOX 22.1 Equipment needed for emergency needle thoracocentesis

---

- IV cannula (12–14 g) with over-the-needle catheter attached
- Heimlich valve, or a finger cut from a large sterile surgical glove
- Suture material, or a rubber band to secure the flutter valve
- Povidone-iodine swabs for skin preparation
- Jelonet™, or tincture of Benzoin Compound as an adherent for dressings, to provide a good seal
- Sterile dressings and tape
- Sterile gloves
- Local anaesthetic

The catheter is prepared by inserting it into the finger of the surgical glove and then piercing the finger through its tip. This improvised flutter valve is then secured to the catheter with a suture or rubber band to prevent air leakage. The flutter valve allows air to escape from the pleural space whilst preventing inspiration of air.

The technique used for insertion of the cannula is the same as that for an intercostal needle insertion (see page 79).

Once in place the flutter valve must remain outside the dressing and unobstructed. The patient should then be monitored for signs of improvement, in particular a return of normal respiratory rate, the lessening of anxiety, and little or no use of the accessary muscles of respiration.

☐ (C) Circulation

Once any external haemorrhage has been controlled and two large-bore cannulae have been inserted, blood samples can be taken for haemoglobin, haematocrit and crossmatch. IV therapy is then commenced. A problem arises when laboratory facilities, and possibly blood for transfusion, are not available. In these cases, the blood samples can be sent to a larger hospital simultaneously with the transfer of the patient, once he has been optimally stabilized. It is important to remember, however, to wrap up these samples so that they are not damaged in transit.

Colloids, or crystalloids in adequate volume, should be used initially to correct the patient's hypovolaemia (see Chapter 4). If screened blood is available, it should be used if the patient's response to the crystalloids/colloids infusion is inadequate. Donations from staff members with an O Rh-negative blood type can be used, but only in extreme circumstances because of the risk of transmitting blood-borne infections. Another difficulty that can arise with blood donations is the cultural beliefs of either the volunteer or the patient. This issue must be handled with great tact and diplomacy so that anger and distress are avoided.

At this stage it is extremely important for the trauma nurse to start recording and charting vital signs, especially pulse, blood pressure, respiratory rate and core temperature. An automatic patient-monitoring system is highly unlikely to be available; instead a manual technique is used.

These baseline observations must be accurately recorded and charted at 5-minute intervals during the whole resuscitation period. Vital signs should remain stable (i.e. unchanged and within normal limits) for three 5-minute blocks (i.e. 15 minutes) of monitoring before their frequency is reduced to once per 15 minutes. The importance of this particular aspect of patient care cannot be overstressed. The nursing staff involved will require diligence, insight, and a meticulous attention to detail, along with continuous consultation with the medical team leader.

☐ (D) Dysfunction

In the initial stage, the conscious level of the patient should be assessed using the AVPU system and the pupillary response (size, reaction, equality; see Chapter 1). Later the Glasgow Coma Scale should be recorded and subsequently reassessed at 15-minute intervals. Again strict and accurate documentation of observations is imperative so that signs of deterioration can be detected early and acted upon accordingly.

☐ **(E) Exposure**

This is necessary so that the detailed examination of the secondary survey can be carried out. It is important to remember, however, that care should be taken when cutting clothes not just to prevent further injury but also to limit financial hardship. Ideally, the nurse should cut along the seams whenever possible so that the clothes can be repaired later.

If they are available, thick woollen blankets or pre-heated blankets should be used for covering the patient and to prevent excessive chilling. It must be remembered that throughout the winter months there can be extremes of temperature between day and night. This, coupled with the fact that the victim may often lie at the accident scene for many hours, can give rise to hypothermia. Resuscitation room staff should therefore be aware of and ready to manage this complication (see Chapter 13).

The trauma nurse must remember to remove jewellery, especially rings, and ensure their safekeeping.

At the end of the primary survey, the trauma personnel should carry out an overall reassessment of the patient, ensuring that no aspect of the primary survey has been missed.

Radiological examination of the cervical spine, chest and pelvis can now be carried out if the necessary equipment and personnel are available. If not, the patient's further management is based entirely on the clinical diagnosis, augmented by information on the mechanism of injury, a high index of suspicion, and the patient's response to the initial resuscitative measures.

■ **Secondary survey**

As discussed in Chapter 1, the secondary survey includes the detailed head-to-toe evaluation of the trauma patient with appropriate anticipation and with nursing intervention as indicated by each finding.

Ongoing recording and charting of vital signs, neurological status and IV fluid therapy must continue throughout the secondary survey. In those patients who have a thoracic injury the trauma nurse must also auscultate the chest for decreased air entry. The anterior, posterior, superior and inferior aspects of the thoracic wall should be checked at 15-minute intervals, or following any change in the patient's state. All findings must be recorded and acted upon as necessary.

A urinary catheter and a naso- or orogastric tube should be inserted unless there are contraindications (e.g. a fractured base of skull or urethral injury). Urinalysis can then be carried out, with any abnormalities reported to the team leader. The urine output needs to be measured and charted at 30-minute intervals. Ideally, the output should stabilize to 35–50 ml/hr, but this depends on IV fluid therapy and the injury sustained.

The nurse responsible for these recordings must include nasogastric volume loss (if any) in the 'output' total, and must also observe gastric fluid for colour, contents and smell. Intake and output should correlate; if they do not, a reason must be found.

In the presence of fractures, it is necessary to monitor the peripheral pulses on the affected limb and to assess perfusion. These observations should be taken and charted at 30-minute intervals, as well as before and after the application of any splint. Deviation from the norm must be prepared to the team leader.

The question of when analgesic cover should be prescribed and administered is difficult as it depends on many factors. However, once the life-threatening problems have been dealt with and the secondary surveys almost completed, analgesic cover must be considered. Apart from the patient's distress, severe pain results in restlessness and agitation which make a thorough examination of the trauma victim extremely difficult. It also affects pulse, blood pressure and respiratory rate, and decreases the patient's ability to compensate physiologically for his injuries. This can contribute to a marked deterioration in the trauma victim.

To provide analgesic cover, 15 mg of morphine sulphate can be diluted with 14 ml of sterile normal saline, producing a solution of 1 mg/ml. This should then be administered intravenously at a rate of 1 mg per minute over a 10-minute period. The patient must be reviewed at 1-minute intervals with a 'top-up' dose of 2–3 mg being administered until analgesic cover is adequate. The situation should be reviewed at 30-minute intervals, the aim being to reach and maintain an analgesic peak. An antiemetic will need to be administered intravenously at the same time.

As vital signs are being monitored, any respiratory depression should be observed quickly and appropriately acted upon, as previously discussed. Extreme caution must be exercised in the analgesic cover of head-injured patients so as not to mask any alteration of conscious level.

Reaction and response to injury varies from person to person, but gentle, sympathetic and humane handling of each person is a major aspect of nursing care, both during treatment and later, during definitive care and rehabilitation. Throughout the primary and secondary survey there must therefore be full communication with the patient whatever his level of consciousness. This ensures that he is fully aware of what is happening and is psychologically in tune with and trusts the personnel looking after him. A lot of the patient's fears are thereby alleviated, along with aggressive behaviour and, to a certain extent, pain.

The history (AMPLE) must be obtained from the patient (if he is not unconscious or confused) and witnesses. It is also important to ascertain who are the next-of-kin. This can be achieved in a variety of ways. The patient himself may be able to tell the team, or he may be carrying some form of identification amongst his belongings. In certain areas, a vehicle registration number can be used by the police to determine the owner's name and address from their computerized vehicle records. Commonly someone knows the victim, and by some quirk of communication will come to the hospital looking for their injured friend or relative. Whichever means are used, for compassionate and humane reasons a serious attempt *must* be made to contact and inform the victim's relatives (see Chapter 16).

If operative intervention is necessary, consent has to be obtained, either from the patient himself or from his next-of-kin. If these are not known, in certain countries the medical superintendent may sign the consent form. This administrator can also give consent on behalf of patients who are unconscious or confused or who are unable to speak the local language. In the last case a translator must be found as a matter of urgency so that the patient can give his own consent.

By the end of the secondary survey, overall documentation of the patient's progress or signs of deterioration should be well established. It must be remembered, however, to observe the patient for any signs of distress. For example, a cool, clammy appearance with undue irritability or unconsciousness could indicate internal haemorrhage even though documented observations may be within normal limits.

Once a preliminary diagnosis has been made, with or without the aid of diagnostic and radiological back-up, the need to transfer the patient to a more advanced hospital should also be considered.

■ Definitive care

After the life-threatening problems have been dealt with, in-depth management of all the injuries sustained can be put in the correct priority and dealt with accordingly.

Minor injuries, such as wounds, are treated during this phase of the overall care. All soft-tissue lacerations must be cleaned scrupulously, to prevent infection and to ensure good healing with little scarring (see Chapter 10). Tetanus toxoid prophylaxis should be prescribed and administered where indicated.

☐ Stabilization and transfer

Whether transferring a patient from the resuscitation room to a ward or theatre in the same hospital or to a hospital 500 km away, the basic objectives remain the same. It must first of all be determined whether the injuries sustained warrant transfer and whether the patient is actually fit to travel. Do the severity and extent of the injuries received outweigh the chances of survival? This is particularly important when vast distances are involved, with extremely poor road conditions or with limited transport facilities and no means of aero-medical evacuation.

The actual decision to transfer a patient can be taken on the basis of knowledge of the patient's injuries, the resources of the hospital and the patient's trauma score (see Chapter 21). A patient with a trauma score of 12 or less will require anaesthetic and surgical back-up.

Once the decision has been taken, it is the responsibility of the team leader in charge of the resuscitation to relate concisely and accurately all the relevant details to the receiving physician by radio or telephone (Box 22.2).

BOX 22.2   Essential transfer information: oral account

- Patient's name and address
- Brief history of incident, mechanism of injury
- Relevant pre-hospital information
- Initial resuscitation room findings and vital signs
- Treatment instigated and the patient's response
- Further pre-transfer treatment required by receiving team

Over and above this verbal communication with the physician involved, a written account must accompany the patient. Such a documented account should include the information in Box 22.3.

Prior to actual transfer, the primary and secondary survey must be reassessed to ensure that no life-threatening injuries have been missed or poorly assessed and managed.

Checklist before transfer

Airway

This must be cleared and secured by whichever method is most appropriate for the patient, and achieved by whatever equipment or improvised equipment is available.

Stabilization of the spine

This is carried out in the manner described in Chapter 8. The use of a spinal board is recommended.

Breathing

Ongoing oxygen administration must be carried out at a pre-determined rate and flow. The patency of chest drains should also be checked, and if a

---

BOX 22.3 Essential transfer information: written account

---

1 All relevant patient's details – name, address, age, next-of-kin, address, telephone contact numbers and patient's hospital number.

2 History and mechanism of injury.

3 The patient's condition on admission, including clinical and neurological status.

4 The vital signs, both the overall trend and the last set of observations before transfer.

5 Type and volume of intravenous fluids infused, and urinary output.

6 Specific observations, for example distal pulses.

7 Management of the patient, including medications given and route of administration.

8 Results of blood tests, radiological findings (when available), and the clinical results of any intervention, including vital signs.

9 Any relevant medical history.

10 Name and address of the referring hospital, and the telephone number and name of the referring physician, as well as the receiving hospital's and physician's names.

---

proper intercostal drain has been inserted the fluid level should be determined. Even in cases where an improvised drain has been used, the patency of the flutter valve should be reassessed by ensuring that the valve opens with each expiration. This is particularly important when a haemo- or pneumothorax is present.

Circulation

External haemorrhage must be controlled and intravenous fluids commenced. These fluids should be flowing well with no signs of thrombophlebitis. The nurse must check that the urinary catheters are not blocked by blood and that urine output is adequate. A naso- or orogastric tube must be *in situ* and well secured so that aspiration of stomach contents can be carried out. These tubes should be connected to a closed drainage system.

Exposure

The patient must be adequately covered to prevent the further loss of body heat.

Fractures

All fractures must be immobilized by application of traction and splintage. The peripheral pulses need to be regularly palpated and the findings charted.

Wounds

These need to be cleaned, dressed and securely taped.

Property

The nurse should ensure that the patient's clothing and property have been duly removed and documented in the appropriate valuables hook and transferred with the patient, or given to relatives for safekeeping.

BOX 22.4   Equipment needed for transfer

- Spinal board, with securing straps or triangular bandages
- Cervical collar, with sandbags already in place
- Portable suction, pre-tested to ensure function
- Suction tubing
- Suction catheters plus Yankauer suction
- Self-inflating bag-valve-mask ventilatory system
- Two oxygen cylinders with all attachments:
  - Pressure gauge, checked to ensure full cylinder of oxygen
  - Rotameter
  - Oxygen tubing
  - Oxygen mask
  - Spanner for opening the cylinder valve
- Intravenous fluid (2 litres of Ringer's lactate) plus 4 litres of Haemaccel®
- Two 16 g IV cannulae
- Tape, gauze, gloves
- Two 15 ml syringes of morphine sulphate with normal saline (depending on the length of journey) and antiemetic cover
- Stethoscope and sphygmomanometer
- Pen torch
- Charts for ongoing recording of observations
- Blankets
- Transfer letter, case notes, blood results and x-rays
- Food and fluid for the transfer team accompanying the patient
- Container for rubbish and a sharps bin

Medication

Optimum analgesic cover should have been achieved by this stage. Administration of analgesia can continue during transfer with a bolus dose of morphine sulphate (5 ml/5 mg) being administered prior to the actual moving of the patient. Some form of antiemetic will also be needed to counteract travel sickness and the nausea side-effect of the opiate.

If indicated, a bolus dose of an antibiotic such as cephazolin (1 g) should be prescribed and administered via an intravenous infusion. This is usually reserved for injuries such as compound fractures or lion bites where systemic infection is likely.

Personnel

This usually comprises a nurse alone, only occasionally with a doctor also.

Management during transfer

As far as possible under the difficult circumstances, the transfer team must continue to carry out the care and management already discussed in this book. Adequate knowledge of the patient's injuries will enable them to anticipate and correctly manage any complications likely to arise during transfer. The trauma victim must be as 'stable' as possible before transfer as this will improve his chances of recovery.

In Africa, a highly specialized 'Cas-Evac' team exists, under the auspices of the Medstar Company. This is based in Johannesburg, in the Republic of South Africa. It provides a pressurized aircraft kitted out as a fully-equipped intensive care unit and staffed by an intensive- and trauma-trained nursing sister plus a traumatologist. This service enhances trauma care but it is expensive: it is therefore mainly used by people who have adequate insurance cover or good financial support. However, the company does also offer telephone advice on patient management.

■ Summary

The overall importance and necessity for specialized trauma care in the 'golden hour' is a relatively new concept in developing countries. Many medical specialists and nursing staff are still not aware of the importance of the principles described in this book. It is very important that the standards described are adhered to, no matter where in the world one lives. More patients will then survive, and their pain and distress during trauma care will be reduced.

■ References and further reading

British Red Cross Society 1993. *Practical First Aid Manual*. London: Dorling Kindersley.

Caroline N 1987. *Emergency Care on the Streets*, 3rd edn. Boston: Little, Brown Company.

Lazear S 1992. Aeromedical transport. In Sheehy S, Marvin J & Jimmerson C (eds): *Emergency Nursing, Principles and Practice*, 3rd edn. St. Louis: C V Mosby.

Salvatores S 1992. Interfacility transport. In Sheehy S, Marvin J & Jimmerson C (eds): *Emergency Nursing, Principles and Practice*, 3rd edn. St. Louis: C V Mosby.

Settle J 1987. Burns – The First Five Days. Romford: Smith & Nephew Pharmaceuticals.

Skinner D, Driscoll P & Earlam R 1991. *ABC of Major Trauma*. London: BMJ Publications.

Index

venous return, reduced 113
venous system 103
  trauma 234
ventilation 72–3
  artificial 50, 91
  bag-valve-facemask apparatus 20,
    50, 412
  burns 315
  children 300–1
  endotracheal intubation 56
  equipment 414–15
  flail chest 83
  head trauma 181
  near-drowning 344
  pregnancy 291
  shock 122
  spontaneous 49
ventilation/perfusion ratio 74–7
ventilators, mechanical 414–15
ventricular fibrillation 336, 339
vertebral column *see* spinal column
visual acuity testing 27
vital signs
  children 295
  monitoring 127
  recording 23–4
Volkmann's contracture 246
vomiting
  cervical spine injury 17

epistaxis 198–9

Waterlow pressure-sore scoring
  system 31, 220
whiplash phenomenon 206
wounds
  burns, cleaning 327
  closure 274–9
  compound fractures 30
  débridement 273–4
  dressings 279–80
  examination 266–7
  healing 262–3
  infection 264, 273
  irrigation 272–3
  management stages 268
  open chest 21, 22, 82–3
  preparation 271–4
  radiation accidents 353
  scrubbing 273
  skin adhesive 279
  skin taping 278
  staples 278–9

x-rays *see* radiography

Yankauer suction 46

List of surgical procedures